Handbook of Formulas
in Chinese Medicine

HANDBOOK

— OF —

FORMULAS

— IN —

CHINESE MEDICINE

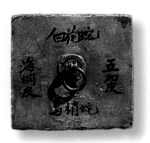

VOLKER SCHEID + ANDREW ELLIS

Illustrations by Bruce Wang

EASTLAND PRESS • SEATTLE

Copyright © 2016 by Eastland Press, Inc.
P.O. Box 99749, Seattle, WA 98139 USA
www.eastlandpress.com

Color images of skin disorders reprinted
with permission of Mazin Al-Khafaji, © 2015

Cover photo © 2016 by John Greim

International Standard Book Number: 978-0-939616-84-8
Library of Congress Control Number: 2016943787
Printed in the United States of America

2   4   6   8   10   9   7   5   3   1

Illustrations by Bruce Wang
Cover design by Patricia O'Connor and Gary Niemeier
Book design by Gary Niemeier

Abbreviated Contents

ACKNOWLEDGEMENTS ••• *xvii*

INTRODUCTION ••• *xix*

   Table 1: Common Methods of Processing Herbs – *xxvi*
   Table 2: Herbs that are Commonly Processed – *xxx*

THE FORMULAS ••• 1–373

INDEX OF FORMULAS BY PINYIN ••• 375

INDEX OF FORMULAS BY ENGLISH COMMON NAME ••• 383

INDEX OF PATTERNS AND KEY SYMPTOMS ••• 391

Table of Contents: Formulas

► FORMULAS BY *PINYIN*

bā zhēn tāng (Eight-Treasure Decoction) ······ 2

bā zhèng săn (Eight-Herb Powder for Rectification) ······ 4

băi hé gù jīn tāng (Lily Bulb Decoction to Preserve the Metal) ······ 6

bái hŭ tāng (White Tiger Decoction) ······ 8

bái tóu wēng tāng (Pulsatilla Decoction) ······ 10

bàn xià bái zhú tiān má tāng (Pinellia, White Atractylodes, and Gastrodia Decoction) ······ 12

bàn xià hòu pò tāng (Pinellia and Magnolia Bark Decoction) ······ 14

bàn xià xiè xīn tāng (Pinellia Decoction to Drain the Epigastrium) ······ 16

băo chăn wú yōu fāng (Worry-Free Formula to Protect Birth) ······ 18 *băo hé wán* (Preserve Harmony Pill) ······ 20

bèi mŭ guā lóu săn (Fritillaria and Trichosanthes Fruit Powder) ······ 22

bì xiè fēn qīng yĭn/bēi xiè fēn qīng yĭn (Tokoro Drink to Separate the Clear) ······ 24

bīng péng săn (Borneal and Borax Powder) ······ 26

bŭ fèi tāng (Tonify the Lungs Decoction) ······ 28

bŭ yáng huán wŭ tāng (Tonify the Yang to Restore Five [-Tenths] Decoction) ······ 30

bŭ zhōng yì qì tāng (Tonify the Middle to Augment the Qi Decoction) ······ 32

cāng ér zĭ săn (Xanthium Powder) ······ 34

chái gé jiĕ jī tāng (Bupleurum and Kudzu Decoction to Release the Muscle Layer) ······ 36

chái hú guì jiāng tāng (Bupleurum, Cinnamon Twig, and Ginger Decoction) ······ 38

chái hú jiā lóng gŭ mŭ lì tāng (Bupleurum Plus Dragon Bone and Oyster Shell Decoction) ······ 40

chái hú qīng gān tāng (Bupleurum Decoction to Clear the Liver) ······ 42

chái hú shū gān săn (Bupleurum Powder to Dredge the Liver) ······ 44

chuān xiōng chá tiáo săn (Chuanxiong Powder to Be Taken with Green Tea) ······ 46

cōng bái qī wèi yĭn (Scallion Drink with Seven Ingredients) ······ 48

cōng chĭ tāng (Scallion and Prepared Soybean Decoction) ······ 50

dà bŭ yīn wán (Great Tonify the Yin Pill) ······ 52

dà chái hú tāng (Major Bupleurum Decoction) ······ 54

dà chéng qì tāng (Major Order the Qi Decoction) ······ 56

dà huáng fù zĭ tāng (Rhubarb and Aconite Accessory Root Decoction) ······ 58

dà huáng mŭ dān tāng (Rhubarb and Moutan Decoction) ······ 60

dà qín jiāo tāng (Major Large Gentian Decoction) ······ 62

dà qīng lóng tāng (Major Bluegreen Dragon Decoction) ······ 64

dá yuán yĭn (Reach the Source Drink) ······ 66

dān shēn yĭn (Salvia Drink) ······ 68

dāng guī bŭ xuè tāng (Tangkuei Decoction to Tonify the Blood) ······ 70

dāng guī lóng huì wán (Tangkuei, Gentian, and Aloe Pill) ······ 72

dāng guī niān tòng tāng (Tangkuei Decoction to Pry Out Pain) ······ 74

dāng guī sháo yào săn (Tangkuei and Peony Powder) ······ 76

dāng guī sì nì tāng (Tangkuei Decoction for Frigid Extremities) ······ 78

dăo chì săn (Guide Out the Red Powder) ······ 80

dì huáng yĭn zi (Rehmannia Drink) ······ 82

dìng chuăn tāng (Arrest Wheezing Decoction) ······ 84

dìng zhì wán (Settle the Emotions Pill) ······ 86

dú huó jì shēng tāng (Pubescent Angelica and Taxillus Decoction) ······ 88

èr chén tāng (Two-Aged Herb Decoction) ······ 92

èr miào sǎn (Two-Marvel Powder) ······ 94

èr xiān tāng (Two-Immortal Decoction) ······ 96

èr zhì wán (Two-Solstice Pill) ······ 98

fáng fēng tōng shèng sǎn (Saposhnikovia Powder that Sagely Unblocks) ······ 100

fáng jǐ huáng qí tāng (Stephania and Astragalus Decoction) ······ 104

fú líng wán (Poria Pill) ······ 106

gān cǎo gān jiāng fú líng bái zhú tāng (Licorice, Ginger, Poria, and White Atractylodes Decoction) ······ 108

gān lù xiāo dú dān (Sweet Dew Special Pill to Eliminate Toxin) ······ 110

gān mài dà zǎo tāng (Licorice, Wheat, and Jujube Decoction) ······ 112

gé gēn huáng qín huáng lián tāng (Kudzu, Scutellaria, and Coptis Decoction) ······ 114

gé gēn tāng (Kudzu Decoction) ······ 116

gé huā jiě chéng sǎn (Kudzu Flower Powder to Relieve Hangovers) ······ 118

gé xià zhú yū tāng (Drive Out Stasis Below the Diaphragm Decoction) ······ 120

gù chòng tāng (Stabilize Gushing Decoction) ······ 122

gù jīng wán (Stabilize the Menses Pill) ······ 124

guī pí tāng (Restore the Spleen Decoction) ······ 126

guì zhī fú líng wán (Cinnamon Twig and Poria Pill) ······ 128

guì zhī tang (Cinnamon Twig Decoction) ······ 130

gǔn tán wán (Flushing Away Roiling Phlegm Pill) ······ 132

hāo qín qīng dǎn tāng (Sweet Wormwood and Scutellaria Decoction to Clear the Gallbladder) ······ 134

hòu pò wēn zhōng tāng (Magnolia Bark Decoction for Warming the Middle) ······ 136

hǔ qían wán (Hidden Tiger Pill) ······ 138

huáng lián jiě dú tāng (Coptis Decoction to Resolve Toxicity) ······ 140

huáng qí guì zhī wǔ wù tāng (Astragalus and Cinnamon Twig Five-Substance Decoction) ······ 142

huáng qín tāng (Scutellaria Decoction) ······ 144

huò xiāng zhèng qì sǎn (Patchouli/Agastache Powder to Rectify the Qi) ······ 146

jì chuān jiān (Benefit the River [Flow] Decoction) ······ 148

jī míng sǎn (Powder to Take at Cock's Crow) ······ 150

jiā wèi xiāng sū sǎn (Augmented Cyperus and Perilla Leaf Powder) ······ 152

jiàn pí wán (Strengthen the Spleen Pill) ······ 154

jīn huáng săn/jīn huáng gāo (Golden-Yellow Plaster) ······ 156

jīn líng zǐ săn (Melia Toosendan Powder) ······ 158

jīn suŏ gù jīng wán (Metal Lock Pill to Stabilize the Essence) ······ 160

jiŭ wèi qiāng huó tāng (Nine-Herb Decoction with Notopterygium) ······ 162

jú pí zhú rú tāng (Tangerine Peel and Bamboo Shavings Decoction) ······ 164

juān bì tāng (Remove Painful Obstruction Decoction) ······ 166

kŭ shēn tāng (Sophora Root Wash) ······ 168

lǐ zhōng wán (Regulate the Middle Pill) ······ 170

lián pò yǐn (Coptis and Magnolia Bark Drink) ······ 172

líng guì zhú gān tāng (Poria, Cinnamon Twig, Atractylodes, and Licorice Decoction) ······ 174

líng jiăo gōu téng tāng (Antelope Horn and Uncaria Decoction) ······ 176

liù jūn zǐ tāng (Six-Gentlemen Decoction) ······ 178

liù wèi dì huáng wán (Six-Ingredient Pill with Rehmannia) ······ 180

liù yī săn (Six-to-One Powder) ······ 182

lóng dăn xiè gān tāng (Gentian Decoction to Drain the Liver) ······ 184

má huáng tāng (Ephedra Decoction) ······ 186

má huáng xì xīn fù zǐ tāng (Ephedra, Asarum, and Aconite Accessory Root Decoction) ······ 188

má xìng shí gān tāng (Ephedra, Apricot Kernel, Gypsum, and Licorice Decoction) ······ 190

má zǐ rén wán (Hemp Seed Pill) ······ 192

mài mén dōng tāng (Ophiopogonis Decoction) ······ 194

mŭ lì săn (Oyster Shell Powder) ······ 196

mù xiāng bīng láng wán (Aucklandia and Betel Nut Pill) ······ 198

píng wèi săn (Calm the Stomach Powder) ······ 200

pŭ jì xiāo dú yǐn (Universal Benefit Drink to Eliminate Toxin) ······ 202

qiān zhèng săn (Lead to Symmetry Powder) ······ 204

qiāng huó shèng shī tāng (Notopterygium Decoction to Overcome Dampness) ······ 206

qīng dài săn (Indigo Powder) ······ 208

qīng hāo biē jiă tang (Sweet Wormwood and Soft-Shelled Turtle Shell Decoction [Version 1]) ······ 210

qīng qì huà tán wán (Clear the Qi and Transform Phlegm Pill) ······ 212

qīng shŭ yì qì tāng (Clear Summerheat and Augment the Qi Decoction) ······ 214

qīng wèi săn (Clear the Stomach Powder) ······ 216

qīng yíng tāng (Clear the Nutritive Level Decoction) ······ 218

qīng zào jiù fèi tāng (Clear Dryness and Rescue the Lungs Decoction) ······ 220 *rén shēn bài dú sǎn* (Ginseng Powder to Overcome Pathogenic Influences) ······ 222

rùn cháng wán (Moisten the Intestines Pill from *Master Shen's Book*) ······ 224

sān rén tāng (Three-Seed Decoction) ······ 226

sān zǐ yǎng qīn tāng (Three-Seed Decoction to Nourish One's Parents) ······ 228

sāng jú yǐn (Mulberry Leaf and Chrysanthemum Drink) ······ 230

sāng xìng tāng (Mulberry Leaf and Apricot Kernel Decoction) ······ 232

shā shēn mài mén dōng tāng (Glehnia and Ophiopogonis Decoction) ······ 234

shào fù zhú yū tāng (Drive Out Stasis from the Lower Abdomen Decoction) ······ 236

sháo yào gān cǎo tāng (Peony and Licorice Decoction) ······ 238

shēn fù tang (Ginseng and Aconite Accessory Root Decoction) ······ 240

shēn líng bái zhú sǎn (Ginseng, Poria, and White Atractylodes Powder) ······ 242

shèn qì wán (Kidney Qi Pill) ······ 244

shēn tōng zhú yū tāng (Drive Out Stasis from a Painful Body Decoction) ······ 246

shēng huà tāng (Generating and Transforming Decoction) ······ 248

shēng mài sǎn (Generate the Pulse Powder) ······ 250

shí quán dà bǔ tāng (All-Inclusive Great Tonifying Decoction) ······ 252

shí wèi bài dú sǎn (Ten-Ingredient Powder to Overcome Toxicity) ······ 254

shī xiào sǎn (Sudden Smile Powder) ······ 256

sì jūn zǐ tāng (Four-Gentlemen Decoction) ······ 258

sì nì sǎn (Frigid Extremities Powder) ······ 260

sì nì tāng (Frigid Extremities Decoction) ······ 262

sì shén wán (Four-Miracle Pill) ······ 264

sì wù tāng (Four-Substance Decoction) ······ 266

suān zǎo rén tāng (Sour Jujube Decoction) ······ 268

táo hé chéng qì tāng (Peach Pit Decoction to Order the Qi) ······ 270

tiān má gōu téng yǐn (Gastrodia and Uncaria Drink) ······ 272

tiān wáng bǔ xīn dān (Emperor of Heaven's Special Pill to Tonify the Heart) ······ 274

tōng guān wán (Open the Gate Pill) ······ 276

tòng xiè yào fāng (Important Formula for Painful Diarrhea) ······ 278

tuō lǐ xiāo dú yǐn (Support the Interior and Eliminate Toxin Drink) ······ 280

wěi jīng tāng (Reed Decoction) ······ 282

wēn dǎn tāng (Warm Gallbladder Decoction) ······ 284

wēn jīng tāng (Flow-Warming Decoction) ······ 286

wēn pí tāng (Warm the Spleen Decoction) ······ 288

wǔ lín sǎn (Powder for Five Types of Painful Urinary Dribbling) ······ 290

wǔ líng sǎn (Five-Ingredient Powder with Poria) ······ 292

wū méi wán (Mume Pill) ······ 294

wǔ pí sǎn (Five-Peel Powder) ······ 298

wǔ wèi xiāo dú yǐn (Five-Ingredient Drink to Eliminate Toxin) ······ 300

wú zhū yú tāng (Evodia Decoction) ······ 302

xiān fāng huó mìng yǐn (Immortals' Formula for Sustaining Life) ······ 304

xiāng shā liù jūn zǐ tāng (Six-Gentlemen Decoction with Aucklandia and Amomum) ······ 306

xiǎo chái hú tāng (Minor Bupleurum Decoction) ······ 308

xiāo fēng sǎn (Eliminate Wind Powder from *Orthodox Lineage*) ······ 310

xiǎo huó luò dān (Minor Invigorate the Collaterals Special Pill) ······ 312

xiǎo jiàn zhōng tāng (Minor Construct the Middle Decoction) ······ 314

xiǎo qīng lóng tāng (Minor Bluegreen Dragon Decoction) ······ 316

xiǎo xiàn xiōng tāng (Minor Decoction [for Pathogens] Stuck in the Chest) ······ 318

xiǎo xù mìng tāng (Minor Extend Life Decoction) ······ 320

xiāo yáo sǎn (Rambling Powder) ······ 322

xiè bái sǎn (Drain the White Powder from *Craft of Medicinal Treatment for Childhood Disease Patterns*) ······ 324

xiè huáng sǎn (Drain the Yellow Powder) ······ 326

xīn yí qīng fèi yǐn (Magnolia Flower Drink to Clear the Lungs) ······ 328

xìng sū sǎn (Apricot Kernel and Perilla Leaf Powder) ······ 330

xuān bì tāng (Disband Painful Obstruction Decoction) ······ 332

xuè fǔ zhú yū tāng (Drive Out Stasis from the Mansion of Blood Decoction) ······ 334

yī guàn jiān (Linking Decoction) ······ 336

yīn chén hāo tāng (Virgate Wormwood Decoction) ······ 338

yín qiáo sǎn (Honeysuckle and Forsythia Powder) ······ 340

yòu guī wán (Restore the Right [Kidney] Pill) ······ 342

yù píng fēng sǎn (Jade Windscreen Powder) ······ 344

yù quán wán (Jade Spring Pill) ······ 346

yuè jū wán (Escape Restraint Pill) ······ 348

zài zào sǎn (Renewal Powder) ······ 350

zēng yè tāng (Increase the Fluids Decoction) ······ 352

zhèn gān xī fēng tāng (Sedate the Liver and Extinguish Wind Decoction) ······ 354

zhēn wǔ tāng (True Warrior Decoction) ······ 356

zhì gān cǎo tāng (Prepared Licorice Decoction) ······ 358

zhǐ shí dǎo zhì wán (Unripe Bitter Orange Pill to Guide Out Stagnation) ······ 360

zhǐ shí xiāo pǐ wán (Unripe Bitter Orange Pill to Reduce Focal Distention) ······ 362

zhǐ shí xiè bái guì zhī tāng (Unripe Bitter Orange, Chinese Garlic, and Cinnamon Twig Decoction) ······ 364

zhǐ sòu sǎn (Stop Coughing Powder) ······ 366

zhū líng tāng (Polyporus Decoction) ······ 368

zhú yè shí gāo tang (Lophatherum and Gypsum Decoction) ······ 370

zuǒ guī wán (Restore the Left [Kidney] Pill) ······ 372

▶ FORMULAS BY ENGLISH COMMON NAME

All-Inclusive Great Tonifying Decoction (*shí quán dà bǔ tāng*) ······ 252

Antelope Horn and Uncaria Decoction (*líng jiǎo gōu téng tāng*) ······ 176

Apricot Kernel and Perilla Leaf Powder (*xìng sū sǎn*) ······ 330

Arrest Wheezing Decoction (*dìng chuǎn tāng*) ······ 84

Astragalus and Cinnamon Twig Five-Substance Decoction (*huáng qí guì zhī wǔ wù tāng*) ······ 142

Aucklandia and Betel Nut Pill (*mù xiāng bīng láng wán*) ······ 198

Augmented Cyperus and Perilla Leaf Powder (*jiā wèi xiāng sū sǎn*) ······ 152

Benefit the River [Flow] Decoction (*jì chuān jiān*) ······ 148

Borneal and Borax Powder (*bīng péng sǎn*) ······ 26

Bupleurum and Kudzu Decoction to Release the Muscle Layer (*chái gé jiě jī tāng*) ······ 36

Bupleurum, Cinnamon Twig, and Ginger Decoction (*chái hú guì jiāng tāng*) ······ 38

Bupleurum Decoction to Clear the Liver (*chái hú qīng gān tāng*) ······ 42

Bupleurum Plus Dragon Bone and Oyster Shell Decoction (*chái hú jiā lóng gǔ mǔ lì tāng*) ······ 40

Bupleurum Powder to Dredge the Liver (*chái hú shū gān sǎn*) ······ 44

Calm the Stomach Powder (*píng wèi sǎn*) ······ 200

Chuanxiong Powder to Be Taken with Green Tea (*chuān xiōng chá tiáo sǎn*) ······ 46

Cinnamon Twig and Poria Pill (*guì zhī fú líng wán*) ······ 128

Cinnamon Twig Decoction (*guì zhī tang*) ······ 130

Clear Dryness and Rescue the Lungs Decoction (*qīng zào jiù fèi tāng*) ······ 220

Clear Summerheat and Augment the Qi Decoction (*qīng shǔ yì qì tāng*) ······ 214

Clear the Nutritive Level Decoction (*qīng yíng tāng*) ······ 218

Clear the Qi and Transform Phlegm Pill (*qīng qì huà tán wán*) ······ 212

Clear the Stomach Powder (*qīng wèi sǎn*) ······ 216

Coptis and Magnolia Bark Drink (*lián pò yǐn*) ······ 172

Coptis Decoction to Resolve Toxicity (*huáng lián jiě dú tāng*) ······ 140

Disband Painful Obstruction Decoction (*xuān bì tāng*) ······ 332

Drain the White Powder from *Craft of Medicinal Treatment
    for Childhood Disease Patterns* (*xiè bái sǎn*) ······ 324

Drain the Yellow Powder (*xiè huáng sǎn*) ······ 326

Drive Out Stasis Below the Diaphragm Decoction (*gé xià zhú yū tāng*) ······ 120

Drive Out Stasis from a Painful Body Decoction (*shēn tōng zhú yū tāng*) ······ 246

Drive Out Stasis from the Lower Abdomen Decoction (*shào fù zhú yū tāng*) ······ 236

Drive Out Stasis from the Mansion of Blood Decoction (*xuè fǔ zhú yū tāng*) ······ 334

Eight-Herb Powder for Rectification (*bā zhèng sǎn*) ······ 4

Eight-Treasure Decoction (*bā zhēn tāng*) ······ 2

Eliminate Wind Powder from *Orthodox Lineage* (*xiāo fēng sǎn*) ······ 310

Emperor of Heaven's Special Pill to Tonify the Heart (*tiān wáng bǔ xīn dān*) ······ 274

Ephedra, Apricot Kernel, Gypsum, and Licorice Decoction (*má xìng shí gān tāng*) ······ 190

Ephedra, Asarum, and Aconite Accessory Root Decoction (*má huáng xì xīn fù zǐ tāng*) ······ 188

Ephedra Decoction (*má huáng tāng*) ······ 186

Escape Restraint Pill (*yuè jū wán*) ······ 348

Evodia Decoction (*wú zhū yú tāng*) ······ 302

Five-Ingredient Drink to Eliminate Toxin (*wǔ wèi xiāo dú yǐn*) ······ 300

Five-Ingredient Powder with Poria (*wǔ líng sǎn*) ······ 292

Five-Peel Powder (*wǔ pí sǎn*) ······ 298

Flow-Warming Decoction (*wēn jīng tāng*) ······ 286

Flushing Away Roiling Phlegm Pill (*gǔn tán wán*) ······ 132

Four-Gentlemen Decoction (*sì jūn zǐ tāng*) ······ 258

Four-Miracle Pill (*sì shén wán*) ······ 264

Four-Substance Decoction (*sì wù tāng*) ······ 266

Frigid Extremities Decoction (*sì nì tāng*) ······ 262

Frigid Extremities Powder (*sì nì sǎn*) ······ 260

Fritillaria and Trichosanthes Fruit Powder (*bèi mǔ guā lóu sǎn*) ······ 22

Gastrodia and Uncaria Drink (*tiān má gōu téng yǐn*) ······ 272

Generate the Pulse Powder (*shēng mài sǎn*) ······ 250

Generating and Transforming Decoction (*shēng huà tāng*) ······ 248

Gentian Decoction to Drain the Liver (*lóng dǎn xiè gān tāng*) ······ 184

Ginseng and Aconite Accessory Root Decoction (*shēn fù tang*) ······ 240

Ginseng, Poria, and White Atractylodes Powder (*shēn líng bái zhú sǎn*) ······ 242

Ginseng Powder to Overcome Pathogenic Influences (*rén shēn bài dú sǎn*) ······ 222

Glehnia and Ophiopogonis Decoction (*shā shēn mài mén dōng tāng*) ······ 234

Golden-Yellow Plaster (*jīn huáng sǎn/jīn huáng gāo*) ······ 156

Great Tonify the Yin Pill (*dà bǔ yīn wán*) ······ 52

Guide Out the Red Powder (*dǎo chì sǎn*) ······ 80

Hemp Seed Pill (*má zǐ rén wán*) ······ 192

Hidden Tiger Pill (*hǔ qían wán*) ······ 138

Honeysuckle and Forsythia Powder (*yín qiáo sǎn*) ······ 340

Immortals' Formula for Sustaining Life (*xiān fāng huó mìng yǐn*) ······ 304

Important Formula for Painful Diarrhea (*tòng xiè yào fāng*) ······ 278

Increase the Fluids Decoction (*zēng yè tāng*) ······ 352

Indigo Powder (*qīng dài sǎn*) ······ 208

Jade Spring Pill (*yù quán wán*) ······ 346

Jade Windscreen Powder (*yù píng fēng sǎn*) ······ 344

Kidney Qi Pill (*shèn qì wán*) ······ 244

Kudzu Decoction (*gé gēn tāng*) ······ 116

Kudzu Flower Powder to Relieve Hangovers (*gé huā jiě chéng sǎn*) ······ 118

Kudzu, Scutellaria, and Coptis Decoction (*gé gēn huáng qín huáng lián tāng*) ······ 114

Lead to Symmetry Powder (*qiān zhèng sǎn*) ······ 204

Licorice, Ginger, Poria, and White Atractylodes Decoction (*gān cǎo gān jiāng fú líng bái zhú tāng*) ······ 108

Licorice, Wheat, and Jujube Decoction (*gān mài dà zǎo tāng*) ······ 112

Lily Bulb Decoction to Preserve the Metal (*bǎi hé gù jīn tāng*) ······ 6

Linking Decoction (*yī gùan jiān*) ······ 336

Lophatherum and Gypsum Decoction (*zhú yè shí gāo tang*) ······ 370

Magnolia Bark Decoction for Warming the Middle (*hòu pò wēn zhōng tāng*) ······ 136

Magnolia Flower Drink to Clear the Lungs (*xīn yí qīng fèi yǐn*) ······ 328

Major Bluegreen Dragon Decoction (*dà qīng lóng tāng*) ······ 64

Major Bupleurum Decoction (*dà chái hú tāng*) ······ 54

Major Large Gentian Decoction (*dà qín jiāo tāng*) ⸱⸱⸱⸱⸱⸱ 62

Major Order the Qi Decoction (*dà chéng qì tāng*) ⸱⸱⸱⸱⸱⸱ 56

Melia Toosendan Powder (*jīn líng zǐ sǎn*) ⸱⸱⸱⸱⸱⸱ 158

Metal Lock Pill to Stabilize the Essence (*jīn suǒ gù jīng wán*) ⸱⸱⸱⸱⸱⸱ 160

Minor Bluegreen Dragon Decoction (*xiǎo qīng lóng tāng*) ⸱⸱⸱⸱⸱⸱ 316

Minor Bupleurum Decoction (*xiǎo chái hú tāng*) ⸱⸱⸱⸱⸱⸱ 308

Minor Construct the Middle Decoction (*xiǎo jiàn zhōng tāng*) ⸱⸱⸱⸱⸱⸱ 314

Minor Decoction [for Pathogens] Stuck in the Chest (*xiǎo xiàn xiōng tāng*) ⸱⸱⸱⸱⸱⸱ 318

Minor Extend Life Decoction (*xiǎo xù mìng tāng*) ⸱⸱⸱⸱⸱⸱ 320

Minor Invigorate the Collaterals Special Pill (*xiǎo huó luò dān*) ⸱⸱⸱⸱⸱⸱ 312

Moisten the Intestines Pill from *Master Shen's Book* (*rùn cháng wán*) ⸱⸱⸱⸱⸱⸱ 224

Mulberry Leaf and Apricot Kernel Decoction (*sāng xìng tāng*) ⸱⸱⸱⸱⸱⸱ 232

Mulberry Leaf and Chrysanthemum Drink (*sāng jú yǐn*) ⸱⸱⸱⸱⸱⸱ 230

Mume Pill (*wū méi wán*) ⸱⸱⸱⸱⸱⸱ 294

Nine-Herb Decoction with Notopterygium (*jiǔ wèi qiāng huó tāng*) ⸱⸱⸱⸱⸱⸱ 162

Notopterygium Decoction to Overcome Dampness (*qiāng huó shèng shī tāng*) ⸱⸱⸱⸱⸱⸱ 206

Open the Gate Pill (*tōng guān wán*) ⸱⸱⸱⸱⸱⸱ 276

Ophiopogonis Decoction (*mài mén dōng tāng*) ⸱⸱⸱⸱⸱⸱ 194

Oyster Shell Powder (*mǔ lì sǎn*) ⸱⸱⸱⸱⸱⸱ 196

Patchouli/Agastache Powder to Rectify the Qi (*huò xiāng zhèng qì sǎn*) ⸱⸱⸱⸱⸱⸱ 146

Peach Pit Decoction to Order the Qi (*táo hé chéng qì tāng*) ⸱⸱⸱⸱⸱⸱ 270

Peony and Licorice Decoction (*sháo yào gān cǎo tāng*) ⸱⸱⸱⸱⸱⸱ 238

Pinellia and Magnolia Bark Decoction (*bàn xià hòu pò tāng*) ⸱⸱⸱⸱⸱⸱ 14

Pinellia Decoction to Drain the Epigastrium (*bàn xià xiè xīn tāng*) ⸱⸱⸱⸱⸱⸱ 16

Pinellia, White Atractylodes, and Gastrodia Decoction (*bàn xià bái zhú tiān má tāng*) ⸱⸱⸱⸱⸱⸱ 12

Polyporus Decoction (*zhū líng tāng*) ⸱⸱⸱⸱⸱⸱ 368

Poria, Cinnamon Twig, Atractylodes, and Licorice Decoction (*líng guì zhú gān tāng*) ⸱⸱⸱⸱⸱⸱ 174

Poria Pill (*fú líng wán*) ⸱⸱⸱⸱⸱⸱ 106

Powder for Five Types of Painful Urinary Dribbling (*wǔ lín sǎn*) ⸱⸱⸱⸱⸱⸱ 290

Powder to Take at Cock's Crow (*jī míng sǎn*) ⸱⸱⸱⸱⸱⸱ 150

Prepared Licorice Decoction (*zhì gān cǎo tāng*) ⸱⸱⸱⸱⸱⸱ 358

Preserve Harmony Pill (*bǎo hé wán*) ⸱⸱⸱⸱⸱⸱ 20

Pubescent Angelica and Taxillus Decoction (*dú huó jì shēng tāng*) ⸱⸱⸱⸱⸱⸱ 88

Pulsatilla Decoction (*bái tóu wēng tāng*) ······ 10

Rambling Powder (*xiāo yáo sǎn*) ······ 322

Reach the Source Drink (*dá yuán yǐn*) ······ 66

Reed Decoction (*wěi jīng tāng*) ······ 282

Regulate the Middle Pill (*lǐ zhōng wán*) ······ 170

Rehmannia Drink (*dì huáng yǐn zi*) ······ 82

Remove Painful Obstruction Decoction (*juān bì tāng*) ······ 166

Renewal Powder (*zài zào sǎn*) ······ 350

Restore the Left [Kidney] Pill (*zuǒ guī wán*) ······ 372

Restore the Right [Kidney] Pill (*yòu guī wán*) ······ 342

Restore the Spleen Decoction (*guī pí tāng*) ······ 126

Rhubarb and Aconite Accessory Root Decoction (*dà huáng fù zǐ tāng*) ······ 58

Rhubarb and Moutan Decoction (*dà huáng mǔ dān tāng*) ······ 60

Salvia Drink (*dān shēn yǐn*) ······ 68

Saposhnikovia Powder that Sagely Unblocks (*fáng fēng tōng shèng sǎn*) ······ 100

Scallion and Prepared Soybean Decoction (*cōng chǐ tāng*) ······ 50

Scallion Drink with Seven Ingredients (*cōng bái qī wèi yǐn*) ······ 48

Scutellaria Decoction (*huáng qín tāng*) ······ 144

Sedate the Liver and Extinguish Wind Decoction (*zhèn gān xī fēng tāng*) ······ 354

Settle the Emotions Pill (*dìng zhì wán*) ······ 86

Six-Gentlemen Decoction (*liù jūn zǐ tāng*) ······ 178

Six-Gentlemen Decoction with Aucklandia and Amomum (*xiāng shā liù jūn zǐ tāng*) ······ 306

Six-Ingredient Pill with Rehmannia (*liù wèi dì huáng wán*) ······ 180

Six-to-One Powder (*liù yī sǎn*) ······ 182

Sophora Root Wash (*kǔ shēn tāng*) ······ 168

Sour Jujube Decoction (*suān zǎo rén tāng*) ······ 268

Stabilize Gushing Decoction (*gù chōng tāng*) ······ 122

Stabilize the Menses Pill (*gù jīng wán*) ······ 124

Stephania and Astragalus Decoction (*fáng jǐ huáng qí tāng*) ······ 104

Stop Coughing Powder (*zhǐ sòu sǎn*) ······ 366

Strengthen the Spleen Pill (*jiàn pí wán*) ······ 154

Sudden Smile Powder (*shī xiào sǎn*) ······ 256

Support the Interior and Eliminate Toxin Drink (*tuō lǐ xiāo dú yǐn*) ······ 280

Sweet Dew Special Pill to Eliminate Toxin (*gān lù xiāo dú dān*) ······ 110

Sweet Wormwood and Scutellaria Decoction to Clear the Gallbladder (*hāo qín qīng dǎn tāng*) ······ 134

Sweet Wormwood and Soft-Shelled Turtle Shell Decoction [Version 1] (*qīng hāo biē jiǎ tang*) ······ 210

Tangerine Peel and Bamboo Shavings Decoction (*jú pí zhú rú tāng*) ······ 164

Tangkuei and Peony Powder (*dāng guī sháo yào sǎn*) ······ 76

Tangkuei Decoction for Frigid Extremities (*dāng guī sì nì tāng*) ······ 78

Tangkuei Decoction to Pry Out Pain (*dāng guī niān tòng tāng*) ······ 74

Tangkuei Decoction to Tonify the Blood (*dāng guī bǔ xuè tāng*) ······ 70

Tangkuei, Gentian, and Aloe Pill (*dāng guī lóng huì wán*) ······ 72

Ten-Ingredient Powder to Overcome Toxicity (*shí wèi bài dú sǎn*) ······ 254

Three-Seed Decoction (*sān rén tāng*) ······ 226

Three-Seed Decoction to Nourish One's Parents (*sān zǐ yǎng qīn tāng*) ······ 228

Tokoro Drink to Separate the Clear (*bì xiè fēn qīng yǐn/bēi xiè fēn qīng yǐn*) ······ 24

Tonify the Lungs Decoction (*bǔ fèi tāng*) ······ 28

Tonify the Middle to Augment the Qi Decoction (*bǔ zhōng yì qì tāng*) ······ 32

Tonify the Yang to Restore Five [-Tenths] Decoction (*bǔ yáng huán wǔ tāng*) ······ 30

True Warrior Decoction (*zhēn wǔ tāng*) ······ 356

Two-Aged Herb Decoction (*èr chén tāng*) ······ 92

Two-Immortal Decoction (*èr xiān tāng*) ······ 96

Two-Marvel Powder (*èr miào sǎn*) ······ 94

Two-Solstice Pill (*èr zhì wán*) ······ 98

Universal Benefit Drink to Eliminate Toxin (*pǔ jì xiāo dú yǐn*) ······ 202

Unripe Bitter Orange, Chinese Garlic, and Cinnamon Twig Decoction (*zhǐ shí xiè bái guì zhī tāng*) ······ 364

Unripe Bitter Orange Pill to Guide Out Stagnation (*zhǐ shí dǎo zhì wán*) ······ 360

Unripe Bitter Orange Pill to Reduce Focal Distention (*zhǐ shí xiāo pǐ wán*) ······ 362

Virgate Wormwood Decoction (*yīn chén hāo tāng*) ······ 338

Warm Gallbladder Decoction (*wēn dǎn tāng*) ······ 284

Warm the Spleen Decoction (*wēn pí tāng*) ······ 288

White Tiger Decoction (*bái hǔ tāng*) ······ 8

Worry-Free Formula to Protect Birth (*bǎo chǎn wú yōu fāng*) ······ 18

Xanthium Powder (*cāng ér zǐ sǎn*) ······ 34

Acknowledgements

THE INSPIRATION FOR COMPILING THIS HANDBOOK arose from teaching Chinese medicine formulas and strategies in Munich, London, and elsewhere in the world. I am most grateful to the many students who attended the courses and lectures for allowing me the space to explore and develop different concepts and ideas, for their patience and good will, and for their many-faceted feedback. At a later stage, when the handbook had started to acquire a distinctive shape and form, we benefitted from the input of individual students and focus groups in Seattle and London. I am particularly grateful to Giusi Pezzotta, who spent many hours extracting information from *Chinese Herbal Medicine: Formulas & Strategies* (2nd edition), compiled the original version of the formula diagrams, and was helpful in many other ways. Mary Beddoe also worked on integrating the information from *Formulas & Strategies* with that of Chinese sources. Without them this handbook would not exist. The same holds true for the diverse inputs provided by the Eastland Press team. Dan Bensky's role as editor was crucial in making the book cohere in a way that it would not otherwise have done. Gary Niemeier, with the help of Lilian Bensky and illustrator Bruce Wang, patiently and expertly turned ideas into visible shapes. John and Patricia O'Connor shepherded the book from the conceptual stage into a usable handbook. Last but not least, I want to thank Andy Ellis for being the perfect yin to my yang (or vice versa) on this project. It's been a privilege and a pleasure to work with all of you. — VS

CHINESE MEDICINE IS AN ACCUMULATION OF KNOWLedge that is handed forward generation to generation. Without the kindness of my teachers I would not have been in a position to participate in this project. Thus, I would like to acknowledge the generosity of all my teachers, and particularly Shi Neng-Yun, Gan Zu-Wang, Xu Fu-Su, Chen Jun-Ming, Zhou Sen, Yu Guo-Jun, Dr. James Tin Yau So, and Zhang Guang-Cai, all of whom were so willing to share their experience and knowledge. Finally, I was honored to be invited by Dan Bensky and Volker Scheid to work with them on this book. My appreciation for their unending patience with my idiosyncratic approach to grammar, composition, and erudite minutiae is second only to my respect for their knowledge and work ethic. — AE

Introduction

FORMULAS ARE ARGUABLY THE CORE OF ALL CHINESE herbal medical practice. While they are made up of specific ingredients, and it is the medicinal effects of these ingredients that gives a formula its healing powers, in Chinese medicine it is almost always the formula, and not an individual herb or mineral, that addresses the patient's underlying disease mechanisms. Behind the formulas stand strategies and theories about how the human body works, and while theories come and go, are contested and rarely agreed upon by the entire Chinese medical community, the formulas themselves endure and their appeal extends beyond the narrow boundaries of specific medical currents. One needn't be an expert on cold damage theory to successfully use cold damage formulas, or an expert on warm disorder theory to use warm disorder formulas. Indeed, a formula like Tonify the Middle to Augment the Qi Decoction (*bǔ zhōng yì qì tāng*) has long transcended its origin in the Spleen and Stomach current. This is not to say that engagement with the ideas that went into a formula's original composition does not help us to prescribe it more effectively, or that studying strategies and materia medica is not essential. However, when it comes to writing a prescription in the clinic, Chinese medicine invariably seeks to match a diagnosis, pattern, or condition with a corresponding formula, or at least components of formulas. This book seeks to make that job easier.

Goals of this Handbook

This book is a clinical handbook that is intended to be used as a reference text while seeing patients. To that end, we include only information that is immediately relevant to decision making under conditions where time is usually of the essence. Ideally, readers would already be familiar with the vast majority of this information. Possessing this background knowledge will allow users to exploit the book's intended function as a handbook most effectively.

We all utilize and remember information in different ways and focus on different sensory channels to access it. We have taken this into account in the way we present information in this handbook. Textual content is presented in lists or short sentences to facilitate memorization and recall. In addition, we have used a number of diagrams and color coding schemes for those whose memories and minds work better with images than with text.

Throughout, we emphasize the tools that allow us to match diagnoses, patterns, and conditions to formulas and vice versa. These are the tools of Chinese medical diagnosis: the eight parameters, patterns, and pulse and tongue diagnosis. Further, our inclusion of abdominal diagnosis recognizes the use of non-Chinese influences in modern practice.

To further enhance the clinical usefulness of the handbook, we have identified key signs and symptoms, and, where relevant, important clinical markers, for each formula. These are drawn from our familiarity with the literature, and therefore involve some measure of personal judgment. Though each of the authors has more than thirty years of clinical experience, we do not deem these judgments to be the final word in the matter; we do hope, however, that you will find them useful in your own practice.

We have presented different versions of the diagrams, tables, and textual information in this handbook to focus groups of practitioners and students. This has helped us fine tune how the information is presented. We feel confident that regular use of the handbook will assist in the memorization of important information and increase understanding of the formulas.

Limitations of this Handbook

This handbook is not intended to replace a textbook such as our *Formulas & Strategies*, from which much of the information in this text is drawn. On the contrary, this book aims to complement formula textbooks by providing concisely stated and clinically relevant information that can be easily accessed to quickly lead the practitioner toward a correct formula .

How to Use this Handbook

Once you have made a diagnosis, you will often have two, three, or even more formulas in mind that might match the pattern or disorder. This handbook allows you to quickly check and compare the formulas and their range of indications. Or perhaps you have a particular formula in mind but want to be sure it is really indicated for this specific case. You may recall a formula that is not quite right, but cannot remember what other formulas treat this condition or pattern. You may know the formula you want to use but have forgotten some of its ingredients. Or you may simply want to look up the dosages. By including only clinically relevant material, this handbook allows you to do all of these things with ease.

Though novice, and even experienced, practitioners face the problems listed above, the situation is even more extreme for students who are just starting out in the clinic or preparing for exams. Here, too, our handbook may be useful. It can serve as a review guide, allowing you to quickly look up ingredients, indications, and contraindications. It concisely presents the essentials for how to use a formula in the clinic: what the pulse or abdomen might feel like; what the tongue might look like; or how you might want to modify the formula to address specific symptoms. It will also lead you to consider other formulas that treat similar conditions and in this way help you learn precisely what the formula does and does not do.

Introduction to Each Section

Name of formula and why this book is arranged by pinyin

For each formula we provide the Chinese name in traditional and simplified characters and pinyin transliteration. We also provide an English translation of the Chinese name. The translations are taken from *Chinese Herbal Medicine: Formulas & Strategies* (2nd ed). Please refer to that text for more details on the formula names.

The formulas are listed alphabetically by their pinyin names. We chose this mode of organization for two reasons. First, because people memorize and translate formulas differently, the pinyin name is the one that is least ambiguous to our audience. Second, alphabetical pinyin listing facilitates quick access to the formulas. Organizing a handbook in the traditional fashion of functional category is problematic. This is because the reader may not know under which category a specific formula is listed, a problem that is compounded by the absence of any standard criteria for including a formula in one or another category.

Graphic: why it is there and how to use it

Below the name of each formula you will find a graphic or image depicting a typical patient for whom this formula is indicated. The graphic is intended to imprint in the reader's mind the type of person for whom the formula is appropriate. But it is unavoidably a generalization and should not be taken too literally; it is suggestive but not exclusive. A graphic that depicts a thin, young woman should not preclude the formula's use for an overweight, aging man as long as he presents with the pattern the formula addresses. If nothing else, the graphic can serve as a reminder to double-check your conclusions.

In selecting the graphics we have been guided by the following considerations. For the sake of consistency and to assist in learning by repetition, we chose a limited repertoire of approximately 40 graphics. Each graphic seeks to highlight one or more of the following patient characteristics: age, gender, body type or constitution, the site where symptoms characteristically occur if relevant, and any distinctive behavioral signs such as irritability.

Each graphic is labeled with the key signs and symptoms for the pattern in question. These too are neither exhaustive nor exclusive, but serve as a reminder of what to look for in the classic presentation of the formula.

For the formulas that primarily deal with skin issues, instead of an illustration of a typical patient, we provide a photograph showing a characteristic skin lesion for which that formula is indicated. We have done this because for many skin conditions it is the skin lesion itself that is the key to proper usage, rather than a typical patient. We are grateful to our colleague and friend, Mazin al-Khafaji, for use of these photographs.

Ingredients & dosage

The list of ingredients for each formula is taken from *Formulas & Strategies,* with one group of exceptions. For the handbook we have deleted all obsolete substances, making substitutions when they exist, and deleting them when there are no commonly-used substitutions.

Dosing is an aspect of Chinese medicine that is clearly part of the art and will vary for individual patients based on their particular circumstances. However, there are "normal" amounts that can be referenced and a handbook should include them to be of any use. We have therefore based the dosages used in this book on three Chinese text-

books that were published during the last 20 years.[1] Where they all agree, we have listed a single dosage; where they do not, we have listed a range of dosages. Where none of the texts include dosages for decoctions, although decoctions based on these formulas are commonly used, we have consulted several other representative sources.[2] While the dosages suggested should be sufficient for quick clinical reference, we do encourage readers to use their judgment and tailor the dosages to the needs of their patients.

Problematic substances

This book includes formulas that contain ingredients that can be difficult, for legal and other reasons, to obtain in the West. As noted above, when the related ingredient is undeniably toxic or obsolete for other reasons, we have followed the common practice nowadays of simply deleting it, as in the case of Minium (*qiān dān*) in Bupleurum plus Dragon Bone and Oyster Shell Decoction (*chái hú jiā lóng gǔ mǔ lì tāng*), or substituting another substance for the troublesome item, such as Bubali Cornu (*shuǐ niú jiǎo*) for Rhinocerotis Cornu (*xī jiǎo*) in Rhinoceros Horn and Rehmannia Decoction (*xī jiǎo dì huáng tāng*). When such cases, no special note of these changes is made in the text. Discussions of these issues can be found in *Chinese Herbal Medicine: Materia Medica* (the chapter on obsolete substances) and also in the formula discussion sections of *Formulas & Strategies.*

There is another class of substances, however, that is a bit trickier to handle. These are ingredients that are difficult to obtain in the West because of perceived safety issues that, at least in China, are not considered significant *if* the herbs are chosen and prepared properly and used at the correct

1. Xu Ji-Qun 許濟群, Wang Mian-Zhi 王綿之 (eds.) *Formulas* 方濟學. Beijing: People's Medical Publishing House, 1995; Li Fei 李飛 (ed.) *Formulas* 方劑學. Beijing: People's Medical Publishing House, 2002; Lian Jian-Wei 連建偉, Li Yi 李翼 (ed.) *Formulas* 方劑學. Beijing: Science Press, 2007.

2. Chen Chao-Zu 陳潮祖 (ed.) *Chinese Medicine Treatment Strategies and Formulas*, 4th edition (中醫治法與方). Beijing: People's Medical Publishing House, 2005; Liu Gong-Wang 劉公望 (ed.) *Formulas* 方劑學. Beijing: Huaxia Publishing House, 2002; Ni Cheng 倪誠 (ed.) *New Edition of Formulas* 新編方劑學. Beijing: People's Medical Publishing House, 2006.

dosages for limited periods of time. In addition, there are also substances for which no satisfactory substitutes are readily available. The main herbs in this category are Ephedrae Herba (*má huáng*), Aconiti Radix lateralis praeparata (*zhì fù zǐ*), and Asari Radix et Rhizoma (*xì xīn*). We have chosen to retain these ingredients when they are listed, as the formulas will work best if they are included, but have footnoted them and identified commonly-used substitutes. Where there is no suitable substitute, the practitioner will have to adapt the formula as best she can to the needs of her patient.

Preparation notes

The standard preparation of formulas in Chinese medicine remains the decoction, although concentrated granules and patent medicines in the form of pills, tablets, and tinctures are becoming increasingly common. The dosages listed in this handbook for almost all formulas reflect those for decoctions; the ratios will remain basically the same for granule formulations (for more detail, see *Formulas & Strategies*, xxxiii-xxxix). When a formula requires special instructions regarding duration of decoction, preparation of the herbs, etc., this will be found in the section entitled *Preparation notes*.

Actions

This is a brief summary of what the formula does. It should match what is required by your diagnosis.

Main patterns

This section outlines the main pattern or patterns for which a formula is used. In addition, here we differentiate between key symptoms, those which should normally be present when the formula is prescribed, and secondary symptoms, which may be present and make the diagnosis clearer, but need not necessarily be present. We have limited ourselves to four or five key symptoms, and sometimes fewer. In practice, you should check these key symptoms against the pulse, tongue, or abdomen. If those indicators suggest a different pattern, it would be wise to reevaluate the diagnosis.

Tongue & pulse

The information about the tongue and pulse provided in these sections is both clinical and didactic. For instance, a patient with Liver qi stagnation will often have a wiry pulse. Thus a formula like Rambling Powder (*xiāo yáo sǎn*), which is indicated to treat this problem, will have a wiry pulse listed rather than a deficient, thin, or slippery one. In practice, however, the deficiency that this formula also treats may dominate the pulse picture and alter the pulse. In that case, knowing that a wiry pulse is an important part of the clinical picture for this formula remains useful as it helps one remember the core issues that the formula addresses, even if that aspect of the pulse is not easily palpable. The same reasoning applies to information regarding the tongue. For instance, if a patient for whom we are thinking of prescribing Honeysuckle and Forsythia Powder (*yín qiào sǎn*) has a red tongue tip (as stated in the text), this helps to confirm the diagnosis. While the tongue that we suggest for the pattern may not be the one that the patient presents, it is still useful to know what the typical tongue would be because it reveals a lot about the formula and the pattern it treats.

Clinical notes

This is a brief bullet-point review of how the formula is typically used. It further defines the list of patterns by relating each one to specific symptoms or diseases. Where feasible, this section also provides clinical pointers intended to help the reader arrive at a decision about the suitability of the formula. We may also list possible modifications for adjusting the core formula to meet different clinical presentations.

Contraindications

This section contains a brief summary of contraindications that one should consider before prescribing the formula. Of course, all formulas are, in a sense, contraindicated for situations for which they are not designed. Thus, if a formula tonifies and warms, it is contraindicated for cases of excess heat and is unsuitable for cases that lack cold and deficiency. While this may be obvious, it is important that practitioners, especially those relatively new to this work, keep this in mind and not prescribe formulas based on symptoms alone.

How to use formulas with similar indications

Appended to most formulas is a list of other formulas that might be considered in patients with similar presentations. This list is far from exhaustive. We have focused the comparisons on both the differences in the disease pattern as well as in key symptoms. Focusing on both the underlying cause as well as distinguishing manifestations is the key to discovering the proper use of formulas. Some formulas that are not otherwise discussed as main entries in this handbook may be listed in this section, and are marked with an asterisk (*).

Introduction to Abdominal Diagnosis (腹診 *fù zhěn/fukushin*)

We have included some basic abdominal diagnostic information for many of the formulas in this handbook even though it not an essential and widely taught aspect of modern Chinese medicine in either China or the West. We have done so because abdominal diagnosis can provide important information to help us differentiate patterns and select the proper formula. For those readers who already know abdominal diagnosis as applied to herbal formulas, our handbook will provide a useful additional resource. Other readers may be tempted to learn more about this diagnostic tool. While it emerged historically in Japan and remains widely associated with Japanese-style Kampo medicine, as practitioners of Chinese medicine in the West, we need not be constrained by this.

Abdominal diagnosis has a number of useful aspects. First, it is easier to learn than pulse diagnosis and, in our experience, easier to reach consensus among practitioners about the findings observed. Second, there exist a number of widely agreed upon markers to a range of commonly used formulas, specifically those that are commonly used in Japanese Kampo medicine. Third, changes in abdominal findings can both help us ascertain the efficacy of our formula choice as well as indicate when a formula may need to be changed in the course of treatment.

For those readers who have never studied abdominal diagnosis in relation to formula patterns, we list below the basic terms that are used in this handbook to denote various abdominal findings and their range of meanings. While this information is no substitute for hands-on study of abdominal diagnosis, it will at least provide context and demonstrate why such study may be useful.

- *Full and/or weak and soft abdomen:* The strength of the abdominal wall and, by extension, excess and deficiency.

- *Tension in the hypochondrium:* Tension under the ribs upon palpation that may be experienced as uncomfortable or painful by the patient.

- *Discomfort in the epigastrium:* A subjective feeling of discomfort or even pain in the epigastrium. Pressing on the area may or may not be uncomfortable or painful, and this differentiation provides useful clinical information.

- *Discomfort or distention of the abdomen:* Fullness, distention, and discomfort that may involve the entire upper abdomen above the umbilicus. Pressing on the area may or may not be uncomfortable or painful, and this differentiation provides useful clinical information.

- *Splashing sounds:* These are elicited by tapping the epigastrium and left hypochondriac region. They indicate stagnating fluids.

- *Tension of the rectus abdominus muscle:* This refers to a rectus abdominus that is tense and easily palpable. It may occur on one or both sides, above and below the umbilicus.

- *Pulsations:* Pulsations felt when palpating around the midline and the umbilicus.

- *Lax or weak lower abdomen:* This refers to palpable weakness of the lower abdomen. It is often accompanied by a tense rectus abdominus in the lower abdomen.

- *Pain or resistance to pressure in the lower abdomen:* Pain elicited on (deep) palpation, generally in one or both inguinal regions.

- *Tension in the lower abdomen:* Subjectively felt tension in the lower abdomen and discomfort felt upon palpating the supra-pubic region.

- *Pencil line:* A palpable thickening of the linea alba, either above or below the umbilicus.

Our main sources for the abdominal findings used in this text were found in the literature on Japanese abdominal diagnosis. Because the range of formulas used in Japanese Kampo medicine is significantly smaller than that used in Chinese medicine, where we could not find referenced information on a particular formula, none has been provided.

Explanation of Composition Graphic

In addition to presenting information about the composition of the formula in a conventional format that lists ingredients with their dosage, we have added a composition graphic for each formula. A simple list, while useful, does not put the ingredients in full context and leaves out important information, such as temperature and taste, that are supplied later in the textbook entries.

The advantage of a graphic in a handbook such as this is twofold. First, it condenses key information into a single, small space. Second, it provides an image of the formula as a whole. In a sense, conventional lists and explanations introduce each separate note of a chord, leaving it to the reader to reconstitute the chord in their own imagination. A graphic, on the other hand, makes the chord come alive. For each ingredient we have included color representations of their temperature and taste.

We have chosen not to include information on channels/organs entered as there is a wide variety of opinion on this question, it is not always relevant, and it would clutter up the graphic. Nor have we listed all the functions of the ingredients, but have limited ourselves to those relevant to the given formula.

Herb Preparation

It is not standard for a formula text to include detailed information on processing and preparation of individual substances. In part, this is because different versions of the same formula will often list different modes of preparation for the same ingredient. In addition, herbal pharmacies in the West, as in China today, rarely carry the full range of prepared herbs that were available to a physician in, say, 18th century Suzhou. Some practitioners spend

▶ KEY TO FORMULA COLORS

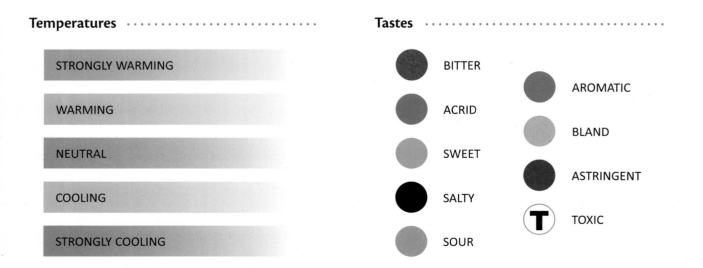

Temperatures ·

STRONGLY WARMING

WARMING

NEUTRAL

COOLING

STRONGLY COOLING

Tastes ·

BITTER

ACRID

SWEET

SALTY

SOUR

AROMATIC

BLAND

ASTRINGENT

(T) TOXIC

a lot of effort on this aspect of their practice. Others do not. For these reasons, we usually do not provide specific preparation information for the herbs in the list of ingredients. However, because we believe that this information can be clinically important, it occurred to us that a brief discussion of the subject here would be useful to the reader. This conclusion was reached when we realized that most of our formula descriptions either omitted information about processing and preparation of individual herbs, or only mentioned it in general terms. This leaves the reader without the proper information needed to make a decision about the preparation of a particular herb in a formula that is most suited to the goals of that formula.

In source texts the subject of processing and preparation of individual herbs is often omitted. Presumably this is because the author assumed that the practitioner was well versed in the subject and could choose the properly treated herb based on the functions and qualities that he or she required for the case at hand. Modern texts, on the other hand, often simply lack specificity when describing the treatment of a particular herb. For example, the term Pinelliae Rhizoma praeparatum (*zhì bàn xià*) provides no clue as to whether treatment should be with alum, ginger, or limestone.

In the tables below, we present a brief outline of processing information in the hope that it provides the practitioner with enough information to make a decision according to the requirements of the situation for which he or she is prescribing. To return to our example, if a formula calls for Pinelliae Rhizoma praeparatum (*zhì bàn xià*), the practitioner can consult the table below and deduce that, in most instances, Lung phlegm patterns call for the use of clear Pinelliae Rhizoma praeparatum (*qīng bàn xià*) or standard Pinelliae Rhizoma praeparatum (*fǎ bàn xià*), while middle burner damp-stagnation patterns are best addressed with ginger-fried Pinelliae Rhizoma praeparatum (*jiāng bàn xià*).

Because it is beyond the scope of this book to catalogue the treatment of a large number of herbs, we have taken the approach of providing one table that discusses the most common methods of processing and preparation, and a second table that discusses the treatment of a small number of commonly-used herbs.

The first table describes the method of treatment, function, and common examples of herbs that receive that particular treatment. It should be noted that in these discussions, the description is stated in general terms; in practice, preparation is an art which accounts for the uniqueness of each herb. Also, the functions resulting from a particular mode of preparation vary somewhat depending on the herb to which the treatment is applied. The functions listed here are general ones and are provided only as a guide.

The second table below outlines common forms of treatment for commonly-treated herbs. Again, because this is a clinical handbook, only the most important information is listed, and in no way is this intended to be an exhaustive discussion of the subject. We list only the most common treatments for each herb, and the brief discussion of functions and examples is intended to provide the practitioner with enough information to make an informed decision regarding the form of the herb that he or she wishes to include in a formula.

Lastly, it should be noted that although one form of an herb may be more ideal than another to address a given problem, in most cases the type of preparation affects only the *degree* to which a function acts, rather than the presence of the function itself. For example, a wine-treated herb is thought to be more able to move blood than the untreated agent. However, in the case of blood-moving herbs, the untreated agent also possesses that function to some degree, and if the wine-fried item is not available, or if it is considered too warm or dispersing for the patient, it is fine to use the untreated herb.

▶ **Table 1:** Common Methods of Processing Herbs

Treatment	*Pīnyīn* (字)	Description	Function	Examples	Comments
Dry-frying	*chǎo* (炒)	Herbs are heated and stirred in a wok using a moderate heat until the herb darkens slightly and gives off the herb's characteristic aroma.	Reduces cold, bitter or toxic natures of herbs, lessens bad tastes, and makes the herb's ingredients more available for extraction in decoctions.	Gardeniae Fructus *(zhī zǐ)*, Vaccariae Semen *(wáng bù liú xíng)*, Paeoniae Radix rubra *(chì sháo)*, Paeoniae Radix alba *(bái sháo)*, Cassiae Semen *(jué míng zǐ)*, Cannabis Semen *(huǒ má rén)*, Ziziphi spinosae Semen *(suān zǎo rén)*, Coicis Semen *(yì yǐ rén)*, Euryales Semen *(qiàn shí)*, Crataegi Fructus *(shān zhā)*	Most seeds are dry-fried to cause them to crack open and allow their ingredients to be released during decoction. In some cases herbs are dry-fried to give them longer shelf-life.
Wine-frying	*jiǔ chǎo* (酒炒)	Two methods: 1. Herbs are first soaked in rice wine and then stir-fried over a moderate heat. 2. Herbs are stir-fried over a moderate heat as rice wine is spritzed onto them.	Same functions as dry-frying with the additional functions of increasing the blood-moving and collateral-freeing function of the treated herb.	Rhei Radix et Rhizoma *(dà huáng)*, Pheretima *(dì lóng)*, Salviae miltiorrhizae Radix *(dān shēn)*, Paeoniae Radix alba *(bái sháo)*, Paeoniae Radix rubra *(chì sháo)*, Angelicae sinensis Radix *(dāng guī)*, Clematidis Radix *(wēi líng xiān)*	Wine travels to the upper body and thus wine-treated herbs are usually applied to treatment of upper body disorders.
Vinegar-frying	*cù chǎo* (醋炒)	Two methods: 1. Herbs are first soaked in rice vinegar and then stir-fried over a moderate heat. 2. Herbs are stir-fried over a moderate heat as rice vinegar is spritzed onto them.	Same functions as dry-frying with the additional functions of increasing an herb's ability to invigorate blood and relieve pain.	Sparganii Rhizoma *(sān léng)*, Curcumae Rhizoma *(é zhú)*, Kansui Radix *(gān suì)*, Bupleuri Radix *(chái hú)*, Cyperi Rhizoma *(xiāng fù)*, Corydalis Rhizoma *(yán hú suǒ)*, Curcumae Radix *(yù jīn)*, Myrrha *(mò yào)*, Olibanum *(rǔ xiāng)*	Vinegar is sour and thus is used to guide herbs to the Liver channel.

Treatment	*Pīnyīn* (字)	Description	Function	Examples	Comments
Brine-frying	*yán chǎo* (鹽炒)	Two methods: 1. Herbs are first soaked in salted water and then stir-fried over a moderate heat. 2. Herbs are stir-fried over a moderate heat as salted water is spritzed onto them.	Guides herbs to the lower burner and increases an herb's function of nourishing yin and directing fire downward.	Anemarrhenae Rhizoma *(zhī mǔ)*, Phellodendri Cortex *(huáng bǎi)*, Foeniculi Fructus *(xiǎo huí xiāng)*, Eucommiae Cortex *(dù zhòng)*, Psoraleae Fructus *(bǔ gǔ zhī)*, Astragali complanati Semen *(shā yuàn zǐ)*	This method of treatment is mostly applied to herbs that tonify the Kidneys, secure essence, treat bulging disorders, promote urination, or drain ministerial fire.
Honey-frying	*mì zhì* (蜜炙)	The herbs are mix-fried with refined honey. Usually the honey is diluted with water and heated before adding the herbs.	Honey-frying increases the ability of cough-relieving herbs to moisten the Lung and relieve cough. For tonifying herbs, it increases their function of tonifying the Spleen and augmenting qi.	Glycyrrhizae Radix *(gān cǎo)*, Astragali Radix *(huáng qí)*, Ephedrae Herba *(má huáng)*, Stemonae Radix *(bǎi bù)*, Cynanchi stauntonii Rhizoma *(bái qián)*, Mori Cortex *(sāng bái pí)*, Mori Folium *(sāng yè)*, and Trichosanthis Pericarpium *(guā lóu pí)*	When applied to herbs that are dispersing in nature, honey-frying moderates the dispersing nature. It also can decrease side effects and improve the flavor of treated herbs.
Bran-frying	*fū chǎo* (麩炒)	Wheat bran is added to a heated wok and cooked over medium heat until it begins to smoke. The herbs are then added and continually stirred until they darken slightly.	Same functions as dry-frying with the additional functions of increasing the tonifying nature of tonifying herbs and moderating the dispersing or drying nature of dispersing or drying herbs.	Aurantii Fructus immaturus *(zhǐ shí)*, Aurantii Fructus *(zhǐ ké)*, Atractylodis Rhizoma *(cāng zhú)*, Codonopsis Radix *(dǎng shēn)*, Dioscoreae Rhizoma *(shān yào)*, Atractylodis macrocephalae Rhizoma *(bái zhú)*	Bran-frying also decreases the disagreeable smell or taste of foul-smelling or bad-tasting herbs.

Treatment	*Pīnyīn* (字)	Description	Function	Examples	Comments
Wine-steaming	*jiǔ zhēng* (酒蒸)	Herbs are put in a closed container and steamed with rice wine.	Changes the nature of herbs making them warmer and more nourishing.	Rehmanniae Radix *(shēng dì huáng)*, Corni Fructus *(shān zhū yú)*, Cistanches Herba *(ròu cōng róng)*, Polygonati Rhizoma *(huáng jīng)*, Ligustri lucidi Fructus *(nǚ zhēn zǐ)*, Schisandrae Fructus *(wǔ wèi zǐ)*, Siegesbeckiae Herba *(xī xiān cǎo)*	Wine-steaming makes some herbs easier to slice and in some cases is used to preserve herbs. In the case of herbs like Polygonati Rhizoma *(huáng jīng)*, steaming eliminates the herb's tendency to irritate the throat.
Steaming	*zhēng* (蒸)	Herbs are put in a closed container and steamed.	Changes the nature of herbs making them warmer and more nourishing.	Ginseng Radix *(rén shēn)*, Scrophulariae Radix *(xuán shēn)*, and Chaenomelis Fructus *(mù guā)*	Steaming also makes herbs easier to slice.
Calcining	*duàn* (煅)	Different methods are used to heat an agent to a high temperature. Sometimes this is followed by dipping the heated item into vinegar or water.	Makes the agent friable, decreases foul tastes and odors, reduces an agent's cold nature and reduces the water content of the agent.	Ostreae Concha *(mǔ lì)*, Fossilia Ossis Mastodi *(lóng gǔ)*, Alumen dehydratum *(kū fán)*, Gypsum fibrosum *(shí gāo)*, Arcae Concha *(wǎ léng zǐ)*, Meretricis/Cyclinae Concha *(gé qiào)*, Pyritum *(zì rán tóng)*, Haematitum *(dài zhě shí)*, Magnetitum *(cí shí)*	Calcining in general and especially vinegar dip-calcining makes agents more astringent.
Scorching	*jiāo* (焦)	A medium to high heat is used to stir-fry the herbs until they are darkened considerably on the exterior but only slightly on the interior.	Scorching is primarily applied to increase an herb's ability to disperse food stagnation and strengthen the Spleen.	Crataegi Fructus *(shān zhā)*, Gardeniae Fructus *(zhī zǐ)*, Arecae Semen *(bīng láng)*	In some cases scorching is used to reduce an herb's irritating nature.

Treatment	Pīnyīn (字)	Description	Function	Examples	Comments
Charring	*tàn* (炭)	A medium to high heat is used to stir-fry the herbs until they are blackened on the exterior and darkened noticeably on the interior.	Increases or creates an ability to stop bleeding in the treated herb.	Sophorae Fructus *(huái jiǎo)*, Artemisiae argyi Folium *(ài yè)*, Cirsii japonici Herba sive Radix *(dà jì)*, Cirsii Herba *(xiǎo jì)*, Zingiberis Rhizoma *(gān jiāng)*, Mume Fructus *(wū méi)*, Moutan Cortex *(mǔ dān pí)*, Sanguisorbae Radix *(dì yú)*, Rubiae Radix *(qiàn cǎo gēn)*, Typhae Pollen *(pú huáng)*, Schizonepetae Herba *(jīng jiè)*, Saposhnikoviae Radix *(fáng fēng)*	Charring also increases the astringency of the treated herbs and this astringency is usually applied to treating diarrhea or dysentery.
Complex treatments	*fǎn fù zhì fǎ* (反覆 製法)	Generally, these treatments involve multiple soakings of the herbs (often in alum or limestone) and cooking in herb extracts (most commonly of licorice and/or ginger).	Functions vary depending on the treatment.	Pinelliae Rhizoma praeparatum *(zhì bàn xià)*, Aconiti Radix lateralis praeparata *(zhì fù zǐ)*, and Arisaematis Rhizoma praeparatum *(zhì tiān nán xīng)*	

▶ **Table 2:** Herbs that are Commonly Processed

Herb	Pharmaceutical (*Pīnyīn* 字)	Treatment	Function	Examples	Comments
Paeoniae Radix alba *(bái sháo)*	untreated Paeoniae Radix alba *(shēng bái sháo* 生白芍*)*	untreated	Nourishes blood, preserves yin, calms and restrains Liver yang.	Treats menstrual disorders, headache, dizziness, irritability, and spontaneous or night sweating when these are owing to blood deficiency.	
	wine-fried Paeoniae Radix alba *(jiǔ chǎo bái sháo* 酒炒白芍*)*	wine-fried	Treatment renders the herbs less sour and cold so that the herb's function of harmonizing the middle and moderating tension is enhanced.	Treats cramping pain in the abdomen and stomach, rib pain, cramping pain in the limbs and post-partum abdominal pain.	Though uncommon, this herb can also be mix-fried with vinegar. In that case its astringent quality is increased and the treated herb is used in addressing bleeding disorders such as blood in the urine.
	dry-fried Paeoniae Radix alba *(chǎo bái sháo* 炒白芍*)*	dry-fried	Dry-frying moderates the cold nature of the herb and increases its ability to preserve yin and nourish blood.	Treats Liver attacking Spleen deficiency that gives rise to intestinal rumbling, painful cramping diarrhea, or chronic diarrhea with abdominal pain eased by warmth and pressure.	

Herb	Pharmaceutical (*Pīnyīn* 字)	Treatment	Function	Examples	Comments
Atractylodis macrocephalae Rhizoma (*bái zhú*)	untreated Atractylodis macrocephalae Rhizoma (*shēng bái zhú* 生白朮)	untreated	Strengthens the Spleen and dries dampness, promotes water metabolism and disperses swelling.	Treats internal collection of fluids and thin mucus as well as superficial edema and wind-damp painful obstruction.	The untreated herb can be drying.
	earth-fried Atractylodis macrocephalae Rhizoma (*tǔ chǎo bái zhú* 土炒白朮)	earth-fried	Strengthens the Spleen and relieves diarrhea.	Particularly useful for Spleen-deficiency diarrhea or loose stools	
	bran-fried Atractylodis macrocephalae Rhizoma (*fū chǎo bái zhú* 麩炒白朮)	bran-fried	Treatment moderates the herb's drying nature and increases its ability to strengthen the Spleen.	Treats Spleen deficiency that gives rise to digestive weakness or spontaneous sweating.	Tonifies the Spleen without being overly drying.

Herb	Pharmaceutical (*Pīnyīn* 字)	Treatment	Function	Examples	Comments
Pinelliae Rhizoma (*bàn xià*)	untreated Pinelliae Rhizoma (*shēng bàn xià* 生半夏)	untreated	Transforms phlegm and disperses knots.	Treats swellings and toxic bites of insects and snakes.	Toxic. Used externally.
	ginger-fried Pinelliae Rhizoma praeparatum (*jiāng bàn xià* 姜半夏)	alum and ginger treated	Directs rebellious qi downward. Transforms phlegm and dampness.	Treats middle burner rebellious qi seen in nausea and vomiting. It also treats focal distention.	Also used for plum-pit qi.
	clear Pinelliae Rhizoma praeparatum (*qīng bàn xià* 清半夏) or clear-water Pinelliae Rhizoma praeparatum (*qīng shuǐ bàn xià* 清水半夏)	alum-treated	Dries dampness and transforms phlegm.	Treats phlegm-cough and phlegm that gives rise to dizziness.	Also treats vertigo, palpitation and thin mucus.
	standard Pinelliae Rhizoma praeparatum (*fǎ bàn xià* 法半夏)	limestone and licorice treated	Dries dampness and transforms phlegm.	Similar to alum-treated herb but slightly less drying.	Primarily used in prepared products.
Atractylodis Rhizoma (*cāng zhú*)	untreated Atractylodis Rhizoma (*shēng cāng zhú* 生蒼朮)	untreated	Transforms dampness, harmonizes the Stomach and dispels exterior wind-damp.	Treats wind-damp painful obstruction, external contractions with dampness, damp-warmth, and pain in the legs and knees.	
	bran-fried Atractylodis Rhizoma (*fū chǎo cāng zhú* 麸炒蒼朮)	bran-fried	Treatment imparts the bran's fragrance to the herb and makes it better able to strengthen the Spleen.	Treats damp obstruction or thin mucus stagnation in the middle burner, various eye disorders, and damp-heat downpour to the legs and knees.	Because treatment moderates the herb's drying nature, and reduces irritating oils the bran-fried herb is well suited for middle burner disorders and patients who tend to yin deficiency.

Herb	Pharmaceutical (*Pīnyīn* 字)	Treatment	Function	Examples	Comments
Bupleuri Radix (*chái hú*)	untreated Bupleuri Radix (*shēng chái hú* 生柴胡)	untreated	The untreated herb is uplifting and dispersing.	Treats exterior patterns and qi fall patterns.	Many practitioners also feel that the untreated herb is preferred for dredging the Liver especially if the Liver stagnation has caused heat.
	vinegar-fried Bupleuri Radix (*cù chái hú* 醋炒柴胡)	vinegar-fried	Vinegar-frying decreases the herb's ability to uplift and disperse and increases its ability to dredge the Liver and relieve pain.	Mostly used to treat Liver qi stagnation that results in pain and distention in the ribs, menstrual pain and menstrual irregularity.	
Chuanxiong Rhizoma (*chuān xiōng*)	untreated Chuanxiong Rhizoma (*shēng chuān xiōng* 生川芎)	untreated	Invigorates blood and moves qi. Dispels wind and relieves pain.	Treats blood stasis and qi stagnation that brings about menstrual pain, blocked menses, and irregular menstruation as well as swellings and sores, trauma, headache, head wind, and wind-damp painful obstruction.	In general, the wine-treated herb is used for upper body disorders and the untreated herb treats the lower body. Nonetheless, both forms of the herb can be used for either location.
	wine-fried Chuanxiong Rhizoma (*jiǔ chǎo chuān xiōng* 酒川芎)	wine-fried	Wine leads the herb to the upper body and increases its function of moving blood and qi and relieving pain.	Often used for blood stasis headache and pain in the ribs and chest.	

Herb	Pharmaceutical (*Pīnyīn* 字)	Treatment	Function	Examples	Comments
Rhei Radix et Rhizoma (*dà huáng*)	untreated Rhei Radix et Rhizoma (*shēng dà huáng* 生大黃)	untreated	Strong ability to purge the intestines and drain fire and resolve toxicity.	Used to unblock the bowels and to drain fire and resolve toxicity.	The herb is added near the end (*hòu xià* 後下) to preserve its ability to purge the intestines.
	wine-fried Rhei Radix et Rhizoma (*jiǔ dà huáng* 酒大黃)	wine-fried	Treatment decreases the herb's purgative function and moves the focus of the functions to the upper burner.	Treats upper burner excess heat patterns seen as Lung abscess and other Lung heat disorders.	
	steamed Rhei Radix et Rhizoma (*shú dà huáng* 熟大黃)	wine-steamed	Treatment decreases the herb's purgative function and increases its ability to disperse stasis and invigorate the blood.	Treats abdominal masses, blocked menses and internal static blood.	
	vinegar-fried Rhei Radix et Rhizoma (*cù dà huáng* 醋大黃)	vinegar-fried	Treatment decreases the herb's purgative function and adds an ability to disperse stasis and transform stasis.	Treats food accumulation that presents with fullness and focal distention. It also is used with blood moving herbs to disperse abdominal masses.	

Herb	Pharmaceutical (*Pīnyīn* 字)	Treatment	Function	Examples	Comments
Eucommiae Cortex (*dù zhòng*)	untreated Eucommiae Cortex (*shēng dù zhòng* 生杜仲)	untreated	Tonifies the Liver and Kidneys, strengthens the sinews and bones and quiets the fetus.	Treats wind-damp pain or injury in the lower back and knees in the presence of deficiency of the Liver and Kidneys.	The untreated herb is warm and drying and thus particularly suited for cold-damp deficiency obstruction patterns.
	brine-fried Eucommiae Cortex (*yán chǎo dù zhòng* 鹽炒杜仲) or dry-fried Eucommiae Cortex (*chǎo dù zhòng* 炒杜仲)	brine-fried	Treatment increases the herb's function of tonifying the Liver and Kidneys and decreases its drying nature.	Impotence, back pain and insecure fetus in patients with Liver and Kidney deficiency.	Paradoxically, the brine-fried item is also used to treat high blood pressure. Apparently, the amount of salt imbibed is minimal.
Glycyrrhizae Radix (*gān cǎo*)	untreated Glycyrrhizae Radix (*shēng gān cǎo* 生甘草)	untreated	Drains fire, resolves toxicity, transforms phlegm and relieves cough.	Treats phlegm-heat cough, toxic swellings, sore, swollen throat, and undesirable reactions to food or medicine.	All forms of this herb also are used to harmonize the herbs of a formula.
	Glycyrrhizae Radix praeparata (*zhì gān cǎo* 炙甘草)	honey-fried	Tonifies the Spleen and harmonizes the Stomach, augments qi and restores the pulse.	Deficiency of the middle burner that presents as decreased food intake, fatigue, and pain in the epigastrium and abdomen.	

Herb	Pharmaceutical (*Pīnyīn* 字)	Treatment	Function	Examples	Comments
Polygoni multiflori Radix (*hé shǒu wū)*	untreated Polygoni multiflori Radix (*shēng hé shǒu wū* 生首烏)	untreated	Disperses swellings, resolves toxicity and moistens the intestines.	Treats swelling and sores.	Seldom used in modern times. It is not generally available.
	black bean treated Polygoni multiflori Radix (*hēi dòu zhì shǒu wū)* 黑豆製首烏 or Polygoni multiflori Radix praeparata (*zhì hé shǒu wū)*	black bean treated	Nourish the Liver and Kidneys, augments essence and blood, blackens the hair, and strengthens the sinews and bones.	Treats prematurely greying hair, weakness in the lower back and knees, dizziness, tinnitus and other signs of weakness in the blood and essence and deficiency in the Liver and Kidneys.	Treatment with black-bean extract also eliminates the untreated herb's effect of moving the stool. Some companies use rice wine treatment instead of black bean extract, but black bean treated is preferred.
Phellodendri Cortex (*huáng bǎi)*	untreated Phellodendri Cortex (*shēng huáng bǎi* 生黃柏)	untreated	Drains fire, resolves toxicity and dries dampness.	Treats damp heat especially in the lower body as in dysentery and diarrhea, damp-heat rashes and painful urination.	
	brine-fried Phellodendri Cortex (*yán chǎo huáng bǎi* 鹽炒黃柏)	brine-fried	Brine-frying increases the herbs function of promoting descent of fire, enriching yin and reducing deficiency fevers.	Treats steaming bones, night sweats, seminal emissions, weakness in the knees, and coughing of blood associated with yin-deficiency fire.	A less common treatment for this herb is charring (to treat bleeding).
	wine-fried Phellodendri Cortex (*jiǔ chǎo huáng bǎi* 酒炒黃柏)	wine-fried	Wine-frying reduces the bitter and cold nature of the herb and leads the herb to the upper burner.	Treats red eyes, sore throat or mouth sores. It is also applied to the treatment of vaginal discharge.	Because wine rises to the head, this agent can also be used to treat heat disorders of the head and face.

Herb	Pharmaceutical (*Pīnyīn* 字)	Treatment	Function	Examples	Comments
Astragali Radix (*huáng qí*)	untreated Astragali Radix (*shēng huáng qí* 生黄芪)	untreated	Best for augmenting the protective qi, securing the exterior, drawing out toxicity, generating flesh, promoting urination and reducing swelling.	Treats deficiency sweating, weakness in the defense qi, various stages of toxic swellings and qi-deficiency edema.	
	honey-prepared Astragali Radix (*mì zhì huáng qí* 炙黄芪)	honey-fried	Best for augmenting qi and tonifying the middle.	Treats middle burner deficiency that gives rise to lack of appetite, loose stools, sinking of the middle qi (prolapse of rectum or uterus), qi-deficiency bleeding, fatigue and weakness in the four limbs.	The honey-fried item is also suitable for treating qi-deficiency constipation.
Ephedrae Herba (*má huáng*)	untreated Ephedrae Herba (*má huáng* 生麻黄)	untreated	Induces sweat, releases pathogens from the exterior and promotes water metabolism to disperse swelling. Also calms asthma and diffuses Lung qi.	Treats wind-water edema, wind-cold exterior patterns characterized by absence of sweating and painful wind-damp obstruction patterns.	In the dermatology clinic this herb is used to treat yin sores.
	honey-prepared Ephedrae Herba (*mì zhì má huáng* 蜜炙麻黄)	honey-fried	Treatment renders the herb less dispersing and more moderate. Best for calming asthma and diffusing Lung qi.	Treats cough and asthmatic breathing with copious clear phlegm in patterns where wind-cold fetters the Lungs. Is best suited for patterns where the exterior cold pathogen is not severe.	Often used for children and seniors.

Herb	Pharmaceutical (*Pīnyīn* 字)	Treatment	Function	Examples	Comments
Hordei Fructus germinatus (*mài yá*)	untreated Hordei Fructus germinatus (*shēng mài yá* 生麥芽)	untreated	Disperses food accumulation, dredges the Liver.	Treats food accumulation, especially in the presence of Liver qi stagnation.	All forms of this herb are used to end milk production after breastfeeding has ceased. Most practitioners, however, prefer the dry-fried item for this function.
	dry-fried Hordei Fructus germinatus (*chǎo mài yá* 炒麥芽)	dry-fried	Treatment increases the herb's ability to disperse food accumulation.	Especially suited for food stagnation owing to deficiency.	The scorch-fried herb (*jiāo mài yá* 焦麥芽) is said to be even better than the dry-fried herb at dispersing food accumulation, especially when the pattern includes diarrhea.
Ginseng Radix (*rén shēn*)	Ginseng Radix alba (*bái rén shēn* 白人參) or (*bái shēn* 白參)	untreated	Tonify qi, generate fluids, restore the pulse, secure abandoned disorders, tonify the Spleen and augment the Lung.	Treats constitutional deficiency tending toward abandoned disorders, Spleen deficiency digestive disorders, thirst and wasting and thirsting disorder.	
	Ginseng Radix rubra (*hóng rén shēn* 紅人參) or (*hóng shēn* 紅參)	steamed	Greatly tonifies the source qi, restores the pulse, secures abandoned disorders, augments qi and contains the blood in the vessels.	Treats constitutional deficiency tending toward abandoned disorders, cold limbs, faint pulse, and qi failing to contain blood.	The treated herb is considerably warmer than the untreated item.

Herb	Pharmaceutical (*Pīnyīn* 字)	Treatment	Function	Examples	Comments
Mori Cortex (*sāng bái pí*)	untreated Mori Cortex (*sāng bái pí* 生桑白皮)	untreated	Drains the Lung, calms asthmatic breathing, and relieves cough. Can also move water and disperse swelling.	Treats Lung heat or phlegm-fire cough and asthmatic breathing. Also treats edema of the face and limbs.	The untreated herb also moistens the Lung, but much less than the honey-fried version.
	honey-prepared Mori Cortex (*sāng bái pí* 蜜炙桑白皮) or prepared Mori Cortex (*zhì sāng bái pí* 炙桑白皮)	honey-fried	Moistens the Lung and relieves cough.	Treats lung deficiency cough.	Treatment reduces the cold and draining nature of the herb making it safer for children, old folks and those with a fragile constitution.
Crataegi Fructus (*shān zhā*)	untreated Crataegi Fructus (*shān zhā* 生山楂)	untreated	Invigorates blood and transforms stasis.	Treats blood-stasis menstrual pain and menstrual irregularity.	
	dry-fried Crataegi Fructus (*chǎo shān zhā* 炒山楂)	dry-fried	Transforms food accumulation. Dry-frying reduces the herb's tendency to irritate the stomach.	Treats Spleen deficiency food stagnation.	Similar to scorched but slightly less apt at dispersing stagnation.
	scorched Crataegi Fructus (*jiāo shān zhā* 焦山楂)	scorched	Disperses food stagnation and relieves diarrhea.	Treats Spleen deficiency food stagnation.	Treatment reduces the sour taste of the herb and increases the bitter taste.
	carbonized Crataegi Fructus (*shān zhā tàn* 山楂炭)	charred	Stops bleeding, relieves diarrhea, and disperses food stagnation.	Especially used for Spleen deficiency diarrhea and intestinal wind with signs of food stagnation.	

Herb	Pharmaceutical (*Pīnyīn* 字)	Treatment	Function	Examples	Comments
Ziziphi spinosae Semen (*suān zǎo rén*)	untreated Ziziphi spinosae Semen (*shēng suān zǎo rén* 生酸棗仁)	untreated	Nourishes the Heart, quiets the spirit, and tonifies the Liver.	Insomnia, irritability, palpitations and forgetfulness.	Treated and untreated Ziziphi spinosae Semen (*suān zǎo rén*) look very similar, but taste very different. The untreated herb is un-palatable like uncooked peanuts and the roast-ed herb is much tastier, like roasted peanuts. In addition, the stir-fried herb is much more fragrant than the un-treated one.
	dry-fried Ziziphi spinosae Semen (*chǎo suān zǎo rén* 炒酸棗仁)	dry-fried	Nourishes the Heart, quiets the spirit, inhibits sweating, and fragrantly arouses the Spleen.	Fright palpitations, deficiency insomnia, night sweats and forgetfulness.	The treated herb is warmer and thus usu-ally included in warm-ing formulas. Also, as with most seeds, dry-frying makes the components inside the seed more available during decoction.
Cyperi Rhizoma (*xiāng fù*)	untreated Cyperi Rhizoma (*shēng xiāng fù* 生香附)	untreated	Moves upward and outward to treat exterior conditions; moves qi in the chest.	Used in formulas for treatment of external patterns and also treats focal distention and rib pain.	While this form is called "untreated," it is often quick-fried over a strong heat to remove the fine hairs on the rhizome.
	vinegar-fried Cyperi Rhizoma (*cù zhì xiāng fù* 醋香附)	vinegar-fried	Treatment increases the herb's ability to relieve pain, dredge Liver qi and disperse knots.	Treats abdominal and stomach pain owing to food or qi stagnation.	Quadruple-treatment Cyperi Rhizoma (*sì zhì xiāng fù* 四製香附) is treated with ginger, vinegar, wine and salt. Its function is similar to that of the vinegar treated herb.

Herb	Pharmaceutical (*Pīnyīn* 字)	Treatment	Function	Examples	Comments
Gardeniae Fructus (*zhī zǐ*)	untreated Gardeniae Fructus (*shēng zhī zǐ* 生栀子)	untreated	Drains fire, resolves dampness, dispels irritability and cools the blood and resolves toxicity.	Treats hot sores and swellings, warmth disorders with high fever, damp-heat gallbladder disorders, Liver heat disorders and painful urination.	The untreated herb is preferred also for external application in the treatment of trauma. Also, the charred herb is used to treat blood-heat bleeding.
	dry-fried Gardeniae Fructus (*chǎo zhī zǐ* 炒栀子)	dry-fried	Same functions as the untreated herb but slightly more moderate in qi and flavor.	Same as the untreated herb but preferred for patients for whom the untreated herb is too cold and bitter.	As untreated herb is quite bitter and cold it can disturb the middle burner digestive function and lead to nausea or vomiting. Thus, in patients with Spleen-Stomach weakness the dry-fried agent is preferable.

The Formulas

八珍湯（八珍汤）
Eight-Treasure Decoction
bā zhēn tāng

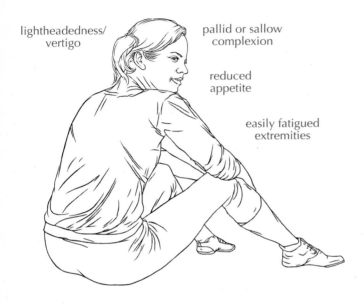

lightheadedness/ vertigo

pallid or sallow complexion

reduced appetite

easily fatigued extremities

INGREDIENTS

Ginseng Radix (*rén shēn*)...3-9g
Atractylodis macrocephalae Rhizoma (*bái zhú*)...................9g
Poria (*fú líng*)...9-15g
Glycyrrhizae Radix praeparata (*zhì gān cǎo*).........................5g
Rehmanniae Radix praeparata (*shú dì huáng*)...................15g
Paeoniae Radix alba (*bái sháo*)...................................9-15g
Angelicae sinensis Radix (*dāng guī*)..................................9g
Chuanxiong Rhizoma (*chuān xiōng*)..................................5g
Zingiberis Rhizoma recens (*shēng jiāng*)...........................9g
Jujubae Fructus (*dà zǎo*).......................................4 pieces

Preparation notes: Originally, the first 8 ingredients were coarsely ground and 9g of the resulting powder was decocted along with 5 slices of Zingiberis Rhizoma recens (*shēng jiāng*) and 1 piece of Jujubae Fructus (*dà zǎo*).

Actions: tonifies and augments the qi and blood

Main pattern: deficiency of both qi and blood

Key symptoms: pallid or sallow complexion • reduced appetite • easily fatigued extremities • lightheadedness/ vertigo

Secondary symptoms: palpitations • anxiety • shortness of breath • laconic speech • lowered vitality

Tongue: pale body • thin, white coating

Pulse: thin, frail • large, deficient, without strength

Abdomen: entire abdomen weak and soft

▶ CLINICAL NOTES

- The root of the qi and blood deficiency that this formula treats is the middle burner: the Spleen and Stomach. This is reflected in the pattern's key signs and symptoms, such as poor appetite, which indicate a weak middle burner that is unable to generate qi and blood.

- Qi and blood deficiency originating in the middle burner can also lead to chills and fever, weight loss, abscesses that neither suppurate nor improve, and continuous spotting from uterine bleeding.

- Best for patients in whom qi and blood are equally deficient.

Contraindications: excess conditions

▶ FORMULAS WITH SIMILAR INDICATIONS

Tangkuei Decoction to Tonify the Blood (*dāng guī bǔ xuè tāng*): For blood deficiency accompanied by floating yang as reflected in a large, deficient pulse, thirst for warm drinks, facial flushing, and sensations of heat.

Restore the Spleen Decoction (*guī pí tāng*): Specific for Spleen qi deficiency leading to Heart blood deficiency. Prominent symptoms are insomnia, palpitations, and anxiety.

All-Inclusive Great Tonifying Decoction (*shí quán dà bǔ tāng*): Also warms the lower burner yang and is therefore a better choice for patients with such symptoms as cold extremities or weakness in the lower body.

COMPOSITION

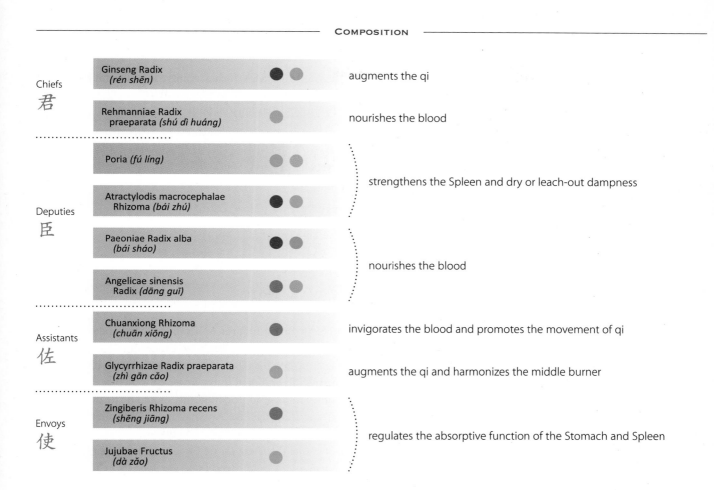

Chiefs 君	Ginseng Radix (*rén shēn*)		augments the qi
	Rehmanniae Radix praeparata (*shú dì huáng*)		nourishes the blood
Deputies 臣	Poria (*fú líng*)		strengthens the Spleen and dry or leach-out dampness
	Atractylodis macrocephalae Rhizoma (*bái zhú*)		
	Paeoniae Radix alba (*bái sháo*)		nourishes the blood
	Angelicae sinensis Radix (*dāng guī*)		
Assistants 佐	Chuanxiong Rhizoma (*chuān xiōng*)		invigorates the blood and promotes the movement of qi
	Glycyrrhizae Radix praeparata (*zhì gān cǎo*)		augments the qi and harmonizes the middle burner
Envoys 使	Zingiberis Rhizoma recens (*shēng jiāng*)		regulates the absorptive function of the Stomach and Spleen
	Jujubae Fructus (*dà zǎo*)		

八正散
Eight-Herb Powder for Rectification
bā zhèng săn

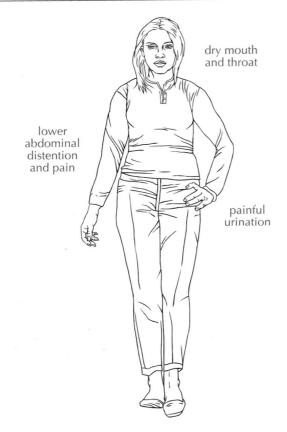

dry mouth
and throat

lower
abdominal
distention
and pain

painful
urination

INGREDIENTS

Akebiae Caulis (*mù tōng*).. 3-6g
Talcum (*huá shí*)... 12-30g
Plantaginis Semen (*chē qián zǐ*) 9-15g
Dianthi Herba (*qú mài*) 6-12g
Polygoni avicularis Herba (*biǎn xù*).............................. 6-12g
Gardeniae Fructus (*zhī zǐ*)... 3-9g
wine-washed Rhei Radix et Rhizoma (*jiǔ xǐ dà huáng*) 6-9g
Junci Medulla (*dēng xīn cǎo*) 3-6g
Glycyrrhizae Radix praeparata (*zhì gān cǎo*) 3-9g

Actions: clears heat • drains fire • promotes urination
• unblocks painful urinary dribbling

Main patterns: Heat heat flowing downward via the Small Intestine and collecting in the lower burner • damp-heat in the Bladder

Key symptoms: dark, turbid, scanty, difficult, and painful urination • in severe cases, urinary retention • lower abdominal distention and pain

Secondary symptoms: dry mouth and throat • thirst with desire for fluids • irritability • restlessness • red eyes • pain in eyeball • dry and painful lips • nosebleed • mouth and tongue ulcers

Tongue: greasy, yellow coating

Pulse: slippery • rapid

Abdomen: lower abdominal tenderness and fullness

▶ CLINICAL NOTES

• This formula focuses on draining damp-heat that constrains the qi transformation function of the Bladder. It is indicated for relatively acute conditions with inhibited urination and pain in the lower abdomen as chief symptoms. More chronic conditions should be treated by modifying formulas like Anemarrhena, Phellodendron, and Rehmannia Pill (*zhī bǎi dì huáng wán*), Tokoro Drink to Separate the Clear (*bì xiè fēn qīng yǐn*), or Clear the Heart Drink with Lotus Seed (*qīng xīn lián zǐ yǐn*). The formula should be further modified to treat the specific presentations of painful urinary dribbling.

• The root cause of acute, excess heat in the lower burner is often excess heat in the Heart or Pericardium. This can present with symptoms of upward flaring of Heart fire such as irritability, restlessness, red eyes, or mouth ulcers. If these symptoms are present, one should add herbs like Coptidis Rhizoma (*huáng lián*) or Lophatheri Herba (*dàn zhú yè*). On the other hand, if upper burner signs are more pronounced, a formula like Guide Out the Red Powder (*dǎo chì săn*) or Drain the Epigastrium Decoction (*xiè xīn tāng*) may be more appropriate.

Contraindications: Long-term use of this formula may cause weakness, lightheadedness, palpitations, and a loss of appetite. Should not be used without significant modification in treating conditions of cold from deficiency, or during pregnancy.

▶ FORMULAS WITH SIMILAR INDICATIONS

Guide Out the Red Powder (*dǎo chì sǎn*): For yin deficiency with pronounced symptoms of upward flaring of Heart fire such as irritability, insomnia, and mouth sores. This formula has a weaker effect on painful urinary dribbling.

Open the Gate Pill (*tong guān wán*): For urinary obstruction due to heat collecting in the lower burner with no signs of upper burner heat or Heart fire.

COMPOSITION

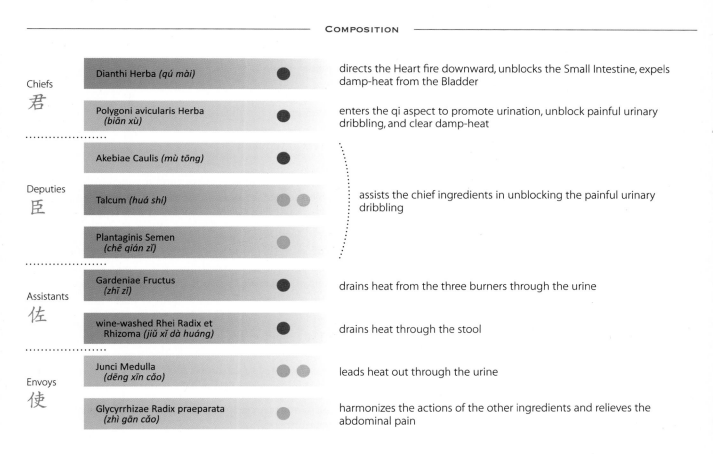

Chiefs 君	Dianthi Herba (*qú mài*)	directs the Heart fire downward, unblocks the Small Intestine, expels damp-heat from the Bladder
	Polygoni avicularis Herba (*biān xù*)	enters the qi aspect to promote urination, unblock painful urinary dribbling, and clear damp-heat
Deputies 臣	Akebiae Caulis (*mù tōng*)	assists the chief ingredients in unblocking the painful urinary dribbling
	Talcum (*huá shí*)	
	Plantaginis Semen (*chē qián zǐ*)	
Assistants 佐	Gardeniae Fructus (*zhī zǐ*)	drains heat from the three burners through the urine
	wine-washed Rhei Radix et Rhizoma (*jiǔ xǐ dà huáng*)	drains heat through the stool
Envoys 使	Junci Medulla (*dēng xīn cǎo*)	leads heat out through the urine
	Glycyrrhizae Radix praeparata (*zhì gān cǎo*)	harmonizes the actions of the other ingredients and relieves the abdominal pain

百合固金湯（百合固金汤）
Lily Bulb Decoction to Preserve the Metal
bǎi hé gù jīn tāng

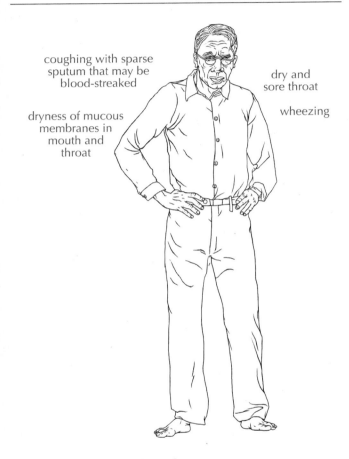

coughing with sparse sputum that may be blood-streaked

dryness of mucous membranes in mouth and throat

dry and sore throat

wheezing

Actions: nourishes the yin • moistens the Lungs • transforms phlegm • relieves coughing

Main pattern: dryness of the Lungs due to Lung and Kidney yin deficiency with deficiency heat

Key symptoms: coughing with sparse sputum that may be blood-streaked • wheezing • a dry and sore throat • dryness of mucous membranes in mouth and throat

Secondary symptoms: hot palms and soles • night sweats • steaming bones • emaciation

Tongue: red body • scanty coating

Pulse: thin • rapid

Abdomen: no specific signs

▶ CLINICAL NOTES

- Primarily for throat pain or chronic cough with or without blood-streaked phlegm from Lung dryness and Kidney yin. May also be used for dry cough without bleeding following an acute infection.

- Because this formula treats heat from deficiency, when using it to treat coughing in the wake of an exterior disorder it is important to ensure that all exterior heat has been cleared as the sour and sticky herbs in this formula will trap any residual pathogen.

- The formula is not indicated for long-term use. Once the heat signs have abated, indicating that the deficiency fire has returned to its source, it is best to switch to a strategy that tonifies middle-burner earth to generate metal.

Contraindications: Spleen deficiency • food stagnation • exterior conditions

▶ FORMULAS WITH SIMILAR INDICATIONS

*Tonify the Lungs Decoction with Ass-Hide Gelatin (*bǔ fèi ē jiāo tāng*): For hemoptysis that has damaged the Lung yin, blood, and qi but with heat from excess rather than from deficiency.

Clear Dryness and Rescue the Lungs Decoction (*qīng zào jiù fèi tāng*): Clears excess heat from the qi aspect as reflected in a rapid, flooding pulse and a yellow tongue coating.

INGREDIENTS

Lilii Bulbus (*bǎi hé*)	4.5g
Rehmanniae Radix (*shēng dì huáng*)	6-9g
Rehmanniae Radix praeparata (*shú dì huáng*)	9g
Ophiopogonis Radix (*mài mén dōng*)	4.5g
Scrophulariae Radix (*xuán shēn*)	2-3g
Fritillariae cirrhosae Bulbus (*chuān bèi mǔ*)	3-4.5g
Platycodi Radix (*jié gěng*)	2-6g
Angelicae sinensis Radix (*dāng guī*)	3-9g
Paeoniae Radix alba (*bái sháo*)	3g
Glycyrrhizae Radix (*gān cǎo*)	3g

Fritillaria and Trichosanthes Fruit Powder (*bèi mǔ guā lóu sǎn*): For transforming phlegm due to heat in the Lungs. It is suited for a situation where the phlegm is severe, dryness is not intense, and the yin has not yet been significantly damaged, marked by deep-seated sputum that is difficult to expectorate and wheezing.

COMPOSITION

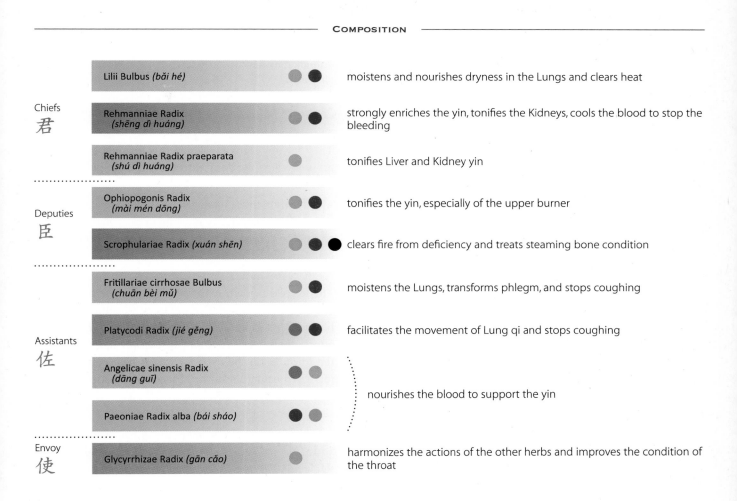

Chiefs 君	Lilii Bulbus (*bǎi hé*)	moistens and nourishes dryness in the Lungs and clears heat
	Rehmanniae Radix (*shēng dì huáng*)	strongly enriches the yin, tonifies the Kidneys, cools the blood to stop the bleeding
	Rehmanniae Radix praeparata (*shú dì huáng*)	tonifies Liver and Kidney yin
Deputies 臣	Ophiopogonis Radix (*mài mén dōng*)	tonifies the yin, especially of the upper burner
	Scrophulariae Radix (*xuán shēn*)	clears fire from deficiency and treats steaming bone condition
Assistants 佐	Fritillariae cirrhosae Bulbus (*chuān bèi mǔ*)	moistens the Lungs, transforms phlegm, and stops coughing
	Platycodi Radix (*jié gěng*)	facilitates the movement of Lung qi and stops coughing
	Angelicae sinensis Radix (*dāng guī*)	nourishes the blood to support the yin
	Paeoniae Radix alba (*bái sháo*)	
Envoy 使	Glycyrrhizae Radix (*gān cǎo*)	harmonizes the actions of the other herbs and improves the condition of the throat

白虎湯（白虎汤）
White Tiger Decoction
bái hǔ tāng

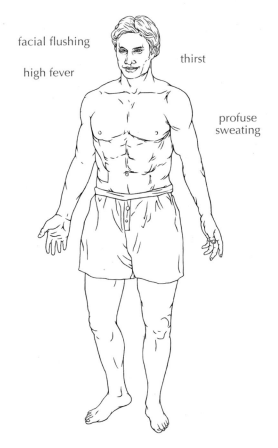

facial flushing

high fever

thirst

profuse sweating

INGREDIENTS

Gypsum fibrosum (*shí gāo*).. 30-48g
Anemarrhenae Rhizoma (*zhī mǔ*) 9-18g
Glycyrrhizae Radix praeparata (*zhì gān cǎo*) 3-6g
Nonglutinous rice (*jīng mǐ*) 9-15g

Actions: clears qi-level heat • drains Stomach fire • generates fluids • alleviates thirst

Main patterns: blazing fire in the yang brightness warp of the six warps of disease or the qi level of the four levels of disease

Key symptoms: high fever • profuse sweating • aversion to heat

• facial flushing • severe thirst • irritability

Secondary symptoms: headache • toothache • bleeding of the gums and nose • confusion

Tongue: red body • dry, yellow coating

Pulse: flooding and forceful • slippery and rapid

Abdomen: may have some focal distention in chest or epigastrium

▶ CLINICAL NOTES

• The four key signs for which this formula is indicated are known as the 'four extremes': a large pulse, severe sweating, severe thirst, and high fever.

• This formula treats damage to the yin-fluids by yang qi excess. The first priority must be to clear the excess heat and fire to control the yang qi. Yin tonification would be contraindicated at this stage.

• As the yang moves outward it takes the fluids with it. This results in such manifestations as severe sweating, a flooding and forceful pulse, facial flushing, and nose bleeds. This same yang pathodynamic, which usually affects the upper body, may also affect urination, thus the formula can be used for excess heat patterns with increased urination in the absence of constipation. The latter mechanism may occur in diabetes, bed wetting, or certain types of heart disease.

• For long-term patterns where the qi has been damaged, add Ginseng Radix (*rén shēn*) or Panacis quinquefolii Radix (*xī yáng shēn*). The pulse in these patients, although large and forceful, is deficient on stronger pressure.

Contraindications: continued presence of obstruction in the exterior with absence of sweating • qi deficiency fevers with sweating and flushing but a large, deficient pulse, no thirst, and worsening of symptoms upon exertion • yin deficiency fevers with a small or thin, rapid pulse and no tongue coating • true cold/false heat patterns

▶ FORMULAS WITH SIMILAR INDICATIONS

Ephedra, Apricot Kernel, Gypsum, and Licorice Decoction

(*má xìng shí gān tāng*): For patterns with slight fever, sweating, and thirst but with cough or wheezing due to the exterior pattern not yet being resolved.

Coptis Decoction to Resolve Toxicity (*huáng lián jiě dú tāng*): For fire that has already entered into the blood aspect (insomnia, irritability and flushing, nosebleeds, vomiting of blood, carbuncles, boils, or petechiae)

Drain the White Powder from *Craft of Medicinal Treatment for Childhood Disease Patterns* (*xiè bái sǎn*): Drains fire from the Lungs, as indicated by cough with absence of fever or thirst.

The skin, particularly at the inside of the forearms, will be hot to the touch but dry.

Tangkuei Decoction to Tonify the Blood (*dāng guī bǔ xuè tāng*): Qi deficiency patterns with fever and flushing but thirst with a desire for warm beverages, sweating aggravated by exertion, and a large but deficient pulse.

Five-Ingredient Powder with Poria (*wǔ líng sǎn*): Although the patient is thirsty, they either do not want to drink or will vomit what has been drunk. This formula also treats a pattern with reduced rather than increased urination.

COMPOSITION

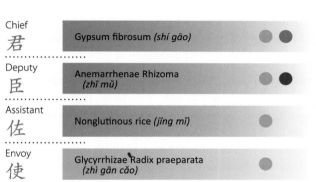

Chief 君	Gypsum fibrosum *(shí gāo)*	clears heat from the interior, vents pathogenic heat to the exterior, releases heat constraint from the muscle layer and skin, and moistens and enriches the yin
Deputy 臣	Anemarrhenae Rhizoma *(zhī mǔ)*	clears heat from the Lungs and Stomach to alleviate irritability, moistens dryness, and enriches the yin
Assistant 佐	Nonglutinous rice *(jīng mǐ)*	benefits the Stomach and protects the fluids, prevents the extremely cold properties of the other ingredients from injuring the middle burner
Envoy 使	Glycyrrhizae Radix praeparata *(zhì gān cǎo)*	

白頭翁湯（白头翁汤）
Pulsatilla Decoction
bái tóu wēng tāng

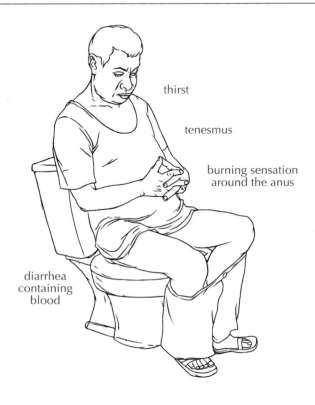

thirst

tenesmus

burning sensation around the anus

diarrhea containing blood

INGREDIENTS

Pulsatillae Radix (*bái tóu wēng*) 12-15g
Coptidis Rhizoma (*huáng lián*) 4-9g
Phellodendri Cortex (*huáng bǎi*) 9-12g
Fraxini Cortex (*qín pí*) 9-12g

Actions: clears heat • resolves toxicity • cools the blood • alleviates dysenteric disorders

Main pattern: hot dysenteric disorder due to heat toxin searing the Stomach and Intestines

Key symptoms: abdominal pain • tenesmus • burning sensation around the anus • thirst

Secondary symptoms: diarrhea containing more blood than pus

Tongue: red body • yellow coating

Pulse: wiry and rapid • slippery, rapid, and forceful

Abdomen: no rebound tenderness

▶ CLINICAL NOTES

• This formula treats heat in the blood aspect or damp-heat in the lower burner manifesting as bleeding and sensations of fullness in the rectum and lower abdomen. While there may be pain, there will be no rebound tenderness or cramping. Although the formula is primarily associated with the treatment of amoebic dysentery, these symptoms may also present in many other disorders such as hemorrhoids, uterine prolapse, pelvic inflammatory disease, or habitual miscarriage.

• Because it treats the Liver channel (which traverses the eyes), this formula is also used to treat Liver channel damp-heat eye disorders presenting with redness, swelling, pain, sensitivity to wind or excessive lacrimation. Generally, one adds herbs such as Chrysanthemi Flos (*jú huā*) and Paeoniae Radix rubra (*chì sháo*) when treating these disorders.

• Combine with Asini Corii Colla (*ē jiāo*) and Glycyrrhizae Radix (*gān cǎo*) when there is concurrent blood deficiency.

Contraindications: diarrhea and dysentery from Spleen yang deficiency

▶ FORMULAS WITH SIMILAR INDICATIONS

*Peony Decoction (*sháo yào tāng*): For conditions with less heat and toxicity (less blood in the stool) but more pronounced qi stagnation (abdominal pain and tenesmus).

Kudzu, Scutellaria, and Coptis Decoction (*gé gēn huáng qín huáng lián tang*): For hot dysenteric disorders where the pathogen is located at the qi level and still present in the upper burner as reflected in symptoms such as neck stiffness or headache. Alternatively, this pattern can be seen as a dual greater yang and yang brightness disorder.

Scutellaria Decoction (*huáng qín tāng*): For dysenteric disorders involving the lesser yang warp as reflected in a bitter taste, fever, and a rapid pulse.

*Yellow Earth Decoction (*huáng tǔ tāng*): For rectal or uterine bleeding from yang deficiency as indicated by a frail pulse and a soft abdomen.

──────────────────────── COMPOSITION ────────────────────────

Chief 君	Pulsatillae Radix *(bái tóu wēng)* ●	clears damp-heat and resolves fire toxicity from the Large Intestine
Deputies 臣	Coptidis Rhizoma *(huáng lián)* ●	clears damp-heat from the Stomach and Intestines
	Phellodendri Cortex *(huáng bǎi)* ●	clears damp-heat from the lower burner
Assistant 佐	Fraxini Cortex *(qín pí)z* ● ●	restrains the diarrhea and enhances the actions of the other herbs

半夏白朮天麻湯（半夏白术天麻汤）
Pinellia, White Atractylodes, and Gastrodia Decoction
bàn xià bái zhú tiān má tāng

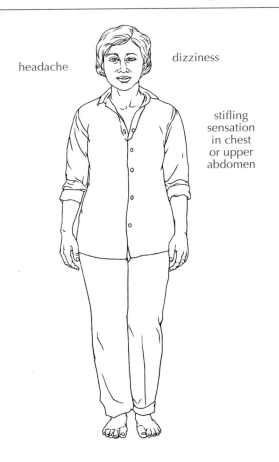

headache   dizziness

stifling sensation in chest or upper abdomen

Actions: strengthens the Spleen • dispels dampness • transforms phlegm • extinguishes wind

Main pattern: upward disturbance by wind-phlegm

Key symptoms: dizziness or vertigo (possibly severe) • headache • stifling sensation in the chest or upper abdomen

Secondary symptoms: nausea or vomiting • copious sputum • tiredness after eating • general fatigue • stiff neck and upper back pain

Tongue: thin, white coating • tooth-marked

Pulse: deep and soft • occasionally wiry • slippery

Abdomen: discomfort in epigastrium • splashing sounds in upper abdomen • soft abdominal wall

▶ CLINICAL NOTES

- This formula is designed to treat dizziness from phlegm clogging the sensory orifices and impeding the qi dynamic. This manifests with a stifling sensation in the chest, distention or nausea in the abdomen, vertigo, and spots in the visual field.

- The primary symptoms of this pattern occur in the upper body and appear intermittently. This indicates the presence of wind. It should be noted that this wind arises from the disturbance of the qi dynamic by phlegm-dampness and is not the Liver wind typically associated with dizziness. Instead, the Spleen and Stomach are the root here.

Contraindications: vertigo from ascendant Liver yang or blood deficiency

▶ FORMULAS WITH SIMILAR INDICATIONS

*Augmented Rambling Powder (*jiā wèi xiāo yáo sǎn*): For dizziness and other signs of constraint of Liver qi. This formula treats patterns with signs of blood deficiency, middle burner weakness, and heat from constraint that is reflected in a wiry but deficient or thin pulse.

Gastrodia and Uncaria Drink (*tiān má gōu téng yǐn*): For dizziness from Liver wind or hyperactivity of Liver yang as

---

─── INGREDIENTS ───

Pinelliae Rhizoma praeparatum (*zhì bàn xià*) 4.5-9g

Gastrodiae Rhizoma (*tiān má*) 3-6g

Atractylodis macrocephalae Rhizoma (*bái zhú*) 9g

Citri reticulatae Exocarpium rubrum (*jú hóng*) 3-6g

Poria (*fú líng*) 3-6g

Glycyrrhizae Radix (*gān cǎo*) 1.5-3g

Zingiberis Rhizoma recens (*shēng jiāng*) .... 1-3 slices

Jujubae Fructus (*dà zǎo*) .... 2-3 pieces

reflected in the irritability, insomnia, and wiry pulse that is strong at the surface and weaker in the deeper positions.

Six-Gentlemen Decoction (*liù jūn zǐ tāng*): For dizziness due to a deficient and dampness-encumbered Spleen that fails to promote the descent of turbid yin and ascent of clear yang. Symptoms in this pattern worsen after expenditure of energy, whereas phlegm predominant patterns tend to worsen with rest and improve with activity.

Six-Ingredient Pill with Rehmannia (*liù wèi dì huáng wán*): For dizziness due to Kidney yin deficiency with flaring of deficiency fire. This is evidenced by difficulty in recovering from activity, signs of dryness in the presence of phlegm, backache, and sweating that is typically worse at night.

Kidney Qi Pill (*shèn qì wán*): For dizziness from Kidney deficiency floating yang. The patient will tend to be cold and have increased urination, backache, and edema.

COMPOSITION

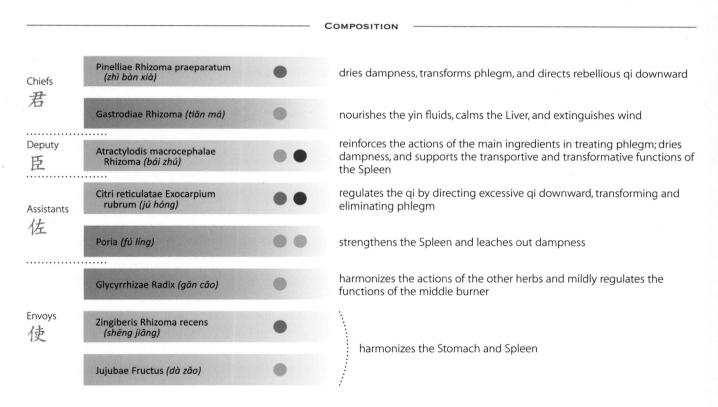

Chiefs 君	Pinelliae Rhizoma praeparatum (*zhì bàn xià*)	●	dries dampness, transforms phlegm, and directs rebellious qi downward
	Gastrodiae Rhizoma (*tiān má*)	●	nourishes the yin fluids, calms the Liver, and extinguishes wind
Deputy 臣	Atractylodis macrocephalae Rhizoma (*bái zhú*)	● ●	reinforces the actions of the main ingredients in treating phlegm; dries dampness, and supports the transportive and transformative functions of the Spleen
Assistants 佐	Citri reticulatae Exocarpium rubrum (*jú hóng*)	● ●	regulates the qi by directing excessive qi downward, transforming and eliminating phlegm
	Poria (*fú líng*)	● ●	strengthens the Spleen and leaches out dampness
	Glycyrrhizae Radix (*gān cǎo*)	●	harmonizes the actions of the other herbs and mildly regulates the functions of the middle burner
Envoys 使	Zingiberis Rhizoma recens (*shēng jiāng*)	●	harmonizes the Stomach and Spleen
	Jujubae Fructus (*dà zǎo*)	●	

半夏厚樸湯（半夏厚朴汤）
Pinellia and Magnolia Bark Decoction
bàn xià hòu pò tāng

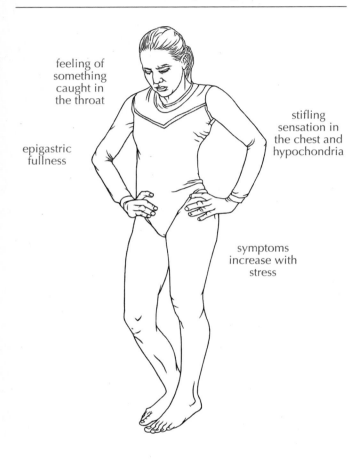

feeling of something caught in the throat

epigastric fullness

stifling sensation in the chest and hypochondria

symptoms increase with stress

INGREDIENTS

Pinelliae Rhizoma praeparatum (*zhì bàn xià*) 9-12g
Magnoliae officinalis Cortex (*hòu pò*) 9g
Poria (*fú líng*) 12g
Zingiberis Rhizoma recens (*shēng jiāng*) 9-15g
Perillae Folium (*zǐ sū yè*) 6g

Actions: promotes the movement of qi • dissipates clumps • directs rebellious qi downward • transforms phlegm

Main patterns: plum-pit qi • clumping of qi and phlegm • rebellious Stomach qi

Key symptoms: a feeling of something caught in the throat that can neither be swallowed nor ejected • stifling sensation in the chest and hypochondria • epigastric fullness • symptoms that tend to worsen when the patient is under emotional stress

Secondary symptoms: breathing difficulty • palpitations • anxiety • irritability • chest pain • nausea • vomiting • dry throat • hiccup • belching • abdominal distention

Tongue: wet body • thin, white coating

Pulse: wiry and slow • wiry and slippery

Abdomen: epigastric focal distention • splashing sound in epigastrium • palpable pulsations in epigastrium • slight distention in lower abdomen even though abdomen generally feels soft

▶ CLINICAL NOTES

• This is the classic formula for plum-pit qi, a sensation of something stuck in the throat that may interfere with breathing or swallowing. While often associated with emotional issues, this feeling can also be caused by physical irritation of the throat characterized by scratching, itching, or persistent coughing. This formula is only indicated if the symptoms are due to clumping of qi and phlegm.

• The formula can also be used to treat other symptoms of qi and fluid stagnation such as abdominal discomfort and bloating, nausea, a tendency to develop edema, expectoration of thin sputum, irregular menstruation or reduced and rough urination. It is particularly suitable if the symptoms are accompanied by emotional constraint with such symptoms as anxiety, feelings of depression, insomnia and/or palpitations.

Contraindications: fire from excess or deficiency presenting with a flushed face, bitter taste, and red tongue

▶ FORMULAS WITH SIMILAR INDICATIONS

Escape Restraint Pill (*yuè jū wán*): For qi constraint of the middle burner leading to a wider variety of secondary pathologies including blood stasis, dampness, phlegm, fire from constraint, and food stagnation.

Pinellia Decoction to Drain the Epigastrium (*bàn xià xiè xīn tāng*): For focal distention due to phlegm-heat in the Stomach accompanied by deficiency cold in the Spleen and marked by

nausea or vomiting, loose stools, and fullness and tightness in the epigastrium.

Licorice, Wheat, and Jujube Decoction (*gān mài dà zǎo tāng*): For loss of control over one's emotions with no signs of clumping of qi or phlegm.

COMPOSITION

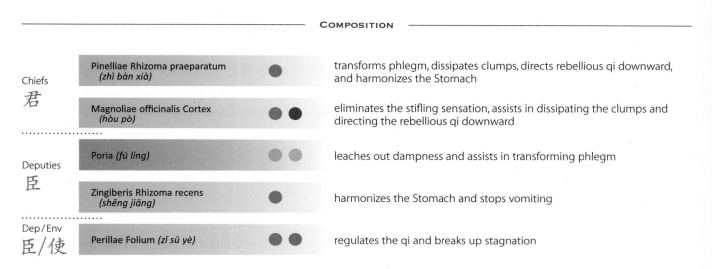

Chiefs 君	Pinelliae Rhizoma praeparatum (*zhì bàn xià*)	transforms phlegm, dissipates clumps, directs rebellious qi downward, and harmonizes the Stomach
	Magnoliae officinalis Cortex (*hòu pò*)	eliminates the stifling sensation, assists in dissipating the clumps and directing the rebellious qi downward
Deputies 臣	Poria (*fú líng*)	leaches out dampness and assists in transforming phlegm
	Zingiberis Rhizoma recens (*shēng jiāng*)	harmonizes the Stomach and stops vomiting
Dep/Env 臣/使	Perillae Folium (*zǐ sū yè*)	regulates the qi and breaks up stagnation

半夏瀉心湯（半夏泻心汤）
Pinellia Decoction to Drain the Epigastrium
bàn xià xiè xīn tāng

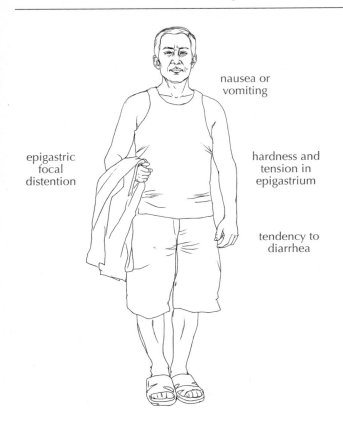

epigastric focal distention

nausea or vomiting

hardness and tension in epigastrium

tendency to diarrhea

INGREDIENTS

Pinelliae Rhizoma praeparatum (*zhì bàn xià*) 9-12g
Zingiberis Rhizoma (*gān jiāng*) 9g
Scutellariae Radix (*huáng qín*) 9g
Coptidis Rhizoma (*huáng lián*) 3g
Ginseng Radix (*rén shēn*) 9g
Jujubae Fructus (*dà zǎo*) .... 4 pieces
Glycyrrhizae Radix praeparata (*zhì gān cǎo*) 9g

Actions: harmonizes the Stomach • directs rebellious qi downward • disperses clumping • eliminates focal distention

Main pattern: Spleen and Stomach deficiency cold with damp-heat obstructing the middle burner

Key symptoms: epigastric focal distention • fullness and tightness with very slight or no pain • nausea or vomiting • tendency to diarrhea

Secondary symptoms: reduced appetite • dry heaves, belching or hiccup • borborygmus • mouth ulcers • fatigue • neck and shoulder stiffness • restlessness • insomnia

Tongue: thin, yellow, and greasy coating • body may be red at the tip

Pulse: wiry • rapid

Abdomen: hardness and tension in epigastrium • tension in rectus abdominis muscle • elastic tension and tenderness on pressure around CV-12 • splashing sounds in upper abdomen

▶ CLINICAL NOTES

- This is a complex pattern with middle burner qi and yang deficiency as well as damp-heat obstructing the qi dynamic of the middle burner so that the clear yang cannot ascend and turbid yin is not directed downward. Deficiency cold here is usually pre-existing or due to external cold entering the interior or inappropriate treatment with bitter, cooling medicinals (including antibiotics). Damp-heat is often caused by long-term overconsumption of rich and greasy foods or alcohol.

- Epigastric focal distention is the chief symptom of this pattern. It reflects the nature and location of the obstruction of the qi dynamic.

- If there are no signs of middle burner deficiency, and focal distention in the epigastrium and obstruction of the middle burner qi dynamic by damp-heat are the main problems, remove Ginseng Radix (*rén shēn*), Glycyrrhizae Radix (*gān cǎo*), Zingiberis Rhizoma (*gān jiāng*), and Jujubae Fructus (*dà zǎo*), and add Aurantii Fructus immaturus (*zhǐ shí*) and Zingiberis Rhizoma recens (*shēng jiāng*) to eliminate the focal distention and relieve the nausea and vomiting.

- For a more pronounced deficiency presentation with restlessness and insomnia, increase the dosage of Glycyrrhizae Radix praeparata (*zhì gān cǎo*).

- The formula may initially cause diarrhea or aggravate any existing diarrhea. If other symptoms improve and the patient feels generally better, continue until the pattern resolves. If the diarrhea becomes worse and watery, and the patient does not feel better or even feels worse, this indicates a middle burner yang deficiency pattern.

Contraindications: This formula is indicated for focal distention caused by clumping of mixed heat and cold in the epigastrium. Where such distention is due to qi stagnation or harbored food, this formula will be ineffective.

▶ FORMULAS WITH SIMILAR INDICATIONS

Calm the Stomach Powder (*píng wèi sǎn*): For damp obstruction of the middle burner with abdominal distention and fullness, loss of taste and appetite, loose stools, and a swollen tongue with a thick, white, and greasy coating. Note that this pattern lacks any marked signs of either heat or cold.

*Coptis Decoction (*huáng lián tāng*): Also for a presentation of mixed heat and cold but with an emphasis on abdominal pain due to blood stasis from cold in the collaterals of the Stomach.

COMPOSITION

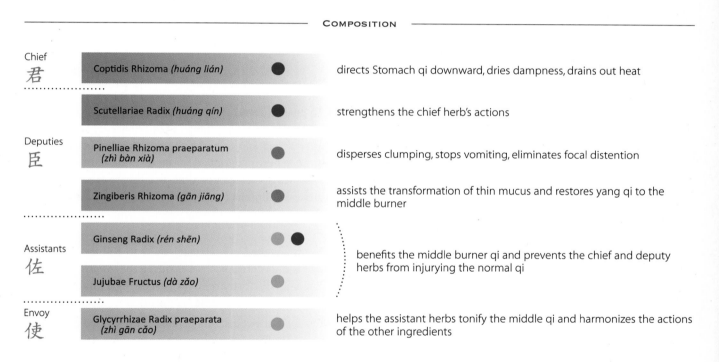

Chief 君	Coptidis Rhizoma (*huáng lián*) ●	directs Stomach qi downward, dries dampness, drains out heat
	Scutellariae Radix (*huáng qín*) ●	strengthens the chief herb's actions
Deputies 臣	Pinelliae Rhizoma praeparatum (*zhì bàn xià*) ●	disperses clumping, stops vomiting, eliminates focal distention
	Zingiberis Rhizoma (*gān jiāng*) ●	assists the transformation of thin mucus and restores yang qi to the middle burner
Assistants 佐	Ginseng Radix (*rén shēn*) ● ●	benefits the middle burner qi and prevents the chief and deputy herbs from injuring the normal qi
	Jujubae Fructus (*dà zǎo*) ●	
Envoy 使	Glycyrrhizae Radix praeparata (*zhì gān cǎo*) ●	helps the assistant herbs tonify the middle qi and harmonizes the actions of the other ingredients

保產無憂方（保产无忧方）
Worry-Free Formula to Protect Birth
bǎo chǎn wú yōu fāng

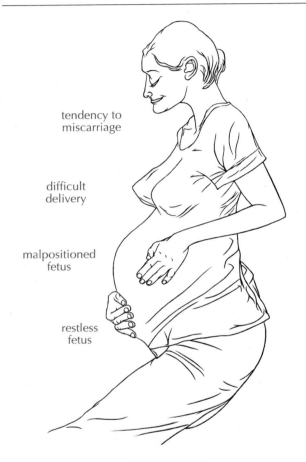

tendency to
miscarriage

difficult
delivery

malpositioned
fetus

restless
fetus

▶ INGREDIENTS

wine-washed Angelicae sinensis Radix (*dāng guī*) 5g
Schizonepetae Spica (*jīng jiè suì*)...................................... 2.5g
honey-prepared Astragali Radix (*mì zhì huáng qí*) 2.5g
Cuscutae Semen (*tù sī zǐ*) .... [wine-fried] 5g
ginger-fried Magnoliae officinalis Cortex (*hòu pò*) 2g
Notopterygii Rhizoma seu Radix (*qiāng huó*).................. 1.5g
Fritillariae cirrhosae Bulbus (*chuān bèi mǔ*) ...... [add at end] 5g
wine-fried Paeoniae Radix alba (*bái sháo*) 4g
Glycyrrhizae Radix (*gān cǎo*).. 1.5g
Chuanxiong Rhizoma (*chuān xiōng*) 5g

vinegar-fried Artemisiae argyi Folium (*ài yè*)............... 1.5g
Zingiberis Rhizoma recens (*shēng jiāng*).................... 3 slices

Actions: tonifies the qi • nourishes the blood • regulates the qi • quiets the fetus • expedites delivery

Main pattern: qi and blood deficiency leading to weakness in the Penetrating and Conception vessels

Key symptoms: restless fetus • tendency to miscarriage • malpositioned fetus • difficult delivery

Tongue: no specific signs

Pulse: no specific signs

Abdomen: no specific signs

▶ CLINICAL NOTES

• To correct fetal malposition, modern texts recommend 4-7 day courses beginning in the 28th week. Alternatively, after 3-5 packets of herbs, the situation can be reassessed and the herbs continued for up to 15 days until the fetus assumes a correct position. For this usage, Fritillariae cirrhosae Bulbus (*chuān bèi mǔ*) may be removed from the formula as its primary role is to provide for a smooth delivery.

• For threatened miscarriage owing to Kidney deficiency, add Kidney tonics such as Taxilli Herba (*sāng jì shēng*) and Eucommiae Cortex (*dù zhòng*). If owing to middle burner heat, add Scutellariae Radix (*huáng qín*) [blackened].

• Once labor begins, the formula is prescribed as needed, and usually 2-4 doses are sufficient. At this time, especially if labor is prolonged, Ginseng Radix (*rén shēn*) is frequently added to the formula to tonify the mother's qi and give her more strength to endure the birthing process. Also, the dose of Fritillariae cirrhosae Bulbus (*chuān bèi mǔ*) can be increased to promote a smooth delivery.

Contraindications: fire from yin deficiency

▶ FORMULAS WITH SIMILAR INDICATIONS

*Taishan Bedrock Powder (*Tàishān pán shí sǎn*): Threatened miscarriage from qi and blood deficiency with heat.

─────────────────── COMPOSITION ───────────────────

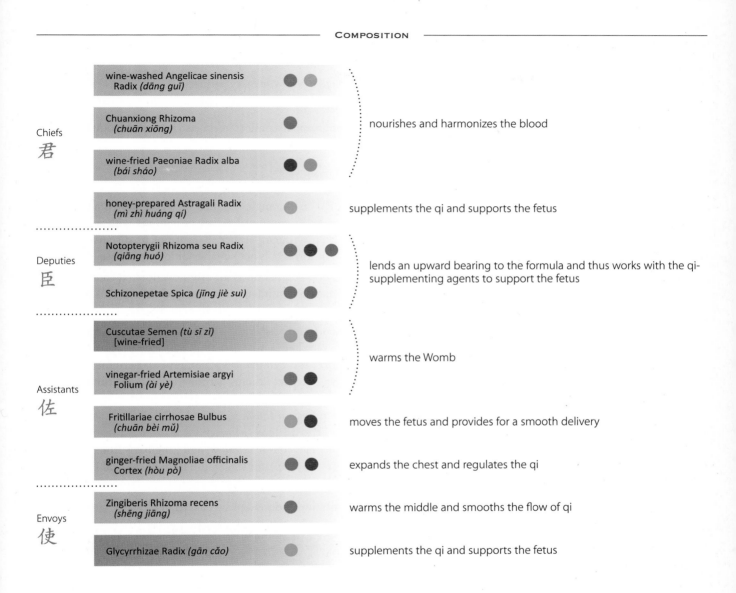

Chiefs
君

wine-washed Angelicae sinensis Radix *(dāng guī)*

Chuanxiong Rhizoma *(chuān xiōng)*

nourishes and harmonizes the blood

wine-fried Paeoniae Radix alba *(bái sháo)*

honey-prepared Astragali Radix *(mì zhì huáng qí)* — supplements the qi and supports the fetus

Deputies
臣

Notopterygii Rhizoma seu Radix *(qiāng huó)*

lends an upward bearing to the formula and thus works with the qi-supplementing agents to support the fetus

Schizonepetae Spica *(jīng jiè suì)*

Assistants
佐

Cuscutae Semen *(tù sī zǐ)* [wine-fried]

vinegar-fried Artemisiae argyi Folium *(ài yè)*

warms the Womb

Fritillariae cirrhosae Bulbus *(chuān bèi mǔ)* — moves the fetus and provides for a smooth delivery

ginger-fried Magnoliae officinalis Cortex *(hòu pò)* — expands the chest and regulates the qi

Envoys
使

Zingiberis Rhizoma recens *(shēng jiāng)* — warms the middle and smooths the flow of qi

Glycyrrhizae Radix *(gān cǎo)* — supplements the qi and supports the fetus

保和丸
Preserve Harmony Pill
bǎo hé wán

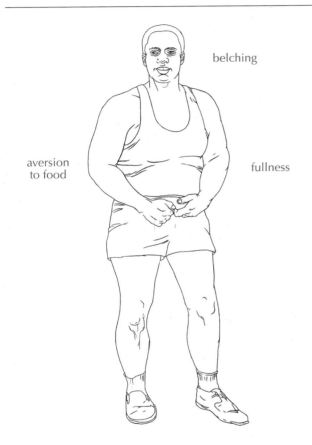

belching

aversion
to food

fullness

INGREDIENTS

Crataegi Fructus (*shān zhā*).. 9-15g
Massa medicata fermentata (*shén qū*) 9-12g
Raphani Semen (*lái fú zǐ*)... 6-9g
Citri reticulatae Pericarpium (*chén pí*)............................. 6-9g
Pinelliae Rhizoma praeparatum (*zhì bàn xià*)................. 9-12g
Poria (*fú líng*) 9-12g
Forsythiae Fructus (*lián qiào*) 3-6g

Actions: reduces food stagnation and harmonizes the Stomach

Main pattern: food stagnation

Key symptoms: fullness or distention in epigastrium or abdomen • foul-smelling belching • aversion to food

Secondary symptoms: abdominal pain • acid regurgitation • nausea and vomiting • diarrhea

Tongue: yellow, greasy coating

Pulse: slippery

Abdomen: discomfort in epigastrium • distention in upper abdomen

▶ CLINICAL NOTES

- This is the main formula for acute food stagnation. It is most commonly used in patients with a history of dietary intemperance. Because of its dispersing nature this formula is not suitable for long-term use.

- Food stagnation is an often overlooked cause of acute diarrhea in infants and young children. This formula is appropriate for treating this condition.

- For food stagnation from meat, increase the dosage of Crataegi Fructus (*shān zhā*); for stagnation from wheat or rice, add Setariae (Oryzae), Fructus germinatus (*gǔ yá*), and Hordei Fructus germinatus (*mài yá*); for stagnation from noodles and other carbohydrates, add fried Raphani Semen (*lái fú zǐ*); for stagnation from alcohol, add Puerariae Flos (*gé huā*); for stagnation from fish, add Perillae Folium (*zǐ sū yè*) and Zingiberis Rhizoma recens (*shēng jiāng*); for stagnation from beans, add fresh radish juice.

Contraindications: Spleen deficiency

▶ FORMULAS WITH SIMILAR INDICATIONS

Strengthen the Spleen Pill (*jiàn pí wán*): For food stagnation with Spleen deficiency and stagnant dampness. This situation generates heat and stagnation and manifests as a generalized sense of fullness and distention throughout the abdomen, reduced appetite, fatigue, deficient pulse, and a greasy, slightly yellow tongue coating.

Three-Seed Decoction to Nourish One's Parents (*sān zǐ yǎng qīn tāng*): For thin mucus obstructing the ability of the Lungs and Stomach to direct downward, which gives rise to cough or wheezing, both of which occur with copious sputum.

*Open the Spleen Pill (*qǐ pí wán*): For treating both the root and branch of middle burner deficiency with food stagnation and dampness marked by no desire to eat or drink, diarrhea, abdominal pain, vomiting, belching that smells rotten or sour, a greasy or turbid tongue coating, and a weak, soggy pulse. Most often used for chronic conditions.

COMPOSITION

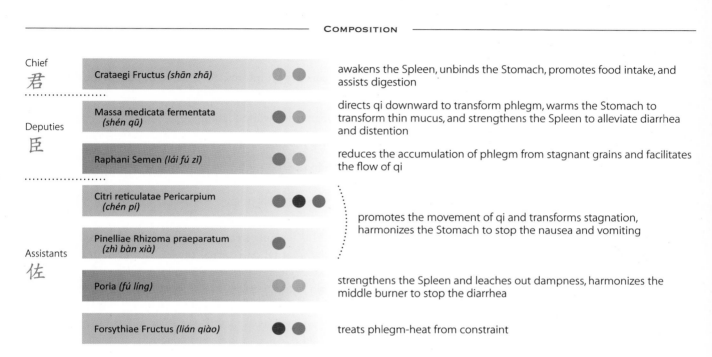

Chief 君	Crataegi Fructus *(shān zhā)*	awakens the Spleen, unbinds the Stomach, promotes food intake, and assists digestion
Deputies 臣	Massa medicata fermentata *(shén qū)*	directs qi downward to transform phlegm, warms the Stomach to transform thin mucus, and strengthens the Spleen to alleviate diarrhea and distention
	Raphani Semen *(lái fú zǐ)*	reduces the accumulation of phlegm from stagnant grains and facilitates the flow of qi
Assistants 佐	Citri reticulatae Pericarpium *(chén pí)*	promotes the movement of qi and transforms stagnation, harmonizes the Stomach to stop the nausea and vomiting
	Pinelliae Rhizoma praeparatum *(zhì bàn xià)*	
	Poria *(fú líng)*	strengthens the Spleen and leaches out dampness, harmonizes the middle burner to stop the diarrhea
	Forsythiae Fructus *(lián qiào)*	treats phlegm-heat from constraint

貝母栝樓散 （贝母栝楼散）
Fritillaria and Trichosanthes Fruit Powder
bèi mǔ guā lóu sǎn

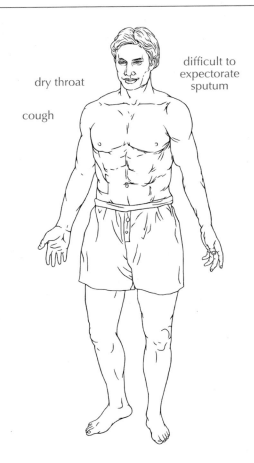

dry throat

difficult to expectorate sputum

cough

Actions: moistens the Lungs • clears heat • regulates the qi • transforms phlegm

Main pattern: dryness in the Lungs that injures the fluids and produces phlegm

Key symptoms: cough with deep-seated sputum that is difficult to expectorate • dry throat

Secondary symptoms: obstruction or pain in the throat • wheezing

Tongue: dry, white coating

Pulse: rough

Abdomen: no specific signs

► CLINICAL NOTES

- This formula treats a Lung disorder that can be caused by internal or external causes. However, in the pattern associated with this formula, exterior symptoms are no longer present. For a concurrent exterior condition, one may add Mori Folium (*sāng yè*), Armeniacae Semen (*xìng rén*), Peucedani Radix (*qián hú*), and Arctii Fructus (*niú bàng zǐ*); for severe coughing and wheezing, add Armeniacae Semen (*xìng rén*), Eriobotryae Folium (*pí pá yè*), and Farfarae Flos (*kuǎn dōng huā*).

- As the formula neither strongly tonifies the fluids nor strongly clears heat, it must be modified if one wishes to simultaneously treat these underlying factors. For severe dryness and sore throat, add Scrophulariae Radix (*xuán shēn*), Ophiopogonis Radix (*mài mén dōng*), and Anemarrhenae Rhizoma (*zhī mǔ*); for hoarseness and blood-streaked sputum, omit Citri reticulatae Exocarpium rubrum (*jú hóng*) and add Glehniae/Adenophorae Radix (*shā shēn*), Ophiopogonis Radix (*mài mén dōng*), Phragmitis Rhizoma (*lú gēn*), and Agrimoniae Herba (*xiān hè cǎo*).

Contraindications: yin deficiency • dryness in the exterior

► FORMULAS WITH SIMILAR INDICATIONS

Mulberry Leaf and Apricot Kernel Decoction (*sāng xìng*

INGREDIENTS

Fritillariae cirrhosae Bulbus (*chuān bèi mǔ*) 9g
Trichosanthis Fructus (*guā lóu*) 9-12g
Trichosanthis Radix (*tiān huā fěn*) 6g
Poria (*fú líng*) 6g
Citri reticulatae Exocarpium rubrum (*jú hóng*) 6g
Platycodi Radix (*jié gěng*) 6g

Preparation notes: Due to its expense, 2g of Fritillariae cirrhosae Bulbus (*chuān bèi mǔ*) is usually ground into a powder and dissolved into each cup of the strained decoction.

tāng): For dryness in the exterior marked by a moderate fever and headache that constrains the Lung qi and causes a dry, hacking cough.

Clear Dryness and Rescue the Lungs Decoction (*qīng zào jiù fèi tāng*): Strongly nourishes the yin and clears heat to treat dryness and heat in the qi aspect presenting as dry cough or coughing with phlegm that is difficult to expectorate, dry throat, fever, and thirst.

Ophiopogonis Decoction (*mài mén dōng tāng*): For deficiency of Lung or Stomach yin and fluids that gives rise to rebellious qi with such symptoms as cough, spitting up of fluids, sticky phlegm, throat discomfort, nausea, and hoarseness .

Lily Bulb Decoction to Preserve the Metal (*bǎi hé gù jīn tāng*): For Lung dryness when it has progressed to Lung and Kidney deficiency marked by a dry mouth and throat, sparse sputum, and signs of yin deficiency.

COMPOSITION

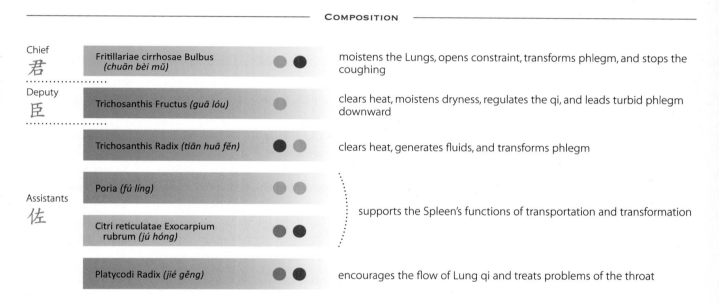

Chief 君	**Fritillariae cirrhosae Bulbus** *(chuān bèi mǔ)*	moistens the Lungs, opens constraint, transforms phlegm, and stops the coughing
Deputy 臣	**Trichosanthis Fructus** *(guā lóu)*	clears heat, moistens dryness, regulates the qi, and leads turbid phlegm downward
	Trichosanthis Radix *(tiān huā fěn)*	clears heat, generates fluids, and transforms phlegm
Assistants 佐	**Poria** *(fú líng)*	supports the Spleen's functions of transportation and transformation
	Citri reticulatae Exocarpium rubrum *(jú hóng)*	
	Platycodi Radix *(jié gěng)*	encourages the flow of Lung qi and treats problems of the throat

萆薢分清飲（萆薢分清饮）
Tokoro Drink to Separate the Clear
bì xiè fēn qīng yǐn/bēi xiè fēn qīng yǐn

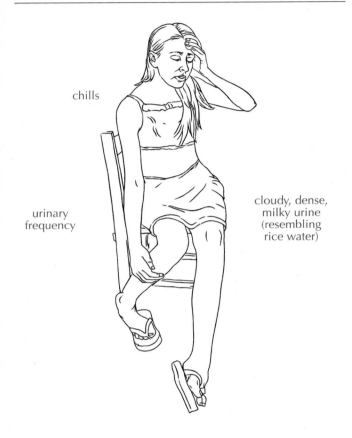

chills

urinary frequency

cloudy, dense, milky urine (resembling rice water)

INGREDIENTS

Dioscoreae hypoglaucae Rhizoma (*bì xiè*) 9g

Alpiniae oxyphyllae Fructus (*yì zhì rén*) 9g

Linderae Radix (*wū yào*) 9g

Acori tatarinowii Rhizoma (*shí chāng pǔ*) 9g

Preparation notes: A pinch of salt should be added to the drained decoction.

Actions: warms the Kidneys • promotes the resolution of dampness • separates out the clear • transforms the turbid

Main pattern: cloudy, painful urinary dribbling due to deficiency cold in the lower burner

Key symptoms: urinary frequency • cloudy, dense, milky urine (resembling rice water) • greasy urine

Secondary symptoms: cold feet • chills

Tongue: pale body • white coating

Abdomen: weak lower abdomen • pencil lines in lower abdomen

▶ CLINICAL NOTES

• The primary marker for this formula is turbid urine due to deficiency cold. This may or may not be accompanied by discomfort in the lower abdomen or painful urination.

• This formula can also be used for chronic white vaginal discharge as well as prostate problems from deficiency cold.

• The presentation treated by this formula commonly arises in the context of either Kidney qi deficiency or sinking of Spleen qi. For Kidney qi deficiency, add herbs that tonify and bind the Kidney qi such as Euryales Semen (*qiàn shí*) and Rubi Fructus (*fù pén zǐ*); for sinking of Speen qi, add Astragali Radix (*huáng qí*), Codonopsis Radix (*dǎng shēn*), Atractylodis macrocephalae Rhizoma (*bái zhú*), and Cimicifugae Rhizoma (*shēng má*).

Contraindications: cloudy painful urinary dribbling characterized by milky, turbid urine due to an accumulation of damp-heat in the Bladder

▶ FORMULAS WITH SIMILAR INDICATIONS

Kidney Qi Pill (*shèn qì wán*): For Kidney deficiency patterns that may manifest with urinary frequency or difficulty. Note, however, that this formula focuses on tonifying Kidney qi and qi transformation and not on transforming dampness. It is thus not indicated for turbid urine unless modified.

*Mantis Egg-Case Powder (*sāng piāo xiāo sǎn*): For Heart and Kidney deficiency leading to failure of fire and water to communicate. This pattern may manifest with urinary frequency and urine that looks like rice water, but is distinguished by a thin and frail pulse as well as signs such as anxiety or difficulty in concentrating.

─── COMPOSITION ───

Chief 君	Dioscoreae hypoglaucae Rhizoma *(bì xiè)*	●	eliminates dampness by promoting the separation of the turbid from the pure fluids and directing the turbid fluids out through the Bladder
Deputy 臣	Alpiniae oxyphyllae Fructus *(yì zhì rén)*	●	warms the Spleen and Stomach to harmonize the middle, and the Kidney yang to secure the lower burner
Assistants 佐	Linderae Radix *(wū yào)*	●	warms the Kidneys and promotes the movement of qi and the transformation of water
	Acori tatarinowii Rhizoma *(shí chāng pǔ)*	● ● ●	transforms turbidity and eliminates dampness and deficiency cold in the Bladder

冰硼散
Borneal and Borax Powder
bīng péng săn

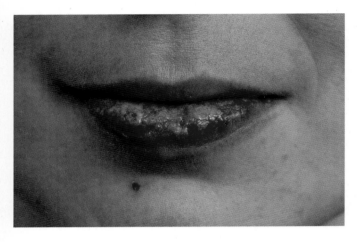

INGREDIENTS

Natrii Sulfas siccatus (*xuán míng fěn*)................................ 15g
Borax (*péng shā*).. 15g
Borneolum (*bīng piàn*) 1.5g

Preparation notes: Grind the first two ingredients into a fine powder and then grind in the last ingredient. Sift the powder in a 100mu (100 openings per inch) sieve. Borneolum (*bīng piàn*) is added last because it contains volatile oils that would be lost during a longer grind and because it is used in a small amount and is less apt to lose volume during the grinding process if added at the end.

Actions: clears heat and resolves toxicity • dispels pus • reduces swelling • relieves pain

Main patterns: sore, swollen throat • swelling or pain in the gums • mouth sores • superficial skin sores • external ear infections

Key symptoms: superficial sores on the skin • irritations or sores in the throat, mouth, or outer ear

► CLINICAL NOTES

• Apply this powder to the nose, mouth, and ears by using a spray bottle. It can be applied to the external female genitals and to sores such as impetigo or herpes simplex by sprinkling on the affected area. For sores, the affected area should be washed with a solution of Alumen dehydratum (*kū fán*) before applying the powder. Apply the powder to the still-moist sores.

• Powdered Indigo naturalis (*qīng dài*) can be added to increase the formula's function of clearing heat and resolving toxicity.

• When treating mouth sores, preceding the application of powder by rinsing the mouth with a decoction of 15g Taraxaci Herba (*pú gōng yīng*) and 15g Portulacae Herba (*mǎ chǐ xiàn*) will increase its efficacy.

• Be sure to use natural Borneolum (*bīng piàn*) for applications to the nose or mouth. The use of autoclaving or some other method to sterilize the material is recommended if applying the formula to mucous membranes or open sores.

Contraindications: none noted

COMPOSITION

Role	Herb			Action
Chief 君	Borneolum *(bīng piàn)*	●	●	reduces swelling and alleviates pain
Deputy 臣	Natrii Sulfas siccatus *(xuán míng fěn)*	●	●	softens hardness and drains fire
Envoy 使	Borax *(péng shā)*	●	●	clears heat, reduces swelling, and disperses clumps

補肺湯（补肺汤）
Tonify the Lungs Decoction
bǔ fèi tāng

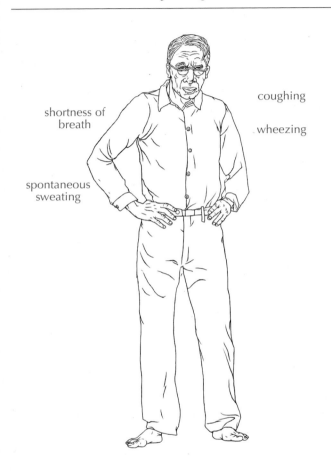

shortness of breath

spontaneous sweating

coughing

wheezing

Key symptoms: shortness of breath • spontaneous sweating • coughing • wheezing

Secondary symptoms: occasional chills and feverishness • fatigue • weak voice

Tongue: pale body

Pulse: frail • deficient and large

Abdomen: weak lower abdomen

► CLINICAL NOTES

- Treats both the root and branches in cases of coughing due to deficiency of both the Lung and Kidney qi.
- This is a very useful formula for treating chronic cough in older patients or in those weakened from other illness or medical treatment.

Contraindications: any acute cough due to invasion of external pathogens

► FORMULAS WITH SIMILAR INDICATIONS

Jade Windscreen Powder (*yù píng fēng sǎn*): For spontaneous sweating and recurrent colds from Lung qi deficiency. Does not treat coughing or Kidney deficiency.

INGREDIENTS

Ginseng Radix (*rén shēn*)... 9g

Astragali Radix (*huáng qí*)... 24g

Rehmanniae Radix praeparata (*shú dì huáng*) 24g

Schisandrae Fructus (*wǔ wèi zǐ*)... 6g

Asteris Radix (*zǐ wǎn*)... 9g

Mori Cortex (*sāng bái pí*).. 12g

Actions: augments the qi • stabilizes the exterior

Main pattern: Lung qi deficiency

───────────────── COMPOSITION ─────────────────

Chiefs
君

Ginseng Radix *(rén shēn)*

Astragali Radix *(huáng qí)*

tonifies the qi and fortifies the protective qi

Schisandrae Fructus *(wǔ wèi zǐ)*

preserves the Lung qi and helps the Kidneys grasp the qi

Deputies
臣

Asteris Radix *(zǐ wǎn)*

moistens the Lungs and stops the coughing

Mori Cortex *(sāng bái pí)*

causes the Lung qi to descend

Assistant
佐

Rehmanniae Radix praeparata
(shú dì huáng)

tonifies the essence; tonifies the lower and basal aspects of the body

補陽還五湯（补阳还五汤）
Tonify the Yang to Restore Five [-Tenths] Decoction
bǔ yáng huán wǔ tāng

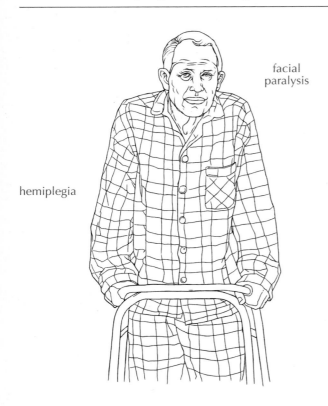

hemiplegia

facial paralysis

INGREDIENTS

Astragali Radix (*huáng qí*) 30-120g
Angelicae sinensis radicis Cauda (*dāng guī wěi*).................... 6g
Chuanxiong Rhizoma (*chuān xiōng*) 3g
Paeoniae Radix rubra (*chì sháo*).. 4.5-6g
Persicae Semen (*táo rén*).. 3g
Carthami Flos (*hóng huā*)... 3g
Pheretima (*dì lóng*) 3g

Actions: tonifies the qi • invigorates the blood • unblocks the channels

Main pattern: qi deficiency leading to static blood obstructing the channels

Key symptoms: hemiplegia • paralysis and atrophy of the lower limbs • facial paralysis

Secondary symptoms: • drooling • slurred speech • dry stools • urinary frequency or incontinence

Tongue: pale, dark body • white coating

Pulse: moderate

Abdomen: no specific signs

▶ CLINICAL NOTES

- The primary purpose of this formula is to treat the sequelae of wind-stroke. It is not indicated for the acute stages. Before using the formula one must be sure that the patient has regained clear consciousness, the body temperature is normal, there is no hemorrhage, and the pulse is moderate.

- If blood pressure is elevated, medicinals such as Gypsum fibrosum (*shí gāo*) and Haematitum (*dài zhě shí*) should be added to this formula to counteract the chief ingredient's effect in raising blood pressure. For very chronic conditions with severe qi and yang deficiency, it is recommended that herbs such as Codonopsis Radix (*dǎng shēn*) or Aconiti Radix lateralis praeparata (*zhì fù zǐ*) be added, and where there is concomitant edema, that the formula be combined with True Warrior Decoction (*zhēn wǔ tāng*).

- The formula can be used in any context where qi deficiency has caused the blood in the channels and collaterals to become static, such as a variety of cardiovascular disorders, diabetes, sciatica, or Bell's palsy.

- It is possible to begin treatment with a lower dosage of Astragali Radix (*huáng qí*) in the range of 30-60g. This can be increased if necessary. The dosage of the blood-invigorating medicinals, on the other hand, may be raised depending on how the formula is used. Adding guiding herbs can help to direct the formula to specific regions of the body: Cinnamomi Ramulus (*guì zhī*) and Mori Ramulus (*sāng zhī*) for the arms and upper extremities; Achyranthis bidentatae Radix (*niú xī*) and Eucommiae Cortex (*dù zhòng*) for the lower extremities; Acori tatarinowii Rhizoma (*shí chāng pǔ*), Polygalae Radix (*yuǎn zhì*), and Curcumae Radix (*yù jīn*) for obstruction of the Heart orifices manifesting as slurred speech.

Contraindications: acute cerebral hemorrhage • wind-stroke with a large and forceful, or firm, wiry, and forceful pulse • yin deficiency • blood heat • pregnancy

▶ FORMULAS WITH SIMILAR INDICATIONS ⇢

*Lindera Powder to Smooth the Flow of Qi (*wū yào shùn qì sǎn*): For post-stroke disorders of recent onset that are not part of a deficiency pattern.

*Construct Roof Tiles Decoction (*jiàn líng tāng*): For ascent of Liver yang and deficiency of yin and blood. It is often applied to patients (including post-stroke patients) who exhibit signs of ascent of Liver yang, such as elevated blood pressure, dizziness, headache, and tinnitus.

—————————————————————— COMPOSITION ——————————————————————

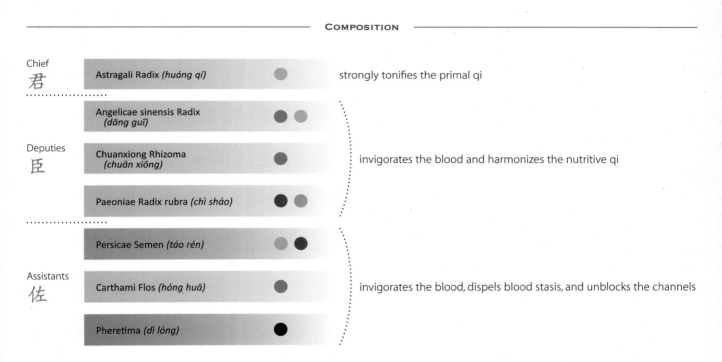

Chief 君	Astragali Radix (*huáng qí*)	strongly tonifies the primal qi
Deputies 臣	Angelicae sinensis Radix (*dāng guī*)	
	Chuanxiong Rhizoma (*chuān xiōng*)	invigorates the blood and harmonizes the nutritive qi
	Paeoniae Radix rubra (*chì sháo*)	
Assistants 佐	Persicae Semen (*táo rén*)	
	Carthami Flos (*hóng huā*)	invigorates the blood, dispels blood stasis, and unblocks the channels
	Pheretima (*dì lóng*)	

補中益氣湯 (补中益气汤)
Tonify the Middle to Augment the Qi Decoction
bǔ zhōng yì qì tāng

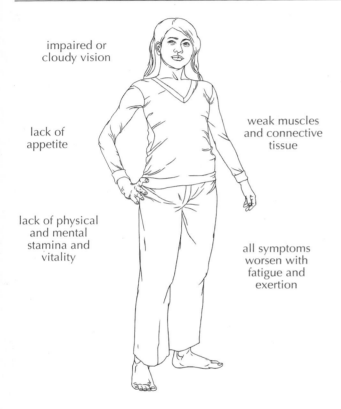

impaired or cloudy vision

lack of appetite

weak muscles and connective tissue

lack of physical and mental stamina and vitality

all symptoms worsen with fatigue and exertion

INGREDIENTS

Astragali Radix (*huáng qí*) 18-30g
Ginseng Radix (*rén shēn*)... 6-9g
Atractylodis macrocephalae Rhizoma (*bái zhú*) 6-9g
Glycyrrhizae Radix praeparata (*zhì gān cǎo*) 9-15g
wine-washed Angelicae sinensis Radix (*jiǔ xǐ dāng guī*) 6g
Citri reticulatae Pericarpium (*chén pí*) 6-9g
Cimicifugae Rhizoma (*shēng má*)..................................... 6-9g
Bupleuri Radix (*chái hú*)... 6-9g

Actions: tonifies the middle burner • augments the qi • raises the yang • lifts what has sunken

Main patterns: Spleen and Stomach deficiency with inability to raise the clear • qi deficiency-type fever • sinking of the middle burner qi

Key symptoms: lack of physical and mental stamina and vitality • all symptoms worsen with fatigue and exertion • weak muscles and connective tissue • impaired or cloudy vision • lack of appetite

Secondary symptoms: dizziness • unsteadiness • deafness • tinnitus • shortness of breath • laconic speech • weak voice • digestive weakness • intermittent fever that is worse upon exertion • spontaneous sweating • aversion to cold • thirst for warm beverages • loose stools • chronic diarrhea or dysentery • hemorrhoids • rectal or uterine prolapse • prolapse of the internal organs • irregular uterine bleeding

Tongue: pale and wet body • scanty or no coating

Pulse: frail • large • forceless

Abdomen: weak and soft • slight tenderness under the ribs • pulsations around the umbilicus • may have pencil-line tension above the umbilicus

► CLINICAL NOTES

- This is an often-used formula with a very wide range of possible indications that all derive from a weakness of the middle burner qi, which is failing to control both yin substance and yang qi. If the yin is not controlled it sinks downward with such symptoms as prolapse, bleeding, diarrhea, bedwetting, increased urination, or discharge. If the yang qi is not controlled it ascends uncontrollably resulting in intermittent fevers, flushing, wheezing, headaches, tinnitus, palpitations, dizziness, or visual disturbances. Accumulation of dampness that is not directed downward can manifest in such symptoms as damp painful obstruction, urinary difficulty, and nasal congestion. All symptoms are brought on or aggravated by effort that consumes the qi.

- A key sign indicating this formula is a large, soft, and weak pulse. This pulse distinguishes the pattern from others with a similar presentation, such as yin or yang deficiency, dampness, or the contraction of external pathogens.

- At present the formula is used to enhance vitality and boost the immune system, often as an adjunct to chemotherapy or radiotherapy or post-operatively. Care should be taken that such treatment does not also support pathogenic qi.

• May also be used during pregnancy for such symptoms as dizziness, edema, palpitations, and fatigue.

• The formula is often tailored to specific indications by adding appropriate draining and clearing herbs where necessary. For example, for ascending yin fire one may add small amounts of salt-fried Phellodendri Cortex (*huáng bǎi*) and Rehmanniae Radix (*shēng dì huáng*); for irritability that does not abate, add a small amount of Coptidis Rhizoma (*huáng lián*); for fire from constraint, add Scutellariae Radix (*huáng qín*), Gypsum fibrosum (*shí gāo*), and Coptidis Rhizoma (*huáng lián*). However, the use of such herbs should only be adjunctive to the main strategy of tonifying middle burner qi and regulating the qi dynamic.

Contraindications: fever due to heat from yin deficiency • contraction of external pathogens • Kidney deficiency patterns

► FORMULAS WITH SIMILAR INDICATIONS

Four-Gentlemen Decoction (*sì jūn zǐ tāng*): Focuses on tonifying the transportive and transformative functions of the Spleen and Stomach marked by a pallid complexion, fatigue, weakness, and sensitive digestion.

Restore the Spleen Decoction (*guī pí tāng*): Used for Spleen and Heart deficiency with palpitations, insomnia, anxiety, withdrawal, reduced appetite, and sometimes chronic bleeding.

COMPOSITION

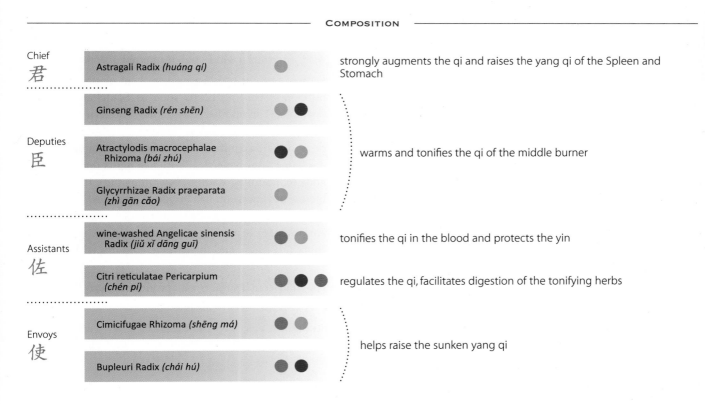

Chief 君	Astragali Radix (*huáng qí*)	strongly augments the qi and raises the yang qi of the Spleen and Stomach
	Ginseng Radix (*rén shēn*)	
Deputies 臣	Atractylodis macrocephalae Rhizoma (*bái zhú*)	warms and tonifies the qi of the middle burner
	Glycyrrhizae Radix praeparata (*zhì gān cǎo*)	
Assistants 佐	wine-washed Angelicae sinensis Radix (*jiǔ xǐ dāng guī*)	tonifies the qi in the blood and protects the yin
	Citri reticulatae Pericarpium (*chén pí*)	regulates the qi, facilitates digestion of the tonifying herbs
Envoys 使	Cimicifugae Rhizoma (*shēng má*)	helps raise the sunken yang qi
	Bupleuri Radix (*chái hú*)	

蒼耳子散（苍耳子散）
Xanthium Powder
cāng ér zǐ săn

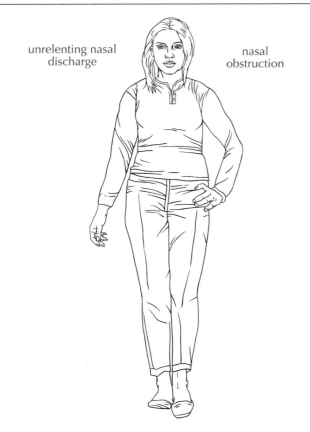

unrelenting nasal discharge

nasal obstruction

INGREDIENTS

Xanthii Fructus (*cāng ěr zǐ*)...6-9g

Magnoliae Flos (*xīn yí*)...3-6g

Angelicae dahuricae Radix (*bái zhǐ*) 6-9g

Menthae haplocalycis Herba (*bò hé*)..........[add near end] 3-6g

Allii fistulosi Bulbus (*cōng bái*).....................................3-6g

Preparation notes: Do not cook for more than 10 minutes. Alternatively, following the original source, 6g of a finely ground powder of the first four herbs can be taken after meals with Allii fistulosi Bulbus (*cōng bái*) and green tea.

Actions: disperses wind • alleviates pain • unblocks the nose

---

Main pattern: nasal congestion and discharge

Key symptoms: unrelenting nasal discharge • nasal obstruction

Secondary symptoms: purulent discharge • frontal headache • migraine headaches • dizziness

Tongue: thin, white coating • greasy, white coating

Pulse: no specific signs

Abdomen: no specific signs

▶ CLINICAL NOTES

• This formula unblocks the nasal orifices with acrid, aromatic, and primarily warming herbs. While originally used for profuse, purulent discharge, in modern practice it is used (with appropriate modifications) to treat nasal congestion regardless of cause. It is most effective, however, if used to address nasal congestion associated with fettering by wind-cold or internal qi constraint.

• If qi constraint produces severe heat or phlegm-heat, bitter and cooling herbs such as Scutellariae Radix (*huáng qín*) should be added. Many modern physicians add Houttuyniae Herba (*yú xīng căo*) because of its demonstrated antibacterial actions. For bloody nasal discharge or nosebleed, add Rubiae Radix (*qiàn căo gēn*) and Rehmanniae Radix (*shēng dì huáng*). In addition, blood-moving agents can be added if the nasal turbinates appear to suffer from stasis or lack of blood flow (as in atrophy). For acute, hot conditions, add Paeoniae Radix rubra (*chì sháo*), and for chronic cold disorders, Lycopi Herba (*zé lán*).

• For wind-cold disorders with pronounced exterior symptoms, the formulas listed below are indicated.

Contraindications: sinus problems due to wind-heat (without modifications) • patients with significant qi, yin, or blood deficiency

▶ FORMULAS WITH SIMILAR INDICATIONS

Kudzu Decoction (*gé gēn tāng*): For wind-cold in the greater yang warp with a floating pulse, chills and fevers, absence of sweating, and stiffness of back and neck.

Cinnamon Twig Decoction (*guì zhī tāng*): For wind attack with floating pulse, chills and fevers, and sweating.

Ephedra, Asarum, and Aconite Accessory Root Decoction (*má huáng xì xīn fù zǐ tāng*): For wind-cold affecting the greater yin warp with a deep pulse and fever.

Chuanxiong Powder to be Taken with Green Tea (*chuān xiōng chá tiáo sǎn*): For headaches and nasal congestion due to external wind.

*Magnolia Flower Powder (*xīn yí sǎn*): For wind-cold leading to nasal congestion and pain, persistent, copious nasal discharge, loss of smell, and headache.

COMPOSITION

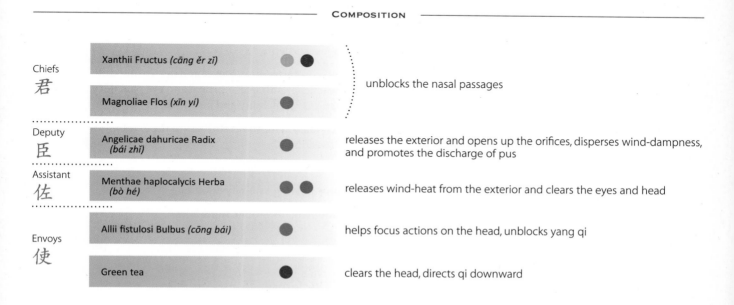

Chiefs 君	Xanthii Fructus (*cāng ěr zǐ*)	unblocks the nasal passages
	Magnoliae Flos (*xīn yí*)	
Deputy 臣	Angelicae dahuricae Radix (*bái zhǐ*)	releases the exterior and opens up the orifices, disperses wind-dampness, and promotes the discharge of pus
Assistant 佐	Menthae haplocalycis Herba (*bò hé*)	releases wind-heat from the exterior and clears the eyes and head
Envoys 使	Allii fistulosi Bulbus (*cōng bái*)	helps focus actions on the head, unblocks yang qi
	Green tea	clears the head, directs qi downward

柴葛解肌湯 （柴葛解肌汤）
Bupleurum and Kudzu Decoction to Release the Muscle Layer
chái gé jiě jī tāng

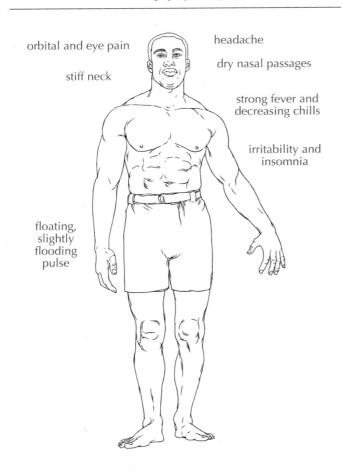

orbital and eye pain

headache

dry nasal passages

stiff neck

strong fever and decreasing chills

irritability and insomnia

floating, slightly flooding pulse

INGREDIENTS

Bupleuri Radix (*chái hú*)... 6g
Puerariae Radix (*gé gēn*)... 9g
Notopterygii Rhizoma seu Radix (*qiāng huó*)...................... 3g
Angelicae dahuricae Radix (*bái zhǐ*) 3g
Scutellariae Radix (*huáng qín*) 6g
Gypsum fibrosum (*shí gāo*)... 5g
Platycodi Radix (*jié gěng*)... 3g
Paeoniae Radix alba (*bái sháo*)... 6g

Glycyrrhizae Radix (*gān cǎo*)... 3g
Zingiberis Rhizoma recens (*shēng jiāng*)................... 3 slices
Jujubae Fructus (*dà zǎo*)...................................... 2 pieces

Preparation notes: Do not cook for more than 20 minutes.

Actions: releases pathogens from the muscle layer • clears interior heat

Main patterns: unresolved, exterior wind-cold that has become constrained and is in the process of transforming into heat • concurrent greater yang and yang brightness stage disorders

Key symptoms: strong fever and decreasing chills • headache • stiff neck • orbital and eye pain • dry nasal passages • irritability and insomnia

Secondary symptoms: stiffness in the extremities • absence of sweating

Tongue: thin, yellow coating

Pulse: floating • slightly flooding

Abdomen: no specific signs

▶ CLINICAL NOTES

• This formula focuses on clearing heat from the yang brightness even though some signs of a greater yang disorder, such as chills and a stiff neck, are still present.

• Can be used not only to treat acute infectious diseases involving the upper respiratory tract, but also to reduce inflammation and pain due to heat constraint along the greater yang channel of the face and neck as seen in trigeminal neuralgia, sinusitis, or inflammatory eye disorders.

• Can be modified to treat the precise location of symptoms and the relative strength of constraint in the yang brightness and greater yang warps. For instance, for severe chills with no sweating, substitute Ephedrae Herba (*má huáng*) for Scutellariae Radix (*huáng qín*), with a large dose in the winter and a smaller one in the spring. During the summer and fall, substitute Perillae Folium (*zǐ sū yè*). For cases without chills, headache, or pain, remove Notopterygii Rhizoma seu Radix (*qiāng huó*) and

Angelicae dahuricae Radix (*bái zhǐ*).

Contraindications: wind-cold disorders that have not transformed into heat • simple exterior wind-heat disorders • yang brightness organ stage disorders with clumping in the interior

▶ FORMULAS WITH SIMILAR INDICATIONS

Kudzu Decoction (*gé gēn tāng*): For more severe constraint, usually marked by significant headache and neck pain, due to cold in the exterior but with fewer signs of heat in the interior.

──── COMPOSITION ────

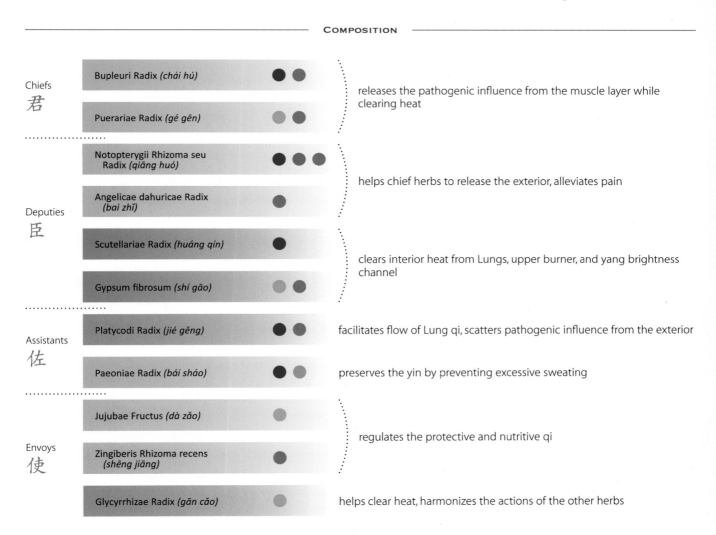

Chiefs 君

Bupleuri Radix (*chái hú*)
Puerariae Radix (*gé gēn*)

releases the pathogenic influence from the muscle layer while clearing heat

Deputies 臣

Notopterygii Rhizoma seu Radix (*qiāng huó*)
Angelicae dahuricae Radix (*bai zhi*)

helps chief herbs to release the exterior, alleviates pain

Scutellariae Radix (*huáng qín*)
Gypsum fibrosum (*shí gāo*)

clears interior heat from Lungs, upper burner, and yang brightness channel

Assistants 佐

Platycodi Radix (*jié gěng*)

facilitates flow of Lung qi, scatters pathogenic influence from the exterior

Paeoniae Radix (*bái sháo*)

preserves the yin by preventing excessive sweating

Envoys 使

Jujubae Fructus (*dà zǎo*)
Zingiberis Rhizoma recens (*shēng jiāng*)

regulates the protective and nutritive qi

Glycyrrhizae Radix (*gān cǎo*)

helps clear heat, harmonizes the actions of the other herbs

柴胡薑湯（柴胡桂姜汤）
Bupleurum, Cinnamon Twig, and Ginger Decoction
chái hú guì jiāng tāng

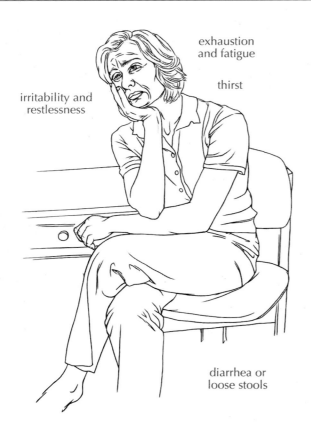

irritability and restlessness

exhaustion and fatigue

thirst

diarrhea or loose stools

Main patterns: constraint of the lesser yang warp with fluids clumping in the interior • Gallbladder heat with Spleen cold

Key symptoms: exhaustion and fatigue (mental and physical) accompanied by irritability and restlessness • diarrhea or loose stools • thirst

Secondary symptoms: headache • pain in the hypochondrium • tachycardia • palpitations • night sweats • insomnia • reduced urination • cold extremities • spontaneous sweating from the head or upper body

Tongue: dry body with thin or thick white coating

Pulse: wiry and tight on the left or wiry and slow on the right, or floating and forceful

Abdomen: tension in hypochondrium • periumbilical pulsations • pressure points on sternum and xiphoid process • no resistance to pressure in abdomen

► CLINICAL NOTES

- Originally for malarial diseases, today the formula is used for mixed excess and deficiency pattern involving the lesser and greater yang (heat constraint) and the lesser yin (deficiency cold) warps. It is used for acute and subacute infections and inflammatory conditions of the digestive system against a background of deficiency cold, as well as for hormonal disorders (thyroid hyperactivity, menopause) and for psycho-emotional disorders and instability.

- This formula often treats patterns that include lesser yang symptoms such as a wiry pulse, dizziness, or a bitter taste.

- Diarrhea or soft stools accompanied by reduced urination or other lesser yang warp signs are viewed by some physicians as key indications for this formula.

Contraindications: pure excess or deficiency patterns

► FORMULAS WITH SIMILAR INDICATIONS

*Bupleurum and Cinnamon Twig Decoction (*chái hú guì zhī tāng*): For simultaneous lesser yang and greater yang warp

───── INGREDIENTS ─────

Bupleuri Radix (*chái hú*)	15g
Cinnamomi Ramulus (*guì zhī*)	12g
Zingiberis Rhizoma (*gān jiāng*)	6g
Trichosanthis Radix (*tiān huā fěn*)	12g
Scutellariae Radix (*huáng qín*)	9g
Ostreae Concha (*mǔ lì*)	21g
Glycyrrhizae Radix praeparata (*zhì gān cǎo*)	3g

Actions: harmonizes and releases the lesser yang • disperses clumping • warms the interior • dispels cold

patterns with joint pain, fever, slight chills, and nausea.

Augmented Rambling Powder (*jiā wèi xiāo yáo sǎn*): Addresses heat constraint with qi and blood deficiency and no signs of cold marked by irritability, possible tidal fevers, dry mouth, and other signs of heat in the upper part of the body.

Bupleurum plus Dragon Bone and Oyster Shell Decoction (*chái hú jiā lóng gǔ mǔ lì tāng*): For a similar presentation, but one that is purely excess such that symptoms are more severe.

Frigid Extremities Powder (*sì nì sǎn*): For qi constraint marked by bloating, abdominal pain, and cold extremities.

—————————————— COMPOSITION ——————————————

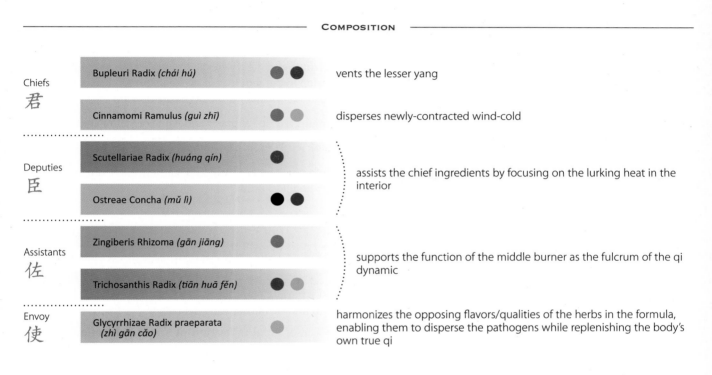

Chiefs
君

Bupleuri Radix *(chái hú)* — vents the lesser yang

Cinnamomi Ramulus *(guì zhī)* — disperses newly-contracted wind-cold

Deputies
臣

Scutellariae Radix *(huáng qín)*

Ostreae Concha *(mǔ lì)*

assists the chief ingredients by focusing on the lurking heat in the interior

Assistants
佐

Zingiberis Rhizoma *(gān jiāng)*

Trichosanthis Radix *(tiān huā fěn)*

supports the function of the middle burner as the fulcrum of the qi dynamic

Envoy
使

Glycyrrhizae Radix praeparata *(zhì gān cǎo)*

harmonizes the opposing flavors/qualities of the herbs in the formula, enabling them to disperse the pathogens while replenishing the body's own true qi

柴胡加龍骨牡蠣湯（柴胡加龙骨牡蛎汤）
Bupleurum Plus Dragon Bone and Oyster Shell Decoction
chái hú jiā lóng gǔ mǔ lì tāng

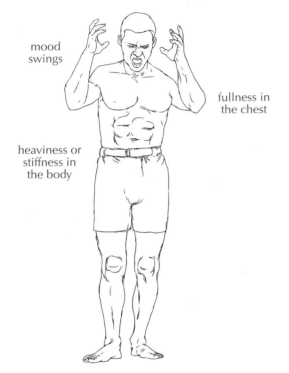

mood swings

fullness in the chest

heaviness or stiffness in the body

INGREDIENTS

Bupleuri Radix (*chái hú*).. 12g
Scutellariae Radix (*huáng qín*) 3g
Pinelliae Rhizoma praeparatum (*zhì bàn xià*)...................... 9g
Ginseng Radix (*rén shēn*)... 4.5g
Zingiberis Rhizoma recens (*shēng jiāng*)............................ 4.5g
Cinnamomi Ramulus (*guì zhī*).. 4.5g
Poria (*fú líng*) 4.5g
Fossilia Ossis Mastodi (*lóng gǔ*) 4.5g
Ostreae Concha (*mǔ lì*)... 4.5g
Rhei Radix et Rhizoma (*dà huáng*) .... [add just before end] 6g
Jujubae Fructus (*dà zǎo*)... 6 pieces

Ingredient notes: Originally this formula also contained Minium (*qiān dān*), a toxic ingredient that is now omitted.

Actions: unblocks the three yang warps via the lesser yang • drains heat • sedates and calms the spirit

Main pattern: constraint in the lesser yang complicated by the presence of heat that often affects the spirit

Key symptoms: fullness in the chest • emotional instability and mood swings involving irritability, fear, and anger • heaviness or stiffness in the body

Secondary symptoms: insomnia • depressive moods • headaches or heavy-headedness • dizziness • pain or tension in the shoulder or neck • palpitations or rapid heartbeat • urinary difficulty • constipation

Tongue: red tip • slippery and white or yellow coating

Pulse: wiry • rapid • forceful

Abdomen: tenderness in hypochondrium • palpable periumbilical pulsations

▶ CLINICAL NOTES

- Although the presentation involves an aspect of deficiency, the overall pattern is one of severe excess of Heart and Liver yang with fluids accumulating in the Stomach due to middle burner yang deficiency.

- The original indication of 'fright palpitations' can be interpreted as symptomatic of an inability of the body to properly respond to certain external stimuli. The formula is thus frequently used in both China and Japan to treat psycho-emotional problems including depression, anxiety, neurosis, and even schizophrenia.

- If constipation is not part of the presentation, omit Rhei Radix et Rhizoma (*dà huáng*). The formula can then be taken for a longer period of time in the treatment of conditions such as hypertension, coronary heart disease, epilepsy, or menopausal syndrome.

Contraindications: deficiency conditions • pregnancy • unsuitable for long-term use

▶ FORMULAS WITH SIMILAR INDICATIONS

Major Bupleurum Decoction (*dà chái hú tāng*): For fullness and heaviness in the flanks and abdomen with constipation, but not widely used for psycho-emotional disorders and even less appropriate for long-term use.

Restrain the Liver Powder (*yì gān sǎn*): For problems with less severe symptoms of excess such as fullness, but with symptoms of Liver wind such as muscle cramps or spasms.

COMPOSITION

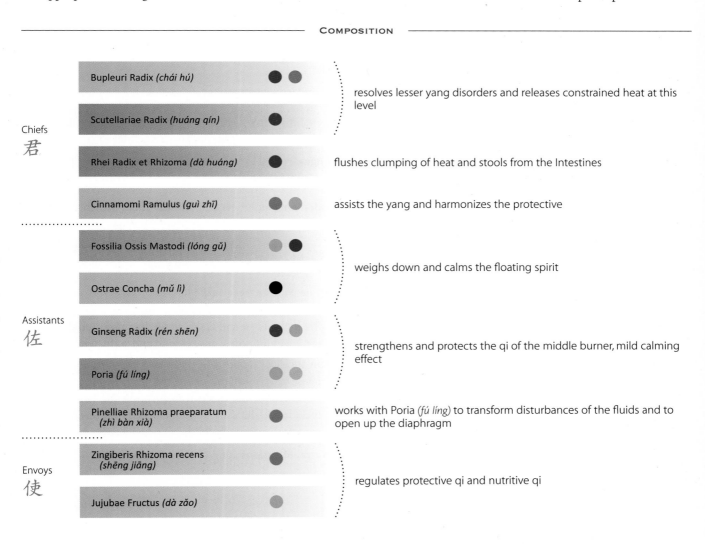

Chiefs
君

Bupleuri Radix (*chái hú*) — resolves lesser yang disorders and releases constrained heat at this level

Scutellariae Radix (*huáng qín*)

Rhei Radix et Rhizoma (*dà huáng*) — flushes clumping of heat and stools from the Intestines

Cinnamomi Ramulus (*guì zhī*) — assists the yang and harmonizes the protective

Assistants
佐

Fossilia Ossis Mastodi (*lóng gǔ*) — weighs down and calms the floating spirit

Ostrae Concha (*mǔ lì*)

Ginseng Radix (*rén shēn*) — strengthens and protects the qi of the middle burner, mild calming effect

Poria (*fú líng*)

Pinelliae Rhizoma praeparatum (*zhì bàn xià*) — works with Poria (*fú líng*) to transform disturbances of the fluids and to open up the diaphragm

Envoys
使

Zingiberis Rhizoma recens (*shēng jiāng*) — regulates protective qi and nutritive qi

Jujubae Fructus (*dà zǎo*)

柴胡清肝湯（柴胡清肝汤）
Bupleurum Decoction to Clear the Liver
chái hú qīng gān tāng

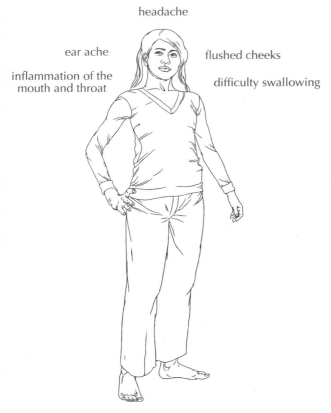

headache

ear ache

flushed cheeks

inflammation of the mouth and throat

difficulty swallowing

Actions: drains fire • resolves toxicity • spreads the Liver qi • cools and invigorates the blood

Main patterns: clumping of fire toxin in mouth and throat, especially along the course of the lesser yang channel

Key symptoms: headache • flushed cheeks • difficulty swallowing • inflammation of the mouth and throat • ear ache

Secondary symptoms: fever • swollen lymph nodes in the neck • bad breath • tinnitus • hearing loss • insomnia • irritability • coughing of thick, viscous sputum • dark urine • nose bleeds • herpes zoster • genital sores

Tongue: red

Pulse: wiry • rapid

Abdomen: tenderness and fullness under the ribcage • hypertonicity of rectus abdominis muscle

▶ CLINICAL NOTES

- The source text indicates that, with respect to ear problems, the formula is indicated for those related to fire in the Liver and Gallbladder. It is also used for herpes sores, genital sores, nose bleeds, and sudden hearing loss.

- In modern Japan this formula is specifically indicated for recurrent inflammatory disorders in the mouth and throat due to fire excess transforming into fire. Examples include tonsillitis and mouth ulcers. These disorders most commonly occur in children and teenagers.

Contraindications: long-term use • pregnancy

INGREDIENTS

Bupleuri Radix (*chái hú*)...................................... 4.5g
Rehmanniae Radix (*shēng dì huáng*)................................ 4.5g
Angelicae sinensis Radix (*dāng guī*) 6g
Paeoniae Radix rubra (*chì sháo*) 4.5
Chuanxiong Rhizoma (*chuān xiōng*) 3g
Forsythiae Fructus (*lián qiào*) 6g
Arctii Fructus (*niú bàng zǐ*) 4.5g
Scutellariae Radix (*huáng qín*) 3g
Gardeniae Fructus (*zhī zǐ*)...................... 4.5g
Trichosanthis Radix (*tiān huā fěn*) 3g
Saposhnikoviae Radix (*fáng fēng*) 3g
Glycyrrhizae Radix (*gān cǎo*)...................... 3g

COMPOSITION

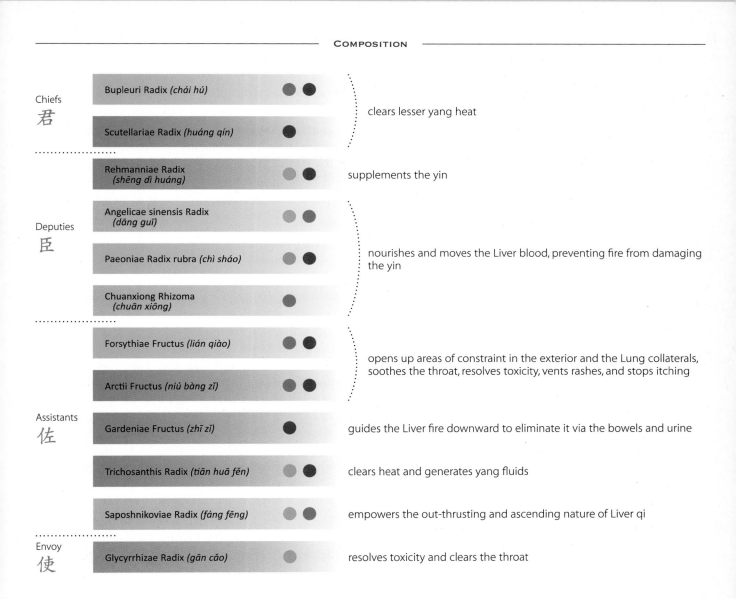

Chiefs
君

Bupleuri Radix *(chái hú)*

Scutellariae Radix *(huáng qín)*

clears lesser yang heat

Deputies
臣

Rehmanniae Radix
(shēng dì huáng)

supplements the yin

Angelicae sinensis Radix
(dāng guī)

Paeoniae Radix rubra *(chì sháo)*

Chuanxiong Rhizoma
(chuān xiōng)

nourishes and moves the Liver blood, preventing fire from damaging the yin

Assistants
佐

Forsythiae Fructus *(lián qiào)*

Arctii Fructus *(niú bàng zǐ)*

opens up areas of constraint in the exterior and the Lung collaterals, soothes the throat, resolves toxicity, vents rashes, and stops itching

Gardeniae Fructus *(zhī zǐ)*

guides the Liver fire downward to eliminate it via the bowels and urine

Trichosanthis Radix *(tiān huā fěn)*

clears heat and generates yang fluids

Saposhnikoviae Radix *(fáng fēng)*

empowers the out-thrusting and ascending nature of Liver qi

Envoy
使

Glycyrrhizae Radix *(gān cǎo)*

resolves toxicity and clears the throat

柴胡疏肝散
Bupleurum Powder to Dredge the Liver
chái hú shū gān sǎn

tendency to sigh or take deep breaths to relieve tension

feelings of frustration that easily give rise to anger

flank pain

Main pattern: constraint and clumping of Liver qi

Key symptoms: flank pain • abdominal distention and fullness • feelings of frustration that easily give rise to anger • muscular tension • tendency to sigh or take deep breaths to relieve tension

Secondary symptoms: belching • nausea • suppressed emotions • fatigue • cold and damp extremities • alternating fever and chills • sensitivity to changes in external environment

Tongue: thin, white coating

Pulse: wiry

Abdomen: tenderness under the ribs • tight rectus abdominis muscle

▶ CLINICAL NOTES

- This is the main formula for stagnation of qi in the Liver channel and thus is most specific for pain in the lower abdomen, abdomen, flanks, and chest. This pain tends to come and go, depending on the patient's emotional state and level of energy. It is generally relieved by activity and accompanied by a forceful, wiry pulse. Typical applications include various types of abdominal pain, belching, premenstrual syndrome, and dysmenorrhea. It is now also used for patterns caused by constrained Liver qi invading other body regions with symptoms like back pain or qi stagnation in the digestive system.

- The formula can be flexibly adapted to treat the many possible variations of this pattern. Thus one can add heat-clearing herbs like Gardeniae Fructus (*zhī zǐ*), Toosendan Fructus (*chuān liàn zǐ*), or Scutellariae Radix (*huáng qín*) when qi stagnation engenders heat; blood-moving herbs like Angelicae sinensis Radix (*dāng guī*) and Curcumae Radix (*yù jīn*) when qi stagnation starts to impact the blood; or Pinelliae Rhizoma praeparatum (*zhì bàn xià*) and Poria (*fú líng*) when Liver qi invades the Stomach to cause vomiting.

Contraindications: long-term use • qi or yin deficiency

─── INGREDIENTS ───

vinegar-fried Citri reticulatae Pericarpium (*cù chǎo chén pí*) . 6g
Bupleuri Radix (*chái hú*)... 6g
Chuanxiong Rhizoma (*chuān xiōng*) 5g
dry-fried Aurantii Fructus (*chǎo zhǐ ké*)............................. 5g
¹Paeoniae Radix (*sháo yào*)... 5g
Glycyrrhizae Radix praeparata (*zhì gān cǎo*) 1.5-3g
Cyperi Rhizoma (*xiāng fù*) 5g

Actions: spreads the Liver qi • harmonizes the blood • relieves pain

_____

1. As the primary function here is to restrain, tonify, or soften, Paeoniae Radix alba *(bái sháo)* is preferred.

▶ FORMULAS WITH SIMILAR INDICATIONS

Frigid Extremities Powder (*sì nì sǎn*): Focuses on constraint of the yang qi in the abdomen failing to reach and warm the extremities, thus it treats a pattern with heat in the abdomen and cold in the extremities.

Rambling Powder (*xiāo yáo sǎn*): For Liver qi constraint associated with deficiency of qi, blood, and dampness. This pattern is marked not only by the presence of hypochondriac tension or pain but also by fatigue, reduced appetite, a pale tongue, and a wiry, deficient pulse.

COMPOSITION

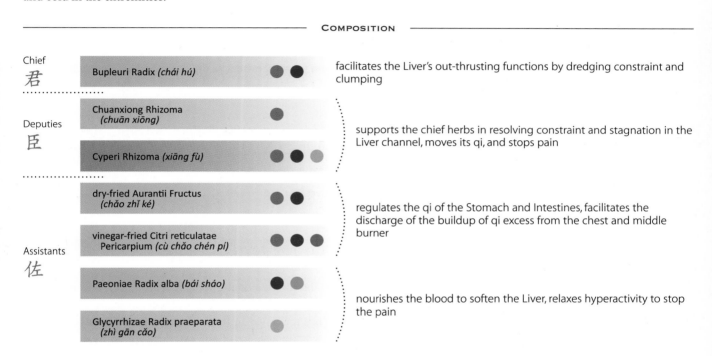

| Chief 君 | Bupleuri Radix *(chái hú)* | facilitates the Liver's out-thrusting functions by dredging constraint and clumping |

| Deputies 臣 | Chuanxiong Rhizoma *(chuān xiōng)* | supports the chief herbs in resolving constraint and stagnation in the Liver channel, moves its qi, and stops pain |
| | Cyperi Rhizoma *(xiāng fù)* | |

Assistants 佐	dry-fried Aurantii Fructus *(chǎo zhǐ ké)*	regulates the qi of the Stomach and Intestines, facilitates the discharge of the buildup of qi excess from the chest and middle burner
	vinegar-fried Citri reticulatae Pericarpium *(cù chǎo chén pí)*	
	Paeoniae Radix alba *(bái sháo)*	nourishes the blood to soften the Liver, relaxes hyperactivity to stop the pain
	Glycyrrhizae Radix praeparata *(zhì gān cǎo)*	

川芎茶調散 （川芎茶调散）
Chuanxiong Powder to Be Taken with Green Tea
chuān xiōng chá tiáo sǎn

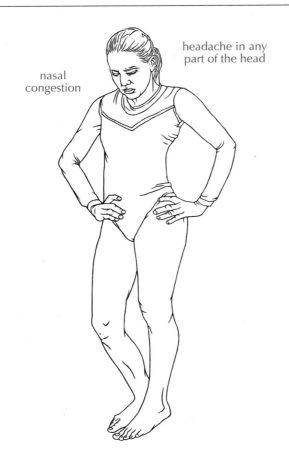

nasal congestion

headache in any part of the head

Menthae haplocalycis Herba (*bò hé*)................................6g
Glycyrrhizae Radix praeparata (*zhì gān cǎo*)..................6g
green tea

Preparation notes: Do not cook for more than 10 minutes. Alternatively, following the original source, 6g of a finely ground powder made of these herbs can be taken after meals with green tea.

Actions: disperses wind • alleviates pain

Main pattern: headache due to externally-contracted wind

Key symptoms: headache in any part of the head • nasal congestion

Secondary symptoms: dizziness • aversion to drafts • fever and chills

Tongue: thin, white coating

Pulse: floating

Abdomen: no specific signs

▶ CLINICAL NOTES

- This formula can be used for acute and chronic headaches due to external wind. It is specific for external wind that has remained in the body for a long time and presents with an absence of any exterior symptoms such as fever or chills.

- With modifications this formula can treat nasal infections, sinusitis, chronic rhinitis, and common colds with headache.

- As wind is 'the chief of the hundred diseases', in practice it will often present with other pathogens. In such cases, the formula can be modified:

  — For pronounced wind-cold, replace Menthae haplocalycis Herba (*bò hé*) with Perillae Folium (*zǐ sū yè*) and Zingiberis Rhizoma recens (*shēng jiāng*).

  — For wind-heat, add Chrysanthemi Flos (*jú huā*), Bombyx batryticatus (*bái jiāng cán*), and Viticis Fructus (*màn jīng zǐ*).

  — For wind-dampness, add Atractylodis Rhizoma (*cāng zhú*) and Ligustici Rhizoma (*gǎo běn*).

INGREDIENTS

Chuanxiong Rhizoma (*chuān xiōng*) 9-12g

Angelicae dahuricae Radix (*bái zhǐ*) 6g

Notopterygii Rhizoma seu Radix (*qiāng huó*)...................... 6g

¹Asari Herba (*xì xīn*) 3g

Schizonepetae Herba (*jīng jiè*) 9-12g

Saposhnikoviae Radix (*fáng fēng*)................................. 6g

---

1. This herb can be difficult to obtain because of legal issues. Clematidis Radix *(wēi líng xiān)* and Liquidambaris Fructus *(lù lù tōng)* may be substituted.

— For very stubborn conditions, increase the dosage of Chuanxiong Rhizoma (*chuān xiōng*) and add Persicae Semen (*táo rén*), Carthami Flos (*hóng huā*), Scorpio (*quán xiē*), and Pheretima (*dì lóng*) to invigorate the blood and unblock the collaterals.

Contraindications: headache from ascendant Liver yang due to Liver or Kidney deficiency • headache due to qi or blood deficiency

▶ FORMULAS WITH SIMILAR INDICATIONS

Xanthium Powder (*cāng ěr zǐ sǎn*): For nasal congestion that may present with headache due to wind-cold fettering the exterior.

Kudzu Decoction (*gé gēn tāng*): For wind-cold transforming into heat with more pronounced exterior symptoms and stiffness of back or neck.

COMPOSITION

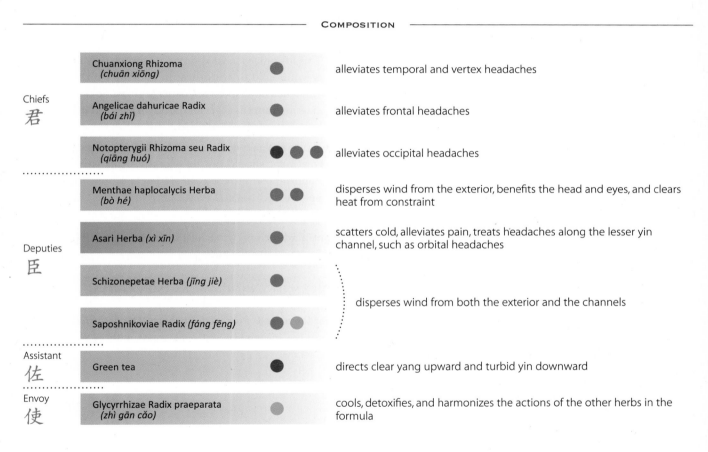

Chiefs 君	Chuanxiong Rhizoma (*chuān xiōng*)	alleviates temporal and vertex headaches
	Angelicae dahuricae Radix (*bái zhǐ*)	alleviates frontal headaches
	Notopterygii Rhizoma seu Radix (*qiāng huó*)	alleviates occipital headaches
Deputies 臣	Menthae haplocalycis Herba (*bò hé*)	disperses wind from the exterior, benefits the head and eyes, and clears heat from constraint
	Asari Herba (*xì xīn*)	scatters cold, alleviates pain, treats headaches along the lesser yin channel, such as orbital headaches
	Schizonepetae Herba (*jīng jiè*)	disperses wind from both the exterior and the channels
	Saposhnikoviae Radix (*fáng fēng*)	
Assistant 佐	Green tea	directs clear yang upward and turbid yin downward
Envoy 使	Glycyrrhizae Radix praeparata (*zhì gān cǎo*)	cools, detoxifies, and harmonizes the actions of the other herbs in the formula

蔥白七味飲（葱白七味饮）
Scallion Drink with Seven Ingredients
cōng bái qī wèi yǐn

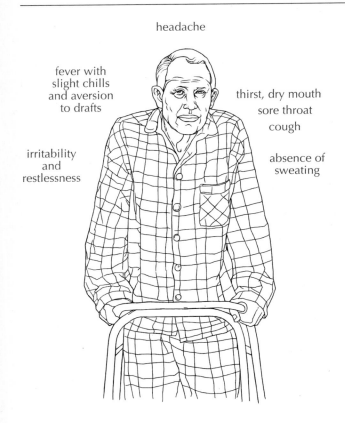

headache

fever with slight chills and aversion to drafts

thirst, dry mouth sore throat cough

irritability and restlessness

absence of sweating

INGREDIENTS

Allii fistulosi Bulbus (*cōng bái*)... 9g
Puerariae Radix (*gé gēn*).. 9g
Sojae Semen praeparatum (*dàn dòu chǐ*) 6g
Zingiberis Rhizoma recens (*shēng jiāng*)............................. 6g
Ophiopogonis Radix (*mài mén dōng*) 9g
Rehmanniae Radix (*shēng dì huáng*).................................... 9g

Actions: nourishes the blood • releases hot or cold wind pathogens from the exterior

Main patterns: externally-contracted wind-cold in patients with constitutional yin deficiency • wind-heat invading the protective qi aspect and Lungs due to damage of yin and fluids

Key symptoms: fever with slight chills and aversion to drafts • dry mouth • sore throat

Secondary symptoms: headache • absence of sweating • cough • irritability and restlessness • thirst

Tongue: red (perhaps only at the tip)

Pulse: rapid

Abdomen: no specific signs

▶ CLINICAL NOTES

- This formula is most appropriate for the very early stages of wind-cold or wind-heat in patients with underlying yin deficiency. It does not damage yin while clearing these exterior patterns that can quickly transform into internal heat patterns in yin-deficient patients.

- While in general any sweating that occurs as a result of treatment should not be excessive, this is particularly important with these patients. Furthermore, they should be covered once they become aware that a sweat is developing to prevent renewed contraction of a pathogen.

Contraindications: wind-heat in the exterior without underlying yin deficiency

▶ FORMULAS WITH SIMILAR INDICATIONS

*Gardenia and Prepared Soybean Decoction (*zhī zǐ chǐ tāng*): For irritability and restlessness without signs of yin deficiency or an exterior condition.

COMPOSITION

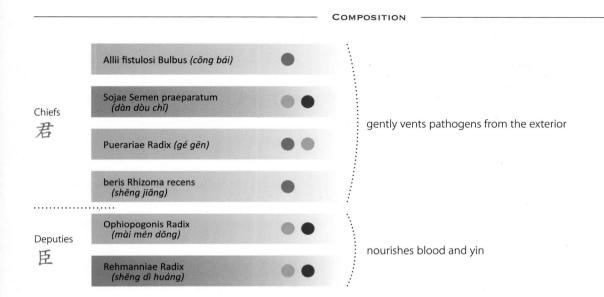

Chiefs
君

Allii fistulosi Bulbus *(cōng bái)*

Sojae Semen praeparatum
(dàn dòu chǐ)

Puerariae Radix *(gé gēn)*

beris Rhizoma recens
(shēng jiāng)

gently vents pathogens from the exterior

Deputies
臣

Ophiopogonis Radix
(mài mén dōng)

Rehmanniae Radix
(shēng dì huáng)

nourishes blood and yin

蔥豉湯（葱豉汤）
Scallion and Prepared Soybean Decoction
cōng chǐ tāng

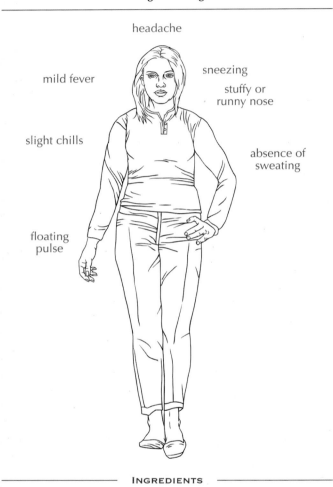

headache

mild fever

sneezing

stuffy or runny nose

slight chills

absence of sweating

floating pulse

INGREDIENTS

Allii fistulosi Bulbus (*cōng bái*)................................ 3-5 stalks
Sojae Semen praeparatum (*dàn dòu chǐ*) 9-30g

Preparation notes: Cook for just 5-10 minutes.

Actions: unblocks the yang (protective) qi in the exterior and induces sweating

Main patterns: early-stage externally-contracted wind-cold or wind-heat disorders

Key symptoms: mild fever • slight chills • absence of sweating

Secondary symptoms: headache • stuffy or runny nose • sneezing

Tongue: thin, white coating

Pulse: floating

Abdomen: no specific signs

▶ CLINICAL NOTES

- A mild formula that is not drying and can be used to resolve both wind-cold and wind-heat in the exterior in the very early stages.
- If there are signs of more severe obstruction, such as pain, this formula is not appropriate.

Contraindications: none noted

▶ FORMULAS WITH SIMILAR INDICATIONS

Cinnamon Twig Decoction (*guì zhī tāng*): For greater yang stage disorders characterized by sweating and a superficial but relaxed pulse. These symptoms are due to disharmony between nutritive and protective qi.

Mulberry Leaf and Chrysanthemum Drink (*sāng jú yǐn*): For wind-heat disorders in the protective aspect with coughing. There may be chills, but the pulse will usually be floating in both distal positions.

Augmented Cyperus and Perilla Leaf Powder (*jiā wei xiāng sū săn*): Suitable for early stage wind-cold exterior patterns in children or weak patients that may be accompanied by digestive symptoms.

———————————————————————————— COMPOSITION ————————————————————————————

Chiefs
君

Allii fistulosi Bulbus *(cōng bái)*	●	unblocks the flow of yang qi in the exterior, induces sweating
Sojae Semen praeparatum *(dàn dòu chǐ)*	● ●	releases externally-contracted pathogenic factors from the exterior, induces sweating

大補陰丸（大补阴丸）
Great Tonify the Yin Pill
dà bǔ yīn wán

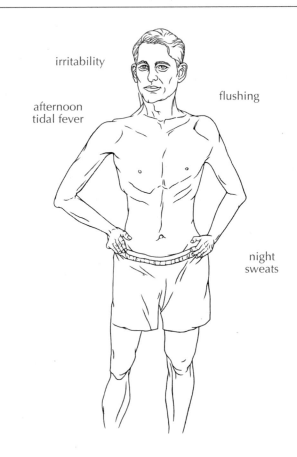

irritability

afternoon
tidal fever

flushing

night
sweats

INGREDIENTS

Rehmanniae Radix praeparata (*shú dì huáng*) 12g

crisp Testudinis Plastrum (*sū guī bǎn*) 12g

dry-fried Phellodendri Cortex (*chǎo huáng bǎi*).................... 9g

wine-fried Anemarrhenae Rhizoma (*jiǔ chǎo zhī mǔ*).......... 9g

Preparation notes: To make into pills, grind the ingredients into a powder and cook with pig's vertebrae, then add honey.

Actions: enriches the yin • directs fire downward

Main pattern: yin deficiency with flourishing deficiency fire

Key symptoms: afternoon tidal fever • night sweats • flushing • irritability

Secondary symptoms: steaming bones • sensation of heat and pain in the knees and legs that is sometimes accompanied by weakness • hunger • cough with blood in the sputum • spontaneous seminal emissions

Tongue: red body • scanty coating

Pulse: thin • rapid • forceful in the proximal position

Abdomen: no specific signs

▶ CLINICAL NOTES

• This is the main formula for flaring of fire associated with yin deficiency. For this reason the fire symptoms will be most pronounced in the afternoon or at night. Flaring fire can manifest in the Stomach (hunger), the Lungs (cough with blood sputum), the Heart (irritability), or the Kidneys (heat in the knees or back).

• Unlike other formulas that tonify the Kidneys to control fire, this one focuses equally on directing fire downward and on tonifying the yin.

Contraindications: Spleen deficiency • fire from excess

▶ FORMULAS WITH SIMILAR INDICATIONS

Six-Ingredient Pill with Rehmannia (*liù wèi dì huáng wán*): A gentler formula that tonifies the Kidney, Liver, and Spleen yin while draining fire and water excess and less directly addressing deficiency fire.

*Anemarrhena, Phellodendron, and Rehmannia Pill (*zhī bái dì huáng wán*): A similar presentation but more generally tonifies the yin rather than intensely focusing on the lower burner yin and essence, along with the resulting flaring of fire from deficiency. It is easier on the digestion, and the proximal position of the pulse will be deep and frail, rather than forceful.

Hidden Tiger Pill (*hǔ qián wán*): For yin deficiency with uncontrolled fire damaging the muscles and blood leading to wasting, obstruction, and wind symptoms.

─────────────── COMPOSITION ───────────────

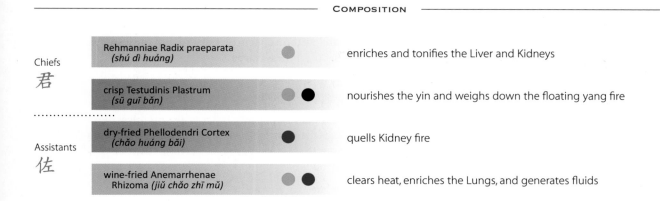

Chiefs
君

Rehmanniae Radix praeparata
(shú dì huáng)

enriches and tonifies the Liver and Kidneys

crisp Testudinis Plastrum
(sū guī bǎn)

nourishes the yin and weighs down the floating yang fire

Assistants
佐

dry-fried Phellodendri Cortex
(chǎo huáng bǎi)

quells Kidney fire

wine-fried Anemarrhenae
Rhizoma (jiǔ chǎo zhī mǔ)

clears heat, enriches the Lungs, and generates fluids

大柴胡湯（大柴胡汤）
Major Bupleurum Decoction
dà chái hú tāng

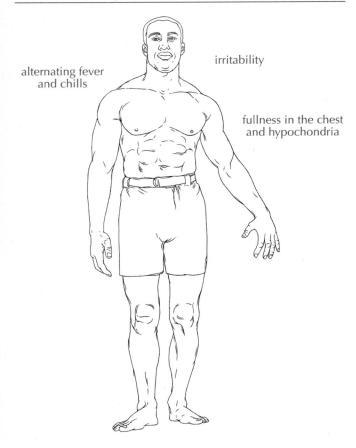

alternating fever and chills

irritability

fullness in the chest and hypochondria

INGREDIENTS

Bupleuri Radix (*chái hú*)	15-24g
Scutellariae Radix (*huáng qín*)	9g
[1]Paeoniae Radix (*sháo yào*)	9g
prepared Aurantii Fructus immaturus (*zhì zhǐ shí*)	9g
Rhei Radix et Rhizoma (*dà huáng*)	6g
Pinelliae Rhizoma praeparatum (*zhì bàn xià*)	9g
Zingiberis Rhizoma recens (*shēng jiāng*)	15g
Jujubae Fructus (*dà zǎo*)	4 pieces

---

1. As the primary function here is to restrain, tonify, or soften, Paeoniae Radix alba *(bái sháo)* is preferred.

Actions: harmonizes and releases the lesser yang • drains internal clumping due to heat

Main pattern: concurrent disorder of the lesser yang and yang brightness warps

Key symptoms: alternating fever and chills • fullness in the chest and hypochondria (with or without pain)

Secondary symptoms: bitter taste • dizziness • temporal headache • tension in neck and shoulder • tinnitus • nausea • vomiting • constipation or burning diarrhea • melancholy • irritability

Tongue: dry and white or yellow coating

Pulse: wiry and forceful • rapid and slippery • deep, excessive, and slow

Abdomen: hard focal distention or fullness and pain in epigastrium extending to flanks and abdomen

▶ CLINICAL NOTES

- This formula can be used for a very wide range of both acute and chronic problems. Typically, patients for whom this formula is appropriate will tend to be overweight and of a robust build and constitution, which differentiates them from patients presenting with a Minor Bupleurum Decoction (*xiǎo chái hú tāng*) pattern. On the other hand, patients for whom one of the Order the Qi Decoctions (*chéng qì tāng*) is more appropriate will lack the typical lesser yang symptoms; or, even if they experience severe abdominal pain, fullness, or distention, their abdomen may not be distended.

- If the patient has neither constipation nor foul-smelling stools, or if these symptoms were present but have abated, Rhei Radix et Rhizoma (*dà huáng*) can be removed from the formula.

Contraindications: deficiency patterns

▶ FORMULAS WITH SIMILAR INDICATIONS

Minor Bupleurum Decoction (*xiǎo chái hú tāng*): For patients who present with a similar pattern of symptoms but without signs of yang brightness warp disorder such as constipation or abdominal fullness.

Bupleurum plus Dragon Bone and Oyster Shell Decoction (*chái hú jiā lóng gǔ mǔ lì tāng*): Treats more complex conditions often involving pronounced psycho-emotional symptoms.

*Bupleurum Decoction plus Mirabilite (*chái hú jiā máng xiāo tāng*): For constipation and fullness in the chest and hypochondria with alternating fever and chills that are more pronounced in the afternoon.

COMPOSITION

Chiefs
君

Bupleuri Radix (*chái hú*) — dredges the lesser yang and releases the exterior

Rhei Radix et Rhizoma (*dà huáng*) — enters the yang brightness to drain heat and open the bowels

Deputies
臣

prepared Aurantii Fructus immaturus (*zhì zhǐ shí*) — breaks up qi stagnation and reduces focal distention and fullness in the chest and abdomen

Scutellariae Radix (*huáng qín*) — clears heat from the lesser yang, drains heat from the bowels

Assistants
佐

Paeoniae Radix alba (*bái sháo*) — relaxes urgency and stops pain

Pinelliae Rhizoma praeparatum (*zhì bàn xià*) — harmonizes the middle burner and directs the rebellious Stomach qi downward, stops vomiting

Envoys
使

Zingiberis Rhizoma recens (*shēng jiāng*)

Jujubae Fructus (*dà zǎo*) — strengthens the ability of Paeoniae Radix (*sháo yào*) to soften the Liver and reduce abdominal spasms

大承氣湯（大承气汤）
Major Order the Qi Decoction
dà chéng qì tāng

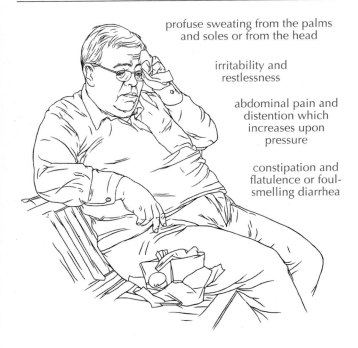

profuse sweating from the palms and soles or from the head

irritability and restlessness

abdominal pain and distention which increases upon pressure

constipation and flatulence or foul-smelling diarrhea

INGREDIENTS

Rhei Radix et Rhizoma (*dà huáng*).......... [add near end] 6-12g
Natrii Sulfas (*máng xiāo*) .... [dissolve in strained decoction] 9g
Aurantii Fructus immaturus (*zhǐ shí*)................................ 12g
Magnoliae officinalis Cortex (*hòu pó*).......................... 15-24g

Actions: vigorously purges heat accumulation

Main pattern: heat excess in the yang brightness organs • heat clumping with circumfluent diarrhea • heat inversion

Key symptoms: constipation and flatulence or foul-smelling diarrhea • abdominal pain and distention which increases upon pressure • irritability and restlessness • profuse sweating from the palms and soles or from the head

Secondary symptoms: tidal fevers • delirious speech • disorientation • cracked lips • dark, scanty urine

Tongue: red body with dry, yellow or black coating, possibly with prickles

Pulse: submerged or excessive and submerged • rapid and slippery

Abdomen: distended and painful abdomen that worsens with pressure • focal distention in epigastrium

► CLINICAL NOTES

• For yang brightness patterns at the organ level where heat has penetrated into the interior and caused clumping and dryness.

• The main intention of the formula is to drain heat from the interior and dispel clumping. While the pattern this formula addresses is characterized by constipation with dry stools, the formula can address any pattern due to internal excess heat in the Stomach and Intestines (such as damp-heat dysentery or diarrhea, severe mental agitation and restlessness, sweating) provided the pulse, tongue, and abdominal signs confirm the pattern.

• The formula and its variants can also be used to regulate the menstrual cycle or treat amenorrhea in constitutionally strong women with matching abdominal presentation or pulse.

Contraindications: This is a very strong formula that may cause vomiting or severe diarrhea. For weak patients it should be used only when absolutely necessary and then with the addition of tonic herbs. Contraindicated during pregnancy.

► FORMULAS WITH SIMILAR INDICATIONS

*Minor Order the Qi Decoction (*xiǎo chéng qì tāng*): For fullness and distention with relatively mild symptoms due to heat and dryness.

Peach Pit Decoction to Order the Qi (*táo hé chéng qì tāng*): For blood accumulation in the lower burner with tenderness in the abdomen and lower abdomen, even on light palpation. There may also be insomnia with nightmares or more severe signs of an agitated spirit.

Major Bupleurum Decoction (*dà chái hú tāng*): For a combined lesser yang/yang brightness pattern with abdominal fullness and pain around the flanks.

Rhubarb and Moutan Decoction (*dà huáng mǔ dān tāng*): For a combination of blood stasis and heat clumping in the lower abdomen with pain and fullness that is aggravated by pressure in the right lower quadrant of the abdomen.

─────────────── COMPOSITION ───────────────

Chief 君	Rhei Radix et Rhizoma *(dà huáng)* ●	attacks accumulation, guides out stagnation, flushes the Intestines and Stomach, drains heat, gets rid of excess
Deputy 臣	Natrii Sulfas *(máng xiāo)* ● ● ●	drains heat, softens areas of hardness, moistens dryness, guides out stagnation
Assistants 佐	Aurantii Fructus immaturus *(zhǐ shí)* ● ●	promotes the movement of qi, unbinds focal distention
	Magnolia officinalis Cortex *(hòu pò)* ● ●	eliminates fullness and reduces distention

大黃附子湯（大黄附子汤）
Rhubarb and Aconite
Accessory Root Decoction
dà huáng fù zǐ tāng

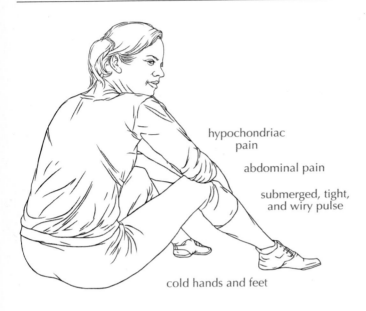

hypochondriac pain

abdominal pain

submerged, tight, and wiry pulse

cold hands and feet

--- INGREDIENTS ---

[1]Aconiti Radix lateralis praeparata (*zhì fù zǐ*) 9-12g
Rhei Radix et Rhizoma (*dà huáng*) 9g
[2]Asari Herba (*xì xīn*) 6g

Actions: warms the interior • disperses cold • unblocks the bowels • alleviates pain

Main pattern: cold excess in the flanks and abdomen causing stagnation of qi and clumping of fluids

Key symptoms: acute abdominal pain • hypochondriac pain • chest pain

Secondary symptoms: constipation • chills • low-grade fever • cold hands and feet

---

1. This herb can be difficult to obtain because of legal issues. A combination of Cinnamomi Cortex *(ròu guì)* and Zingiberis Rhizoma *(gān jiāng)* may be substituted.

2. This herb can be difficult to obtain because of legal issues. Clematidis Radix *(wēi líng xiān)* may be substituted.

Tongue: greasy, white coating

Pulse: submerged, tight, and wiry

Abdomen: pain and tenderness in the hypochondrium and abdomen

▶ CLINICAL NOTES

• Such signs as a white tongue coating, a wet tongue body, or a deep, wiry, and full pulse allow one to differentiate this pattern from similar patterns due to heat.

• If taking the formula is followed by a bowel movement, the prognosis is generally good.

• From a biomedical perspective, the severe pain that is the main indication of this formula can be due to a wide variety of conditions including angina, prolapsed disc, neuralgia including post-herpetic neuralgia, cholecystitis, appendicitis, kidney stones, and sciatica.

Contraindications: interior heat excess patterns

▶ FORMULAS WITH SIMILAR INDICATIONS

*Major Construct the Middle Decoction (*dà jiàn zhōng tāng*): For abdominal pain associated with interior cold from deficiency and visible peristalsis.

Major Bupleurum Decoction (*dà chái hú tāng*): For flank and abdominal pain as part of a combined lesser yang/yang brightness pattern; symptoms are focused on the upper abdomen and accompanied by a bitter taste.

─────────────────────────── COMPOSITION ───────────────────────────

Chief 君	Aconiti Radix lateralis praeparata *(zhì fù zǐ)*	● Ⓣ	warms the yang, dispels cold
Deputy 臣	Rhei Radix et Rhizoma *(dà huáng)*	●	flushes the Intestines, purges accumulation
Assistant 佐	Asari Herba *(xì xīn)*	●	expels cold, disperses accumulation or clumping

大黃牡丹湯（大黃牡丹汤）
Rhubarb and Moutan Decoction
dà huáng mǔ dān tāng

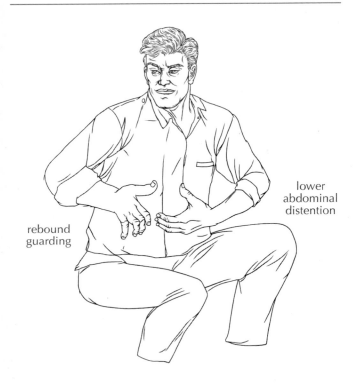

rebound
guarding

lower
abdominal
distention

INGREDIENTS

Rhei Radix et Rhizoma (*dà huáng*).................................... 12g
Natrii Sulfas (*máng xiāo*)[dissolve in strained decoction] 9-12g
Moutan Cortex (*mǔ dān pí*) 3-6g
Persicae Semen (*táo rén*).. 9-15g
Benincasae Semen (*dōng guā zǐ*).................................. 15-30g

Actions: disperses wind • alleviates pain • unblocks the nose

Main pattern: early-stage Intestinal abscess with interior clumping of heat and blood

Key symptoms: lower abdominal distention and pain (usually on right) • pain increases on pressure • rebound tenderness • abdominal guarding

Secondary symptoms: intermittent fever followed by chills and sweating

Tongue: thin, yellow, greasy coating

Pulse: slippery • rapid

Abdomen: rebound tenderness in lower right quadrant

▶ CLINICAL NOTES

• This is an emergency formula for acute pain in the lower right quadrant of the abdomen that overlaps with the biomedical diagnosis of appendicitis. This is a dangerous condition that often requires surgical intervention. In Chinese hospitals the formula is sometimes given to patients who are scheduled for surgery in order to increase the odds of the situation resolving without the need for an operation.

• In addition to acute abdominal pain, this formula can be used for other disorders if they present with constipation, abdominal tenderness, and a yellow tongue coating. Examples include endometriosis, dysentery, diverticulitis, hot disorders of the skin or mucous membranes, and painful menstruation.

Contraindications: This formula is too strong for use during pregnancy or in very weak patients. It should also not be used after the appendix has ruptured.

▶ FORMULAS WITH SIMILAR INDICATIONS

Major Order the Qi Decoction (*dà chéng qì tāng*): For excess in the yang brightness Large Intestine that gives rise to constipation or diarrhea as well as pain in the abdomen. It drains yang brightness excess more powerfully than Rhubarb and Moutan Decoction (*dà huáng mǔ dān tāng*), but it lacks specific herbs to treat abscesses and does not have the blood-moving and stasis-dissipating strength of that formula.

―――――――――――――― **COMPOSITION** ――――――――――――――

Chief
君

Rhei Radix et Rhizoma *(dà huáng)* ● drains heat and breaks up blood stasis

Deputies
臣

Natrii Sulfas *(máng xiāo)* ● ● ● softens the stool, aids in draining heat downward, and unblocks the Intestines

Moutan Cortex *(mǔ dān pí)* ● ● cools the blood and eliminates masses due to blood stasis

Assistants
佐

Persicae Semen *(táo rén)* ● ● breaks up the stasis of blood and has a mild moistening and laxative effect

Benincasae Semen *(dōng guā zǐ)* ● expels pus, eliminates heat, and reduces abscesses in the intestines

大秦艽湯（大秦艽汤）
Major Large Gentian Decoction
dà qín jiāo tāng

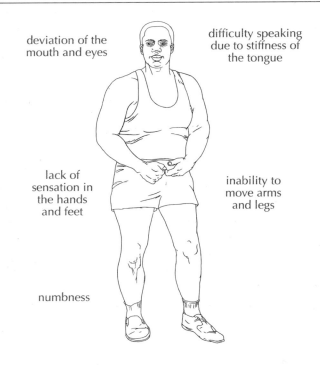

deviation of the mouth and eyes

difficulty speaking due to stiffness of the tongue

lack of sensation in the hands and feet

inability to move arms and legs

numbness

INGREDIENTS

Gentianae macrophyllae Radix (*qín jiāo*) 15g
Angelicae pubescentis Radix (*dú huó*) 12g
Notopterygii Rhizoma seu Radix (*qiāng huó*)...................... 9g
Saposhnikoviae Radix (*fáng fēng*)................................... 90g
Angelicae dahuricae Radix (*bái zhǐ*) 9g
¹Asari Herba (*xì xīn*)... 6g
Atractylodis macrocephalae Rhizoma (*bái zhú*) 12g
Poria (*fú líng*)... 12g
Glycyrrhizae Radix (*gān cǎo*).. 6g
Chuanxiong Rhizoma (*chuān xiōng*) 9g
Angelicae sinensis Radix (*dāng guī*) 9g
Paeoniae Radix alba (*bái sháo*)....................................... 18g
Scutellariae Radix (*huáng qín*)... 9g

1. This herb can be difficult to obtain because of legal issues. Clematidis Radix *(wēi líng xiān)* may be substituted.

Gypsum fibrosum (*shí gāo*)... 18g
Rehmanniae Radix (*shēng dì huáng*).............................. 12g
Rehmanniae Radix praeparata (*shú dì huáng*) 12g

Actions: expels wind • clears heat • nourishes and invigorates the blood

Main pattern: early- or middle-stage wind-stroke in the channels

Key symptoms: deviation of the mouth and eyes • difficulty speaking due to stiffness of the tongue • an inability to move one's arms and legs • numbness • lack of sensation in the hands and feet

Secondary symptoms: chills and fever • muscle spasms • aching joints

Tongue: thin and white or yellow coating

Pulse: floating and tight • wiry and thin

Abdomen: no specific signs

▶ CLINICAL NOTES

- For acute wind-stroke into the channels (channel stroke) as occurs in Bell's palsy. Notably, this presents without signs and symptoms indicating involvement of the organs.
- Because this formula focuses on eliminating wind from the channels as well as promoting qi and blood movement through the channels, it is also used in modern times to treat acute wind-damp painful obstruction.
- One unique aspect of this formula is that it includes Scutellariae Radix (*huáng qín*), Rehmanniae Radix (*shēng dì huáng*), and Gypsum fibrosum (*shí gāo*) to clear heat formed through the acute invasion of a wind pathogen. Its ability to treat internal heat (with the exception of phlegm-heat) differentiates it from most other formulas that dispel wind from the channels.

Contraindications: internal wind • yin deficiency • impaired consciousness • incontinence • phlegm-heat • thick tongue coating

▶ FORMULAS WITH SIMILAR INDICATIONS ⇢

Minor Extend Life Decoction (*xiǎo xù mìng tāng*): For acute channel stroke due to wind-cold with more pronounced cold and more exterior symptoms. This formula contains hot tonifying agents and thus supports the body's normal qi and yang.

Lead to Symmetry Powder (*qiān zhèng sǎn*): For acute wind-phlegm lodging in the greater yang and yang brightness channels and collaterals, resulting in deviation of the mouth and eyes.

COMPOSITION

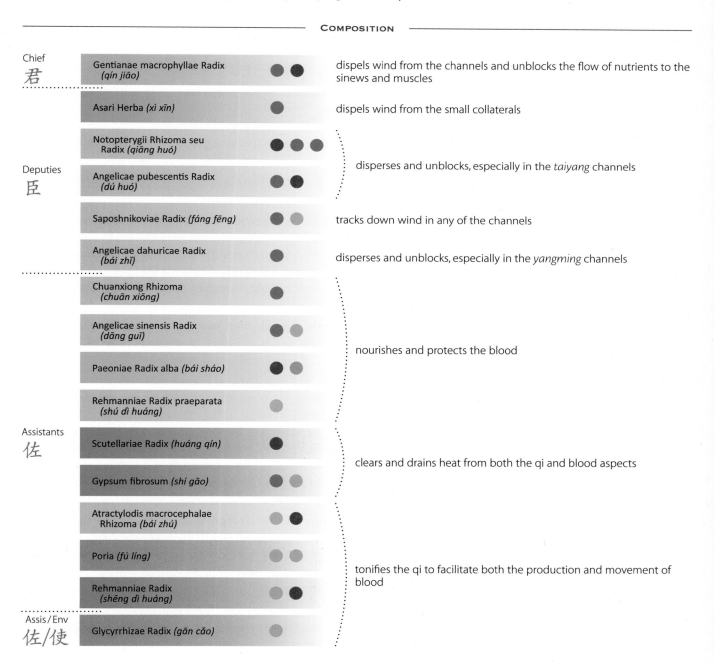

Chief 君	Gentianae macrophyllae Radix (*qín jiāo*)		dispels wind from the channels and unblocks the flow of nutrients to the sinews and muscles
	Asari Herba (*xì xīn*)		dispels wind from the small collaterals
Deputies 臣	Notopterygii Rhizoma seu Radix (*qiāng huó*)		disperses and unblocks, especially in the *taiyang* channels
	Angelicae pubescentis Radix (*dú huó*)		
	Saposhnikoviae Radix (*fáng fēng*)		tracks down wind in any of the channels
	Angelicae dahuricae Radix (*bái zhǐ*)		disperses and unblocks, especially in the *yangming* channels
Assistants 佐	Chuanxiong Rhizoma (*chuān xiōng*)		nourishes and protects the blood
	Angelicae sinensis Radix (*dāng guī*)		
	Paeoniae Radix alba (*bái sháo*)		
	Rehmanniae Radix praeparata (*shú dì huáng*)		
	Scutellariae Radix (*huáng qín*)		clears and drains heat from both the qi and blood aspects
	Gypsum fibrosum (*shí gāo*)		
	Atractylodis macrocephalae Rhizoma (*bái zhú*)		tonifies the qi to facilitate both the production and movement of blood
	Poria (*fú líng*)		
	Rehmanniae Radix (*shēng dì huáng*)		
Assis/Env 佐/使	Glycyrrhizae Radix (*gān cǎo*)		

大青龍湯（大青龙汤）
Major Bluegreen Dragon Decoction
dà qīng lóng tāng

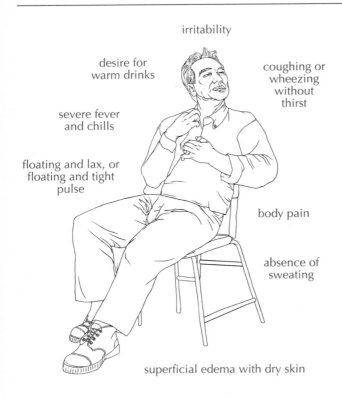

irritability

desire for warm drinks

coughing or wheezing without thirst

severe fever and chills

floating and lax, or floating and tight pulse

body pain

absence of sweating

superficial edema with dry skin

INGREDIENTS

[1]Ephedrae Herba (*má huáng*)... 12g

Armeniacae Semen (*xìng rén*) 6g

Cinnamomi Ramulus (*guì zhī*) 6g

Glycyrrhizae Radix praeparata (*zhì gān cǎo*) 6g

Gypsum fibrosum (*shí gāo*).. 12-18g

Zingiberis Rhizoma (*gān jiāng*).. 9g

Jujubae Fructus (*dà zǎo*)... 3 pieces

Actions: promotes sweating • releases wind-cold from the exterior • clears interior heat

Main patterns: exterior cold with heat from constraint in the

interior • overflowing thin mucus (溢飲 *yì yǐn*) patterns defined by heaviness and aching of the entire body • superficial edema in the extremities

Key symptoms: severe fever and chills • absence of sweating • irritability • body pain • superficial edema with dry skin

Secondary symptoms: sensation of a heavy body that comes and goes • coughing or wheezing without thirst • desire for warm drinks

Tongue: body may be red but coating will often be white

Pulse: floating and lax, or floating and tight

Abdomen: no specific signs

▶ CLINICAL NOTES

• The presentation resembles an Ephedra Decotion (*má huáng tāng*) pattern with one important distinction: in this pattern there is irritability owing to internal heat from interior constraint. If Ephedra Decoction (*má huáng tāng*) is mistakenly prescribed, the irritability will worsen.

• Irritability and heat are the main markers differentiating this formula from lesser yin patterns in the treatment of thin mucus disorders. In lesser yin patterns, body aches and edema will be accompanied by cold.

• Can be used to treat a wide range of disorders in patients with a strong constitution where internal heat, flushing, and irritability are the main symptoms (e.g., heat stroke, hypertension, hemorrhoids, adverse reactions to drugs, nosebleeds), but some signs such as aversion to cold, lack of thirst, a desire for warm drinks, a white tongue coating, or a tight pulse do not fit the presentation of a pure heat pattern.

• Due to its strongly diaphoretic nature this formula should be administered gradually and discontinued once the patient has broken a sweat. This is particularly true when the other signs of a strong exterior pattern have disappeared.

Contraindications: lesser yin patterns • yang deficiency • wind-stroke patterns with deficiency of the exterior • cases where sweating is coupled with an increase in irritability,

---

1. This herb can be difficult to obtain because of legal issues. Perillae Folium (*zǐ sū yè*) may be substituted.

restlessness, and heat • wind-cold fettering the exterior with severe accumulation of fluids in the interior

▶ FORMULAS WITH SIMILAR INDICATIONS

Ephedra Decoction (*má huáng tāng*): For cold constraining the diffusion of yang qi and fluids in the exterior. These patients have no heat in the interior and consequentially are not irritable.

Ephedra, Apricot Kernel, Gypsum, and Licorice Decoction (*má xìng shí gān tang*): For heat constraint at the qi level of the Lungs due to cold. The heat signs are less intense. There is some sweating, but no edema.

Minor Bluegreen Dragon Decoction (*xiǎo qīng lóng tāng*): For wind-cold in the exterior in patients with internal accumulation of phlegm fluids. Signs of heat are very mild or nonexistent.

──────── COMPOSITION ────────

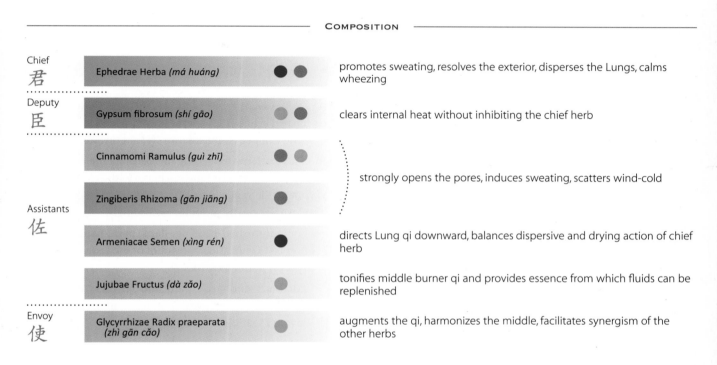

Chief 君	Ephedrae Herba *(má huáng)* ● ●	promotes sweating, resolves the exterior, disperses the Lungs, calms wheezing
Deputy 臣	Gypsum fibrosum *(shí gāo)* ● ●	clears internal heat without inhibiting the chief herb
Assistants 佐	Cinnamomi Ramulus *(guì zhī)* ● ●	strongly opens the pores, induces sweating, scatters wind-cold
	Zingiberis Rhizoma *(gān jiāng)* ●	
	Armeniacae Semen *(xìng rén)* ●	directs Lung qi downward, balances dispersive and drying action of chief herb
	Jujubae Fructus *(dà zǎo)* ●	tonifies middle burner qi and provides essence from which fluids can be replenished
Envoy 使	Glycyrrhizae Radix praeparata *(zhì gān cǎo)* ●	augments the qi, harmonizes the middle, facilitates synergism of the other herbs

達原飲 （达原饮）
Reach the Source Drink
dá yuán yǐn

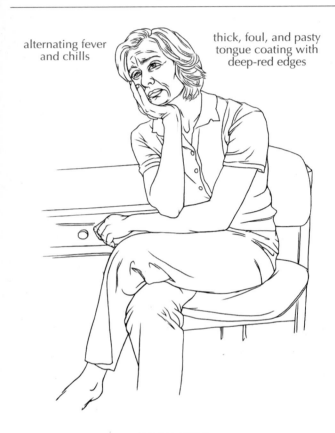

alternating fever and chills

thick, foul, and pasty tongue coating with deep-red edges

Key symptoms: alternating fever and chills (both strong) occurring 1-3 times a day at irregular intervals • fever of unexplained origin

Secondary symptoms: stifling sensation in the chest • nausea or vomiting • headache • irritability • scanty, turbid, and yellow urine

Tongue: deep-red edges • thick, foul, and pasty coating

Pulse: wiry and rapid (neither floating nor submerged)

Abdomen: no specific signs

► CLINICAL NOTES

- A powdery coating on the tongue that looks like rice flour or curdled tofu is a key marker here as it reflects the yang qi being trapped in the interior by foul turbidity.

- In many patterns treated by this formula the pathogenic heat will from time to time discharge to the exterior, often via one of the yang warps where it then causes constraint. The formula can be modified accordingly.

  → For diminished hearing, flank pain, nausea, and a bitter taste indicating constraint of the lesser yang, add Bupleuri Radix (*chái hú*).

  → For back and neck pain and stiffness indicating constraint of the greater yang, add Notopterygii Rhizoma seu Radix (*qiāng huó*).

  → For pain in the orbital and frontal areas with dry nasal passages and insomnia indicating constraint of the greater yang, add Puerariae Radix (*gé gēn*).

- Originally composed to treat epidemic toxins, this formula is used today to treat disorders such as influenza, malaria, and fever of unknown origin.

- Use of this formula must be discontinued once obstruction of the qi dynamic has been cleared and the pathogen is discharged. Such cases will often transmute into a heat pattern as the yang qi that was previously pressed toward the interior now forcefully moves outward.

INGREDIENTS

Tsaoko Fructus (*cǎo guǒ*)	1.5g
Magnoliae officinalis Cortex (*hòu pó*)	3g
Arecae Semen (*bīng láng*)	6g
Scutellariae Radix (*huáng qín*)	3g
Anemarrhenae Rhizoma (*zhī mǔ*)	3g
Paeoniae Radix alba (*bái sháo*)	3g
Glycyrrhizae Radix (*gān cǎo*)	1.5g

Actions: opens the membrane source by thrusting out pathogens • clears away filth • transforms turbidity

Main pattern: foul turbidity entering the body via the nose and mouth to lodge in the membrane source

Contraindications: damp-warm disorders with heat stronger than dampness

▶ FORMULAS WITH SIMILAR INDICATIONS

Bupleurum Drink to Reach the Source (*chái hú dá yuán yǐn*):

For phlegm-dampness obstructing the qi dynamic with less heat signs, more focal distention, and a white tongue coating that looks like curdled cheese.

COMPOSITION

Chiefs 君

Tsaoko Fructus (*cǎo guǒ*) ●●	transforms turbidity, stops vomiting and vents the pathogen lurking in the half-exterior, half-interior level
Magnoliae officinalis Cortex (*hòu pò*) ●●	transforms turbidity, expels dampness, and regulates the qi
Arecae Semen (*bīng láng*) ●●	disperses dampness and reduces stagnation by facilitating the flow of qi, thereby hastening the elimination of the pathogenic influences from the interior

Deputies 臣

Scutellariae Radix (*huáng qín*) ●	clears heat and dries dampness in the Stomach and Gallbladder
Anemarrhenae Rhizoma (*zhī mǔ*) ●●	clears heat, nourishes the yin, and prevents heat from damaging the yin and fluids
Paeoniae Radix alba (*bái sháo*) ●●	prevents the acrid, drying properties of the other herbs from damaging the yin and blood

Envoy 使

Glycyrrhizae Radix (*gān cǎo*) ●	harmonizes the actions of the herbs in the formula

丹參飲（丹参饮）
Salvia Drink
dān shēn yǐn

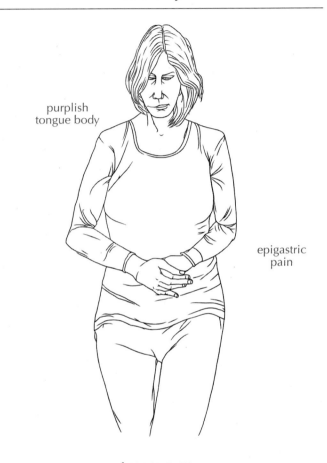

purplish
tongue body

epigastric
pain

Tongue: purplish body • stasis spots • visible sublingual capillaries and/or veins

Pulse: wiry • rough

Abdomen: tenderness in epigastrium, especially with deep pressure

▶ CLINICAL NOTES

- This formula is specifically indicated for epigastric pain from blood stasis and qi stagnation. A key clinical marker is that the pain radiates upward from the epigastrium toward or into the chest.
- This formula can also be used to treat chest pain, dysmenorrhea, and flank pain from qi stagnation and blood stasis.
- This formula is frequently combined with others. For instance, for chest pain it may be combined with Unripe Bitter Orange, Chinese Garlic, and Cinnamon Twig Decoction (*zhǐ shí xiè bái guì zhī tāng*). For qi stagnation with pain in the flanks, nausea, vomiting and a purplish tongue body, it can be combined with Frigid Extremities Powder (*sì nì sǎn*) or Melia Toosendan Powder (*jīn líng zǐ sǎn*).

Contraindications: deficiency patterns

▶ FORMULAS WITH SIMILAR INDICATIONS

Drive Out Stasis Below the Diaphragm Decoction (*gé xià zhú yū tāng*): For blood stasis below the diaphragm accompanied by palpable masses.

Sudden Smile Powder (*shī xiào sǎn*): For chest and epigastric pain due to blood stasis in the channels that is acute, fixed, and does not worsen with pressure.

───── INGREDIENTS ─────

Salviae miltiorrhizae Radix (*dān shēn*).............................30g
Santali albi Lignum (*tán xiāng*)...3g
Amomi Fructus (*shā rén*)..3g

Actions: invigorates the blood • dispels blood stasis • promotes the movement of qi • alleviates pain

Main pattern: blood stasis and qi stagnation in the middle burner

Key symptoms: epigastric pain

Secondary symptoms: dysmenorrhea • flank pain

─────────────── **COMPOSITION** ───────────────

Chief
君
Salviae miltiorrhizae Radix
(dān shēn)
● invigorates the blood, transforms blood stasis, and alleviates pain

Deputy
臣
Santali albi Lignum *(tán xiāng)*
● ● warms the middle burner and regulates the qi

Assistant
佐
Amomi Fructus *(shā rén)*
● ● promotes the movement of qi, relaxes the middle burner, disperses the stifling sensation of constraint in the chest, and alleviates pain

當歸補血湯 （当归补血汤）
Tangkuei Decoction to Tonify the Blood
dāng guī bǔ xuè tāng

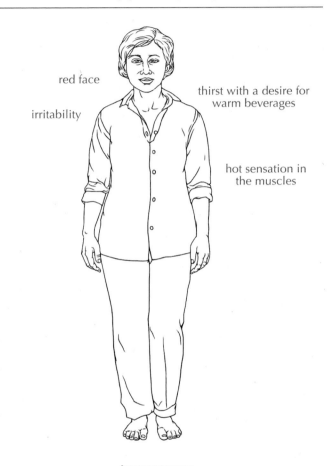

red face

irritability

thirst with a desire for warm beverages

hot sensation in the muscles

Astragali Radix (*huáng qí*) 30g
Angelicae sinensis Radix (*dāng guī*) 6g

Actions: tonifies the qi • generates blood

Main patterns: qi abandonment from loss of blood • blood deficiency from long-term illness

Key symptoms: hot sensation in the muscles • red face • irritability • thirst with a desire for warm beverages

Secondary symptoms: fever • headache • slow healing wounds and sores

Tongue: pale

Pulse: flooding, large, deficient • forceless when pressed hard

Abdomen: weak in depth but may have superficial tightness

▶ CLINICAL NOTES

- The signs of heat in the exterior indicate qi devastation and must not be mistaken for signs of heat excess or yin deficiency. Qi devastation patterns may be seen in postpartum fevers or fevers following surgery.

- The formula may also be used to treat slow-healing wounds and sores, chronic bleeding, or deficiency-type painful obstruction patterns. If it is used to tonify the blood, the dosage of Astragali Radix (*huáng qí*) should be reduced and Ginseng Radix (*rén shēn*) or Codonopsis Radix (*dǎng shēn*) added.

Contraindications: tidal fever from yin deficiency • yang brightness qi aspect heat excess

▶ FORMULAS WITH SIMILAR INDICATIONS

Tonify the Middle to Augment the Qi Decoction (*bǔ zhōng yì qì tāng*): For fever from qi deficiency.

Restore the Spleen Decoction (*guī pí tāng*): For deficiency of Spleen qi and Heart blood that may manifest with chronic bleeding due to the Spleen losing its capacity to govern blood.

*Tonify Spleen-Stomach, Drain Yin Fire, and Raise Yang Decoction (*bǔ pí wèi xiè yīn huǒ shēng yáng tāng*): For relatively severe constraint and fire excess leading to intense heat in the exterior.

*Tangkuei and Six-Yellow Decoction (*dāng guī liù huáng tāng*): For fever and night sweats due to yin deficiency and heat excess.

*Discharge Pus Powder (*tòu nóng sǎn*): For sores where pus has already formed but does not discharge easily.

───────────────────────────── COMPOSITION ─────────────────────────────

Chief
君
| Astragali Radix *(huáng qí)* | ● | tonifies the original qi of the Spleen, secures the exterior |

Deputy
臣
| Angelicae sinensis Radix
(dāng guī) | ● ● | tonifies and invigorates the blood |

當歸龍薈丸（当归龙荟丸）
Tangkuei, Gentian, and Aloe Pill
dāng guī lóng huì wán

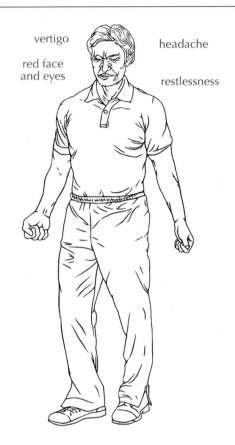

vertigo

red face
and eyes

headache

restlessness

―――――――――――― INGREDIENTS ――――――――――――

Angelicae sinensis Radix (*dāng guī*) 30g

Gentianae Radix (*lóng dǎn cǎo*) 30g

Gardeniae Fructus (*zhī zǐ*) 30g

Coptidis Rhizoma (*huáng lián*) 30g

Phellodendri Cortex (*huáng bǎi*) 30g

Scutellariae Radix (*huáng qín*) 30g

Aloe (*lú huì*) 15g

Indigo naturalis (*qīng dài*) 15g

Rhei Radix et Rhizoma (*dà huáng*) 15g

Aucklandiae Radix (*mù xiāng*) 4.5g

[1]Moschus (*shè xiāng*)... 1.5g

Preparation notes: This formula is almost always taken
with ginger tea in honey pill or granule form with the last
ingredient usually omitted.

Actions: drains Liver and Gallbladder fire excess • unblocks
the stool

Main pattern: constraint and clumping of the Liver and
Gallbladder qi

Key symptoms: headache • vertigo • tinnitus or hearing loss
• restlessness • red face and eyes • propensity to anger

Secondary symptoms: delirious speech • mania and fright
wind in children • spasms • distention and pain in chest and
flanks • dark, rough urination • blockage of the throat with
difficulty swallowing • bitter taste • constipation

Tongue: red sides • yellow coating

Pulse: wiry • rapid • slippery

Abdomen: abdominal distention • distention and resistance
to pressure in the flanks

► CLINICAL NOTES

- This is the main formula for draining fire excess in the
  Liver and Gallbladder channels. Due to the tendency of fire
  to flare upward, symptoms associated with the pattern this
  formula addresses are located primarily in the upper part
  of the body: the head and face. In addition to symptoms
  along the pathways of the Liver and Gallbladder channels,
  the pattern also includes generic signs of fire excess such
  as agitation and restlessness, delirious speech, bitter taste,
  and a rapid, forceful pulse.

- From a six warps perspective, fire excess is invariably
  associated with the yang brightness warp. Thus, upward-
  flaring fire is drained via the bowels. This pattern may
  include abdominal distention and constipation due to
  clumping of fire and stool. These symptoms need not be
  present, however, to justify use of this formula.

―――――――――――――――――――――――――

1. This ingredient can be difficult to obtain because of legal issues.
Angelicae dahuricae Radix *(bái zhǐ)* may be substituted.

Contraindications: fire excess in the Liver and Gallbladder without clumping • Spleen deficiency

▶ FORMULAS WITH SIMILAR INDICATIONS ⇢

Gentian Decoction to Drain the Liver (*lóng dǎn xiè gān tāng*): For Liver and Gallbladder channel damp-heat patterns with downward pouring of Liver channel damp-heat but without clumping or qi stagnation.

COMPOSITION

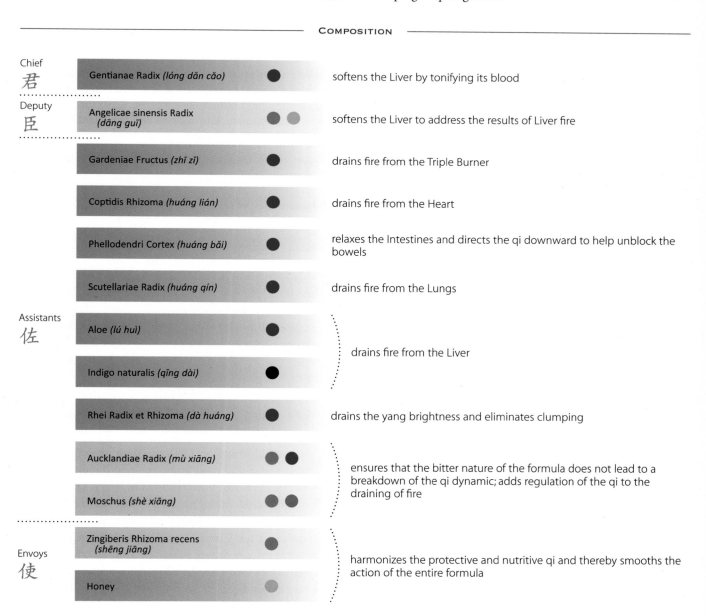

Chief 君	Gentianae Radix *(lóng dǎn cǎo)*	●	softens the Liver by tonifying its blood
Deputy 臣	Angelicae sinensis Radix *(dāng guī)*	● ●	softens the Liver to address the results of Liver fire
	Gardeniae Fructus *(zhī zǐ)*	●	drains fire from the Triple Burner
	Coptidis Rhizoma *(huáng lián)*	●	drains fire from the Heart
	Phellodendri Cortex *(huáng bǎi)*	●	relaxes the Intestines and directs the qi downward to help unblock the bowels
	Scutellariae Radix *(huáng qín)*	●	drains fire from the Lungs
Assistants 佐	Aloe *(lú huì)*	●	drains fire from the Liver
	Indigo naturalis *(qīng dài)*	●	
	Rhei Radix et Rhizoma *(dà huáng)*	●	drains the yang brightness and eliminates clumping
	Aucklandiae Radix *(mù xiāng)*	● ●	ensures that the bitter nature of the formula does not lead to a breakdown of the qi dynamic; adds regulation of the qi to the draining of fire
	Moschus *(shè xiāng)*	● ●	
Envoys 使	Zingiberis Rhizoma recens *(shēng jiāng)*	●	harmonizes the protective and nutritive qi and thereby smooths the action of the entire formula
	Honey	●	

當歸拈痛湯（当归拈痛汤）
Tangkuei Decoction to Pry Out Pain
dāng guī niān tòng tāng

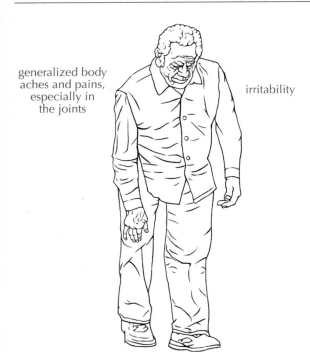

generalized body aches and pains, especially in the joints

irritability

INGREDIENTS

Notopterygii Rhizoma seu Radix (*qiāng huó*) 15g
Saposhnikoviae Radix (*fáng fēng*) 9g
Cimicifugae Rhizoma (*shēng má*) 3-6g
Puerariae Radix (*gé gēn*) 6g
Atractylodis macrocephalae Rhizoma (*bái zhú*) 3-4.5g
Atractylodis Rhizoma (*cāng zhú*) 6-9g
Angelicae sinensis radicis Corpus (*dāng guī shēn*) 9g
Ginseng Radix (*rén shēn*) 6g
Glycyrrhizae Radix (*gān cǎo*) 15g
wine-fried Sophorae flavescentis Radix (*jiǔ chǎo kǔ shēn*) 6g
dry-fried Scutellariae Radix (*chǎo huáng qín*) 3-9g
wine-washed Anemarrhenae Rhizoma (*jiǔ xǐ zhī mǔ*) 9g
Artemisiae scopariae Herba (*yīn chén*) 15g
Polyporus (*zhū líng*) 9g
Alismatis Rhizoma (*zé xiè*) 9g

Actions: resolves dampness • clears heat • disperses wind • relieves pain

Main pattern: constraint from dampness that transforms into heat and pours into the extremities and joints

Key symptoms: generalized body aches and pains, especially in the joints • irritability • swelling and pain of the lower extremities

Secondary symptoms: heavy sensation in the shoulders and back • discomfort or constricted sensation in the chest and diaphragm • multiple sores • carbuncles • furuncles or abscesses accompanied by redness and persistent swelling • itching • pain • fever • thirst

Tongue: greasy, white coating that may have yellow tinge

Pulse: slippery and rapid • soggy and moderate

Abdomen: no specific signs

▶ CLINICAL NOTES

- This formula is specific for painful obstruction with heaviness and stiffness in the back or extremities along with a rapid and soggy or slippery pulse and a greasy tongue coating that may have a yellow tinge. Although the patient may complain of pain, this is typically a sense of annoying discomfort rather than the severe pain caused by cold or blood stasis.

- In the modern clinic this formula is also used for damp-heat skin problems, for hot swelling of the foot, sole, or lower leg, and damp-heat gynecologic disorders.

- The formula's author, Li Dong-Yuan, recommended a number of useful modifications: for pronounced symptoms in the lower body, substitute *fáng jǐ* (Stephaniae/Cocculi/etc. Radix) for Saposhnikoviae Radix (*fáng fēng*); for pronounced sweating, substitute Astragali Radix (*huáng qí*) for Cimicifugae Rhizoma (*shēng má*); for spontaneous sweating, substitute Cinnamomi Ramulus (*guì zhī*) for Atractylodis Rhizoma (*cāng zhú*); for pain characterized by heat, substitute Phellodendri Cortex (*huáng bǎi*) for Anemarrhenae Rhizoma (*zhī mǔ*).

Contraindications: painful obstruction due to wind-cold-dampness

▶ FORMULAS WITH SIMILAR INDICATIONS

*Cinnamon Twig, Peony, and Anemarrhena Decoction (*guì zhī sháo yào zhī mǔ tāng*): For wind-cold-damp painful obstruction with localized swelling and inflammation due to localized constraint.

Disband Painful Obstruction Decoction (*xuān bì tāng*): For more pronounced damp-heat painful obstruction characterized by hot and painful joints, scanty, dark urine, and a gray or yellow, greasy tongue coating.

──── COMPOSITION ────

Chiefs 君	Notopterygii Rhizoma seu Radix (*qiāng huó*)	strongly releases the exterior and disperses externally-contracted pathogenic wind; eliminates dampness, facilitates movement in the joints, and stops pain
	Artemisiae scopariae Herba (*yīn chén*)	clears and resolves damp-heat by leading them out through the urine
Deputies 臣	Saposhnikoviae Radix (*fáng fēng*)	
	Cimicifugae Rhizoma (*shēng má*)	accentuates the wind-dispersing action of Notopterygii Rhizoma seu Radix (*qiāng huó*)
	Puerariae Radix (*gé gēn*)	
	Polyporus (*zhū líng*)	promotes urination and leaches out dampness, while also slightly clearing heat
	Alismatis Rhizoma (*zé xiè*)	
Assistants 佐	Atractylodis macrocephalae Rhizoma (*bái zhú*)	strengthens the Spleen and dries dampness
	Atractylodis Rhizoma (*cāng zhú*)	
	Angelicae sinensis radicis Corpus (*dāng guī shēn*)	tonifies the qi and blood and protects them from all the clearing, draining actions of the other herbs
	Ginseng Radix (*rén shēn*)	
	wine-fried Sophorae flavescentis Radix (*jiǔ chǎo kǔ shēn*)	strongly clears heat and dries dampness
	dry-fried Scutellariae Radix (*chǎo huáng qín*)	
	wine-washed Anemarrhenae Rhizoma (*jiǔ xǐ zhī mǔ*)	clears heat, nourishes the yin, and prevents the main herbs from damaging the yin
Envoy 使	Glycyrrhizae Radix (*gān cǎo*)	adjusts and harmonizes the actions of the various groups of herbs

當歸芍藥散（当归芍药散）
Tangkuei and Peony Powder
dāng guī sháo yào săn

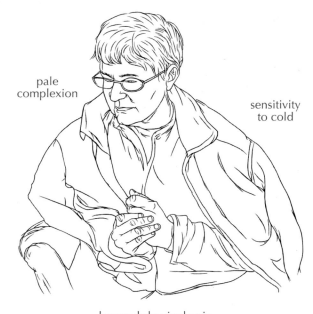

pale complexion

sensitivity to cold

lower abdominal pain

INGREDIENTS

Angelicae sinensis Radix (*dāng guī*) 9g

[1]Paeoniae Radix (*sháo yào*) 9-30g

Poria (*fú líng*) 12g

Atractylodis macrocephalae Rhizoma (*bái zhú*) 12g

Alismatis Rhizoma (*zé xiè*) 12g

Chuanxiong Rhizoma (*chuān xiōng*) 6g

Actions: nourishes the Liver blood • spreads the Liver qi • strengthens the Spleen • resolves dampness

Main patterns: abdominal pain due to disharmony between the Liver and Spleen • blood stasis • qi stagnation • dampness

Key symptoms: lower abdominal pain • sensitivity to cold • pale complexion

Secondary symptoms: dizziness • tinnitus • neck stiffness

---

1. As the primary function here is to restrain, tonify, or soften, Paeoniae Radix alba (*bái sháo*) is preferred.

• palpitations • fatigue • urinary difficulty • slight edema • menstrual irregularity

Tongue: pale body • stasis spots • distended sublingual veins • white coating

Pulse: deep • thin

Abdomen: a generally soft abdomen • hypertonicity of rectus abdominis • pain on deep pressure on either or both sides of lower abdomen • splashing sound in epigastrium

▶ CLINICAL NOTES

• This formula treats a complex yet frequently seen clinical pattern of blood deficiency and stasis accompanied by water buildup and qi deficiency. The presence of both pain and fluid accumulation is the key marker. The pain is often located in the lower abdomen but can occur anywhere. Water buildup may manifest in a wide variety of symptoms such as excessive discharges, dryness, dizziness, nausea, heavy-headedness with reduced urination, increased sweating from the lower body, constipation, and urinary difficulty.

• The main symptoms may be accompanied by cold (either an aversion to cold or cold extremities) from blood deficiency and fatigue from qi deficiency.

• Although widely considered a women's formula used for menstrual problems, infertility, and disorders of pregnancy and postpartum, it can also be used for men who present with the above pattern.

Contraindications: use with caution during pregnancy

▶ FORMULAS WITH SIMILAR INDICATIONS

Rambling Powder (*xiāo yáo săn*): For a similar pattern of blood and qi deficiency with clear Liver qi constraint rather than blood stasis.

Frigid Extremities Powder (*sì nì săn*): For abdominal pain and colic accompanied by symptoms such as bloating and cold extremities due to Liver qi stagnation.

Cinnamon Twig and Poria Pill (*guì zhī fú líng wán*): For blood stasis and water buildup in patients who are not deficient.

───────────────────────────────── COMPOSITION ─────────────────────────────────

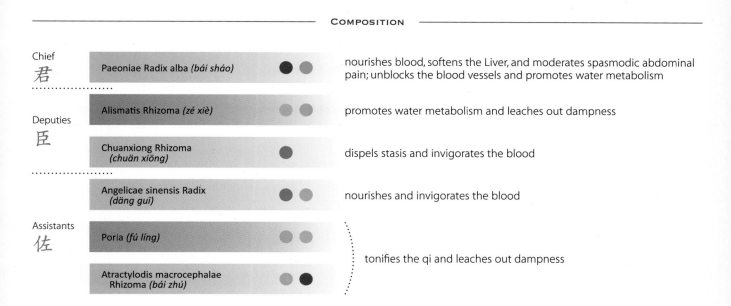

Chief
君 — Paeoniae Radix alba *(bái sháo)* — nourishes blood, softens the Liver, and moderates spasmodic abdominal pain; unblocks the blood vessels and promotes water metabolism

Deputies
臣

Alismatis Rhizoma *(zé xiè)* — promotes water metabolism and leaches out dampness

Chuanxiong Rhizoma *(chuān xiöng)* — dispels stasis and invigorates the blood

Angelicae sinensis Radix *(däng guï)* — nourishes and invigorates the blood

Assistants
佐

Poria *(fú líng)*

Atractylodis macrocephalae Rhizoma *(bái zhú)*

tonifies the qi and leaches out dampness

當歸四逆湯（当归四逆汤）
Tangkuei Decoction for Frigid Extremities
dāng guī sì nì tāng

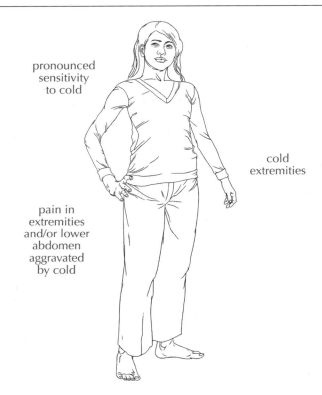

pronounced
sensitivity
to cold

cold
extremities

pain in
extremities
and/or lower
abdomen
aggravated
by cold

INGREDIENTS

Angelicae sinensis Radix (*dāng guī*) 12g

[1]Paeoniae Radix (*sháo yào*) 9g

Cinnamomi Ramulus (*guì zhī*) 9g

[2]Asari Herba (*xì xīn*) 1.5g

Akebiae Caulis (*mù tōng*) 3-6g

Glycyrrhizae Radix praeparata (*zhì gān cǎo*) 6g

Jujubae Fructus (*dà zǎo*) .... 8 pieces

Actions: warms the channels • disperses cold • nourishes the blood • unblocks the blood vessels

1. As the primary function here is to restrain, tonify, or soften, Paeoniae Radix alba *(bái sháo)* is preferred.

2. This herb can be difficult to obtain because of legal issues. Clematidis Radix *(wēi líng xiān)* may be substituted.

Main pattern: cold obstructing circulation of blood in patients with blood deficiency

Key symptoms: pronounced sensitivity to cold • cold extremities • pain in extremities and/or lower abdomen aggravated by cold

Secondary symptoms: numbness • increased urination • migraine-type headaches • nausea • vomiting • lower back pain

Tongue: pale, wet body • little or thin white coating

Pulse: submerged and thin • imperceptible

Abdomen: hypertonicity of rectus abdominis muscle • localized pain on deep pressure in lower abdomen, but the lower abdomen itself is weak

► CLINICAL NOTES

• This formula focuses on cold obstructing the vessels and collaterals in patients with blood deficiency specifically involving the terminal yin warps. Cold leads to constriction of the vessels, causing pain and impairing microcirculation, but there is no damage to the organs. This gives the formula a very wide range of indications including any impairment of circulation caused by cold in patients whose general health is not compromised.

• Key markers for this formula are long-standing cold hands and feet that are both cold to the touch and feel very cold to the patient as well as pain that is aggravated by cold in conjunction with the tongue, pulse, and abdominal signs outlined above.

• Although this formula is often seen as being specifically indicated for women for problems such as migraines, infertility, or menstrual irregularity and dysmenorrhea, it is equally indicated for men to treat impotence, premature ejaculation, and male infertility.

• Many physicians prefer to use the augmented version of this formula, Tangkuei Decoction for Frigid Extremities plus Evodia and Fresh Ginger (*dāng guī sì nì jiā wú zhū yú shēng jiāng tāng*). This is a good option especially if Asari Radix et Rhizoma (*xì xīn*) is unavailable.

Contraindications: blood deficiency patterns with fire

► FORMULAS WITH SIMILAR INDICATIONS

Frigid Extremities Decoction (*sì nì tāng*): For a lesser yin warp pattern where the entire limb or limbs—and not just the extremities—are cold. The patient also presents with lethargy, increased desire to sleep, watery diarrhea, and a submerged pulse. Blood deficiency is not a factor.

Frigid Extremities Powder (*sì nì sǎn*): For a lesser yang warp qi constraint pattern where only the tips of the hands and feet are cold, while the nails and lips are of normal color. The pulse is wiry rather than thin, and most often heat is evident elsewhere in the body presenting as subjective sensations of heat, irritability, insomnia, constipation, dark urine and/or a red tongue with a yellow coating. The pattern often includes a psycho-emotional component.

COMPOSITION

Chiefs 君	Angelicae sinensis Radix (*dāng guī*)	tonifies and invigorates the blood to eliminate cold
	Cinnamomi Ramulus (*guì zhī*)	warms the channels and disperses cold from the nutritive qi
Deputies 臣	Paeoniae Radix alba (*bái sháo*)	tonifies and invigorates the blood to eliminate cold
	Asari Herba (*xì xīn*)	warms the channels and disperses cold from the nutritive qi
Assistants 佐	Glycyrrhizae Radix praeparata (*zhì gān cǎo*)	augments the qi and strengthens the Spleen
	Jujubae Fructus (*dà zǎo*)	
Envoy 使	Akebiae Caulis (*mù tōng*)	facilitates the flow in the channels and vessels and drains the static heat

導赤散（导赤散）
Guide Out the Red Powder
dǎo chì sǎn

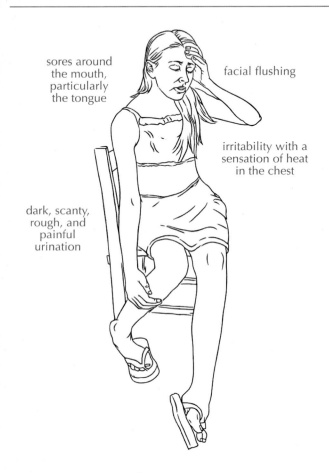

sores around the mouth, particularly the tongue

facial flushing

irritability with a sensation of heat in the chest

dark, scanty, rough, and painful urination

Main patterns: Heart heat

Key symptoms: irritability with a sensation of heat in the chest • facial flushing • sores around the mouth, particularly the tongue • dark, scanty, rough, and painful urination

Secondary symptoms: thirst with a desire to drink cold beverages • blood in the urine • burning urination

Tongue: red tip

Pulse: slippery • rapid

Abdomen: no specific signs

▶ CLINICAL NOTES

• This is heat in the Heart that the body seeks to drain via the Small Intestine. In this case, there will be symptoms of both heat in the Heart such as ulcers on the tongue or insomnia, and urinary symptoms indicating heat in the Small Intestines. Alternatively, one may use this formula to drain heat from the Heart via the Small Intestine, in which case urinary symptoms need not be present.

• The formula is particularly indicated for children and teenagers where symptoms of yang excess arise from the inherent instability of yin and yang rather than from deficiency or contraction of heat from the exterior.

Contraindications: yin deficiency with hyperactive fire • Spleen and Stomach deficiency

▶ FORMULAS WITH SIMILAR INDICATIONS

Eight-Herb Powder for Rectification (*bā zhèng sǎn*): For excess heat in the interior causing acute painful urinary dribbling with pain or bleeding.

*Gardenia and Prepared Soybean Decoction (*zhī zǐ chǐ tāng*): For qi aspect excess heat accumulating in the chest causing irritability and insomnia but without involvement of the Small Intestines or urinary symptoms.

*Clear the Heart Drink with Lotus Seed (*qīng xīn lián zǐ yǐn*): For Heart and Lung qi deficiency patterns accompanied by damp-heat in the Bladder with painful urinary dribbling.

— INGREDIENTS —

Rehmanniae Radix (*shēng dì huáng*) 9-15g
Akebiae Caulis (*mù tong*) 6-9g
Glycyrrhizae Radix tenuis (*gān cǎo shāo*) 3-6g
Lophatheri Herba (*dàn zhú yè*) 3-6g

Preparation notes: Originally, equal amounts of the first three ingredients were ground up and then 9g of the powder taken with 6g of the last ingredient as a draft.

Actions: clears the Heart • promotes urination

─────────────────────── COMPOSITION ───────────────────────

Chief 君	Akebiae Caulis *(mù tōng)*	●	clears heat from the Heart and Small Intestine channels and promotes urination
Deputy 臣	Rehmanniae Radix *(shēng dì huáng)*	● ●	enters the Heart to cool the blood; enters the Kidneys to nourish the yin and generate fluids
Assistant 佐	Lophatheri Herba *(dàn zhú yè)*	● ●	alleviates irritability by clearing heat from the Heart
Envoy 使	Glycyrrhizae Radix tenuis *(gān cǎo shāo)*	●	treats painful urinary dribbling, resolves toxicity, and harmonizes the actions of the other herbs

地黃飲子（地黄饮子）
Rehmannia Drink
dì huáng yǐn zi

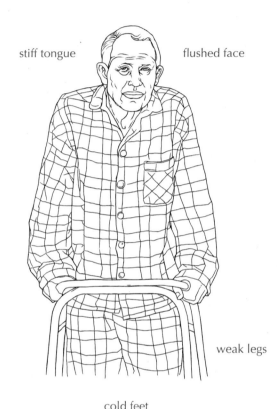

stiff tongue   flushed face

weak legs

cold feet

INGREDIENTS

Rehmanniae Radix praeparata (*shú dì huáng*) 12g

Corni Fructus (*shān zhū yú*)... 9g

wine-prepared Cistanches Herba (*jiǔ cōng róng*)................. 9g

Morindae officinalis Radix (*bā jǐ tiān*)................................ 9g

¹Aconiti Radix lateralis praeparata (*zhì fù zǐ*) ... [cooked first] 6g

Cinnamomi Cortex (*ròu guì*) 6g

Dendrobii Herba (*shí hú*)... 9g

Poria (*fú líng*) 6g

---

1. This ingredient can be difficult to obtain because of legal issues. Psoraleae Fructus *(bǔ gǔ zhī)* may be substituted.

Schisandrae Fructus (*wǔ wèi zǐ*)......................................6g

Ophiopogonis Radix (*zhì mài mén dōng*)...........................6g

Acori tatarinowii Rhizoma (*shí chāng pǔ*) 6g

Polygalae Radix (*yuǎn zhì*)... 6

Zingiberis Rhizoma recens (*shēng jiāng*)...........................6g

Jujubae Fructus (*dà zǎo*)...................................... 4 pieces

Menthae haplocalycis Herba (*bò hé*)......... [add near end] 2g

Actions: enriches the Kidney yin • tonifies the Kidney yang • opens the orifices • transforms phlegm

Main pattern: deficiency of Kidney yin and yang combined with upward-flaring of deficient yang and phlegm turbidity

Key symptoms: stiffness of the tongue with inability to speak • weakness of the lower extremities • cold feet and flushed face • dry mouth with an absence of thirst

Secondary symptoms: fatigue • spontaneous sweating • paralysis of the lower extremities

Tongue: greasy, yellow coating

Pulse: submerged • slow • thin • frail

Abdomen: no specific signs

► CLINICAL NOTES

• Composed originally to treat wind-stroke with inability to speak, use of the formula has been expanded to include patterns of Kidney deficiency below that are accompanied by symptoms of excess (turbid yin) above, with such symptoms as insomnia or edema.

• In order to focus the action of the herbs on the upper burner, it is important that the ingredients not be decocted for too long.

Contraindications: wind-stroke associated with fire excess or external pathogens invading the channels

► FORMULAS WITH SIMILAR INDICATIONS

*Tortoise Shell and Deer Antler Two-Immortal Syrup (*guī lù èr xiān jiāo*): For deficiency patterns with no signs of excess.

COMPOSITION

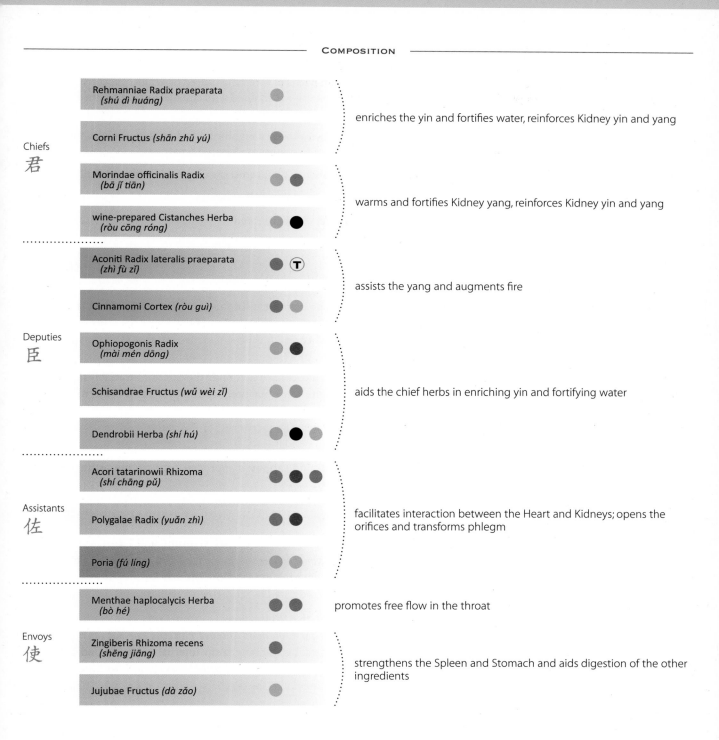

Chiefs 君

Rehmanniae Radix praeparata (shú dì huáng)

Corni Fructus (shān zhū yú)

enriches the yin and fortifies water, reinforces Kidney yin and yang

Morindae officinalis Radix (bā jǐ tiān)

wine-prepared Cistanches Herba (ròu cōng róng)

warms and fortifies Kidney yang, reinforces Kidney yin and yang

Deputies 臣

Aconiti Radix lateralis praeparata (zhì fù zǐ)

Cinnamomi Cortex (ròu guì)

assists the yang and augments fire

Ophiopogonis Radix (mài mén dōng)

Schisandrae Fructus (wǔ wèi zǐ)

aids the chief herbs in enriching yin and fortifying water

Dendrobii Herba (shí hú)

Assistants 佐

Acori tatarinowii Rhizoma (shí chāng pǔ)

Polygalae Radix (yuǎn zhì)

facilitates interaction between the Heart and Kidneys; opens the orifices and transforms phlegm

Poria (fú líng)

Envoys 使

Menthae haplocalycis Herba (bò hé)

promotes free flow in the throat

Zingiberis Rhizoma recens (shēng jiāng)

Jujubae Fructus (dà zǎo)

strengthens the Spleen and Stomach and aids digestion of the other ingredients

定喘湯（定喘汤）
Arrest Wheezing Decoction
dìng chuǎn tāng

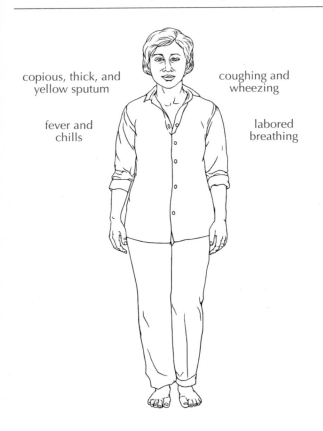

copious, thick, and yellow sputum

coughing and wheezing

fever and chills

labored breathing

INGREDIENTS

dry-fried Ginkgo Semen (*chǎo bái guǒ*) 9-12g
[1]Ephedrae Herba (*má huáng*)...................................... 9g
Perillae Fructus (*zǐ sū zǐ*)... 6g
Glycyrrhizae Radix (*gān cǎo*)...................................... 3g
Farfarae Flos (*kuǎn dōng huā*) 9g
Armeniacae Semen (*xìng rén*) 4.5-6g
prepared Mori Cortex (*zhì sāng bái pí*)...................... 6-9g
dry-fried Scutellariae Radix (*chǎo huáng qín*)............. 4.5-6g
Pinelliae Rhizoma praeparatum (*zhì bàn xià*)................ 9g

1. This herb can be difficult to obtain because of legal issues. Perillae Folium (*zǐ sū yè*) with Platycodi Radix (*jié gěng*) may be substituted.

Actions: disseminates and directs Lung qi downward • arrests wheezing • clears heat • transforms phlegm

Main pattern: wheezing caused by wind-cold constraining the exterior combined with smoldering of phlegm-heat in the interior

Key symptoms: coughing and wheezing • copious, thick, and yellow sputum • labored breathing

Secondary symptoms: simultaneous fever and chills

Tongue: greasy, yellow coating

Pulse: slippery • rapid

Abdomen: no specific signs

▶ CLINICAL NOTES

• The main focus of this formula is to clear and transform phlegm-heat in the Lungs that cause the Lung qi to rebel. Wheezing is the main symptom. This is accompanied by the presence of yellow sputum, indicating phlegm-heat.

• Wind-cold constraining the exterior invariably aggravates symptoms but need not be present in order to use this formula. For patterns where external pathogens are the main factor, other formulas are generally more appropriate.

Contraindications: inappropriate for chronic asthma with qi deficiency

▶ FORMULAS WITH SIMILAR INDICATIONS

Ephedra, Apricot Kernel, Gypsum, and Licorice Decoction (*má xìng shí gān tāng*): For heat in the chest and Lungs and cold fettering the exterior (without the presence of phlegm-heat) indicated by wheezing, irritability, and slight sweating.

Drain the White Powder from *Craft of Medicinal Treatment for Childhood Disease Patterns* (*xiè bái sǎn*): For heat in the Lungs arising from internal causes as indicated by the absence of external symptoms along with skin that feels burning hot to the touch.

Minor Bluegreen Dragon Decoction (*xiǎo qīng lóng tāng*): For thin mucus in the chest and Lungs leading to wheezing and coughing of white, watery sputum.

─────────────── **COMPOSITION** ───────────────

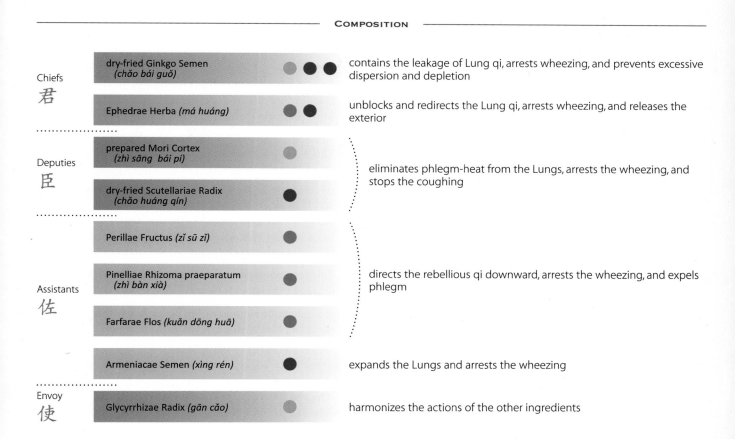

Chiefs
君

dry-fried Ginkgo Semen *(chǎo bái guǒ)* — contains the leakage of Lung qi, arrests wheezing, and prevents excessive dispersion and depletion

Ephedrae Herba *(má huáng)* — unblocks and redirects the Lung qi, arrests wheezing, and releases the exterior

Deputies
臣

prepared Mori Cortex *(zhì sāng bái pí)*

dry-fried Scutellariae Radix *(chǎo huáng qín)*

eliminates phlegm-heat from the Lungs, arrests the wheezing, and stops the coughing

Assistants
佐

Perillae Fructus *(zǐ sū zǐ)*

Pinelliae Rhizoma praeparatum *(zhì bàn xià)*

Farfarae Flos *(kuǎn dōng huā)*

directs the rebellious qi downward, arrests the wheezing, and expels phlegm

Armeniacae Semen *(xìng rén)* — expands the Lungs and arrests the wheezing

Envoy
使

Glycyrrhizae Radix *(gān cǎo)* — harmonizes the actions of the other ingredients

定志丸
Settle the Emotions Pill
dìng zhì wán

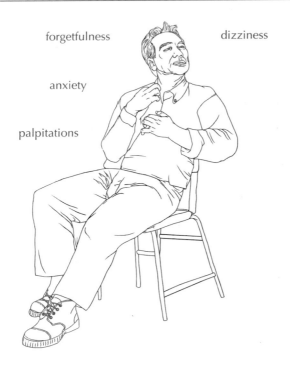

forgetfulness

dizziness

anxiety

palpitations

INGREDIENTS

Ginseng Radix (*rén shēn*).. 9g
Poria (*fú líng*)... 9g
Acori tatarinowii Rhizoma (*shí chāng pǔ*) 6g
Polygalae Radix (*yuǎn zhì*)... 6g

Actions: tonifies the Heart qi • strengthens the resolve • calms the spirit

Main pattern: Heart qi deficiency and constraint caused by phlegm turbidity

Key symptoms: palpitations • forgetfulness • dizziness • anxiety

Secondary symptoms: disorientation • apprehension • worry • incessant laughter and glee • nearsightedness

Tongue: pale body • white coating

Pulse: deep • tight • without force

Abdomen: no specific signs

▶ CLINICAL NOTES

• The main indication of this formula is phlegm-turbidity that produces Heart qi deficiency and Heart qi constraint. This pattern is characterized by anxiety, confusion, forgetfulness, and an inability to concentrate.

• This formula is not specific for insomnia but can treat blood-deficiency insomnia if herbs like Angelicae sinensis Radix (*dāng guī*), Ziziphi spinosae Semen (*suān zǎo rén*), and Platycladi Semen (*bǎi zǐ rén*) are added. If insomnia, anxiety, and apprehension predominate, one can add Fossilia Ossis Mastodi (*lóng gǔ*) or Fossilia Dentis Mastodi (*lóng chǐ*).

• This formula is often used in contemporary practice for nearsightedness with Heart qi deficiency.

Contraindications: blood or yin deficiency without the presence of phlegm-dampness

▶ FORMULAS WITH SIMILAR INDICATIONS

Sour Jujube Decoction (*suān zǎo rén tāng*): For insomnia and anxiety due to a blood-deficient Liver failing to nourish the Heart marked by a pale tongue, lightheadedness, or night sweats.

COMPOSITION

Chief 君	Ginseng Radix (rén shēn)		tonifies the primal qi of all five yin organs, while also benefiting the Heart qi and calming the spirit
Deputy 臣	Poria (fú líng)		quiets the Heart and calms the spirit
Assistants 佐	Acori tatarinowii Rhizoma (shí chāng pǔ)		opens the orifices, dislodges phlegm, removes filth, and quiets the spirit
	Polygalae Radix (yuǎn zhì)		assists in the free movement of the Heart qi, opens constraint, and guides the Kidney qi upward to reach the Heart

獨活寄生湯（独活寄生汤）
Pubescent Angelica and Taxillus Decoction
dú huó jì shēng tāng

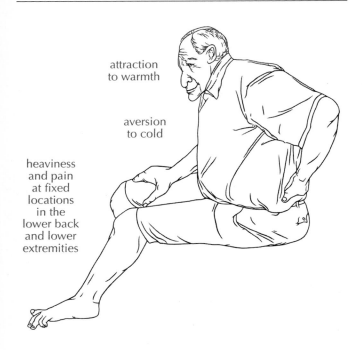

attraction
to warmth

aversion
to cold

heaviness
and pain
at fixed
locations
in the
lower back
and lower
extremities

INGREDIENTS

Angelicae pubescentis Radix (*dú huó*)	9g
[1]Asari Herba (*xì xīn*)	6g
Saposhnikoviae Radix (*fáng fēng*)	6g
Gentianae macrophyllae Radix (*qín jiāo*)	6g
Taxilli Herba (*sāng jì shēng*)	6g
Eucommiae Cortex (*dù zhòng*)	6g
Achyranthis bidentatae Radix (*niú xī*)	6g
Cinnamomi Cortex (*ròu guì*)	6g
Angelicae sinensis Radix (*dāng guī*)	6g
Chuanxiong Rhizoma (*chuān xiōng*)	6g

1. This herb may be difficult to obtain because of legal issues. As a substitute, either Clematidis Radix (*wēi líng xiān*) can be used, the dosage of the yang-fortifying herbs in the formula may be increased, or herbs such as Evodiae Fructus (*wú zhū yú*) and Zingiberis Rhizoma recens (*shēng jiāng*) may be added.

Rehmanniae Radix (*shēng dì huáng*)	6g
Paeoniae Radix alba (*bái sháo*)	6g
Ginseng Radix (*rén shēn*)	6g
Poria (*fú líng*)	6g
Glycyrrhizae Radix (*gān cǎo*)	6g

Actions: expels wind-dampness • disperses painful obstruction • tonifies deficiency

Main pattern: painful obstruction with Liver and Kidney deficiency

Key symptoms: heaviness and pain at fixed locations in the lower back and lower extremities • aversion to cold • attraction to warmth

Secondary symptoms: weakness and stiffness • hypertonicity and immobility • paresthesias or numbness • palpitations

Tongue: pale body • white coating

Pulse: thin • weak • slow

Abdomen: soft and weak lower abdomen • hypertonicity of rectus abdominis muscle in the lower abdomen

▶ CLINICAL NOTES

- This formula treats wind-cold-dampness that has remained in the body for a long time in patients with blood and qi deficiency or combined Kidney and Liver deficiency. One key marker is a weak pulse, and another is the predominance of stiffness over severe pain.

- To be effective, this formula may need to be taken for a long time. It is a useful base formula for all types of painful obstruction and atrophy disorders. More recently, its use has been extended to a large range of disorders that present as blood and qi deficiency complicated by obstruction of the channels and collaterals such as hepatitis, skin conditions, or impotence.

- To enhance the tonifying properties of this formula many physicians replace Rehmanniae Radix (*shēng dì huáng*) with Rehmanniae Radix praeparata (*shú dì huáng*).

- For pronounced cold-type painful obstruction, add Aconiti Radix praeparata (*zhì chuān wū*) and Myrrha (*mò yào*); for pronounced damp-type painful obstruction, omit Rehmanniae Radix (*shēng dì huáng*) and add *fáng jǐ* (Stephaniae/Cocculi/etc. Radix), Coicis Semen (*yì yǐ rén*), and Atractylodis Rhizoma (*cāng zhú*); for less pronounced deficiency patterns, omit Ginseng Radix (*rén shēn*) and Rehmanniae Radix (*shēng dì huáng*); for Spleen deficiency with loose stools, omit Rehmanniae Radix (*shēng dì huáng*); for pain that extends upward along the spine and downward to the knees and ankles, omit Eucommiae Cortex (*dù zhòng*), Chuanxiong Rhizoma (*chuān xiōng*), Ginseng Radix (*rén shēn*), Paeoniae Radix alba (*bái sháo*), and Rehmanniae Radix (*shēng dì huáng*) and add Clematidis Radix (*wēi líng xiān*) and Cibotii Rhizoma (*gǒu jǐ*).

Contraindications: painful obstruction marked by strong excess or damp-heat

▶ **FORMULAS WITH SIMILAR INDICATIONS**

Remove Painful Obstruction Decoction (*juān bì tāng*): This formula primarily treats upper-body painful obstruction with patterns of deficient nutritive and protective qi.

COMPOSITION

Chief 君	Angelicae pubescentis Radix (*dú huó*)	expels wind, dampness, and cold from the lower burner, bones, and sinews
	Asari Herba (*xì xīn*)	scatters cold in the channels and scours out wind-dampness from the sinews and bones to stop the pain
Deputies 臣	Saposhnikoviae Radix (*fáng fēng*)	expels wind and overcomes dampness
	Gentianae macrophyllae Radix (*qín jiāo*)	relaxes the sinews and expels wind-dampness
	Taxilli Herba (*sāng jì shēng*)	expels wind-dampness and tonifies the Liver and Kidneys
	Eucommiae Cortex (*dù zhòng*)	
	Achyranthis bidentatae Radix (*niú xī*)	
	Cinnamomi Cortex (*ròu guì*)	warms and unblocks the channels and fortifies the yang
Assistants 佐	Angelicae sinensis Radix (*dāng guī*)	nourishes and invigorates the blood
	Chuanxiong Rhizoma (*chuān xiōng*)	
	Rehmanniae Radix (*shēng dì huáng*)	
	Paeoniae Radix alba (*bái sháo*)	
	Ginseng Radix (*rén shēn*)	resolves dampness and strengthens the Spleen
	Poria (*fú líng*)	
	Glycyrrhizae Radix (*gān cǎo*)	tonifies the middle qi and harmonizes the actions of the other herbs

[This page intentionally left blank]

二陳湯（二陈汤）
Two-Aged Herb Decoction
èr chén tāng

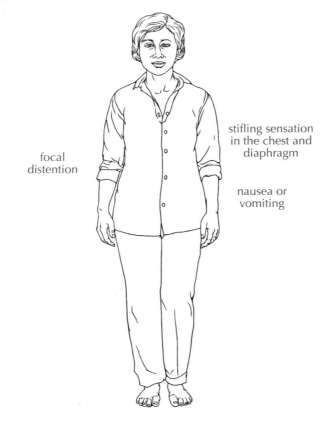

focal distention

stifling sensation in the chest and diaphragm

nausea or vomiting

INGREDIENTS

Pinelliae Rhizoma praeparatum (*zhì bàn xià*) 15g
Citri reticulatae Exocarpium rubrum (*jú hóng*) 9-15g
Poria (*fú líng*) 9-15g
Glycyrrhizae Radix praeparata (*zhì gān cǎo*) 4.5g
Zingiberis Rhizoma recens (*shēng jiāng*) 6-9g
Mume Fructus (*wū méi*) .... 1 piece

Actions: dries dampness • transforms phlegm • regulates the qi • harmonizes the middle burner

Main pattern: phlegm-dampness due to failure of Spleen and Lungs to transform and transport the fluids

Key symptoms: focal distention • nausea or vomiting

Secondary symptoms: coughing with copious white sputum that is easily expectorated • stifling sensation in the chest and diaphragm • palpitations • dizziness • heaviness in limbs

Tongue: white, greasy coating

Pulse: slippery

Abdomen: discomfort in epigastrium • splashing sounds in upper abdomen

▶ CLINICAL NOTES

- This is the basic formula for treating phlegm-dampness. It can be modified in numerous ways to treat almost any manifestation of this pathology irrespective of whether the phlegm manifests with or without form. To treat phlegm disorders on the basis of a more precise manifestation (e.g., wind-phlegm, phlegm-dampness, phlegm-fire, phlegm due to harbored food), one adds herbs that disperse wind, dry dampness, drain fire, etc. For example, for wind-dampness, one can add Clematidis Radix (*wēi líng xiān*), Gentianae macrophyllae Radix (*qín jiāo*), Xanthii Fructus (*cāng ěr zǐ*), and Cinnamomi Ramulus (*guì zhī*); for cough with copious sputum due to phlegm-dampness in the interior complicated by the presence of pathogenic qi in the exterior, add Perillae Folium (*zǐ sū yè*) and Armeniacae Semen (*xìng rén*); for cough with copious sputum due to externally-contracted cold in the Lungs, add Ephedrae Herba (*má huáng*) or Perillae Folium (*zǐ sū yè*) and Armeniacae Semen (*xìng rén*); for vomiting due to cold in the Stomach, add Zingiberis Rhizoma recens (*shēng jiāng*) and Amomi Fructus (*shā rén*); for vomiting of clear fluids, add Atractylodis Rhizoma (*cāng zhú*) and Atractylodis macrocephalae Rhizoma (*bái zhú*); for chronic phlegm in the channels and flesh leading to rubbery nodules, add Ostreae Concha (*mǔ lì*), Scrophulariae Radix (*xuán shēn*), Laminariae Thallus (*hǎi dài*), and Eckloniae Thallus (*kūn bù*); for phlegm-dampness obstructing the womb with irregular menstruation and copious vaginal discharge, add Chuanxiong Rhizoma (*chuān xiōng*) and Angelicae sinensis Radix (*dāng guī*); for concurrent dryness, substitute Trichosanthis Fructus (*guā lóu*) and Fritillariae cirrhosae Bulbus (*chuān bèi mǔ*) for Pinelliae Rhizoma praeparatum (*zhì bàn xià*).

- To treat phlegm disorders on the basis of their location, one can add herbs that guide the formula into specific organs or regions of the body. For example, for damp-heat in the upper burner, add Scutellariae Radix (*huáng qín*), Gardeniae Fructus (*zhī zǐ*), Armeniacae Semen (*xìng rén*), and Platycodi Radix (*jié gěng*); for damp-heat in the middle burner, add Coptidis Rhizoma (*huáng lián*), Pogostemonis/Agastaches Herba (*huò xiāng*), Magnoliae officinalis Cortex (*hòu pò*), and Coicis Semen (*yì yǐ rén*); and for damp-heat in the lower burner, add Sophorae flavescentis Radix (*kǔ shēn*), Phellodendri Cortex (*huáng bǎi*), and Talcum (*huá shí*).

- Because of the formula's sparse composition, it is easily modified to treat phlegm disorders on the basis of a patient's constitution:

  → Such modifications can create commonly used formulas. For example, adding Atractylodis macrocephalae Rhizoma (*bái zhú*) and Codonopsis Radix (*dǎng shēn*) forms Six-Gentlemen Decoction (*liù jūn zǐ tāng*) and addresses those patients whose phlegm is attributed to

Spleen qi deficiency.

  → Other modifications can address specific types of people. For example, one can add Cyperi Rhizoma (*xiāng fù*) and Aurantii Fructus (*zhǐ ké*) to treat those who are obese, who have a tendency to suffer from qi stagnation, or Atractylodis Rhizoma (*cāng zhú*) and Coptidis Rhizoma (*huáng lián*) to treat those who are thin, who have a tendency to develop phlegm-fire.

Contraindications: phlegm-dryness

▶ FORMULAS WITH SIMILAR INDICATIONS

Warm Gallbladder Decoction (*wēn dǎn tāng*): For disharmony between the Gallbladder and Stomach with heat from constraint combining with phlegm with such symptoms as restlessness, insomnia, susceptibility to fright, and timidity.

Pinellia, White Atractylodes, and Gastrodia Decoction (*bàn xià bái zhú tiān má tāng*): For wind-phlegm that rises to block the orifices and cause vertigo and headache often accompanied by spots in the visual field.

──────── COMPOSITION ────────

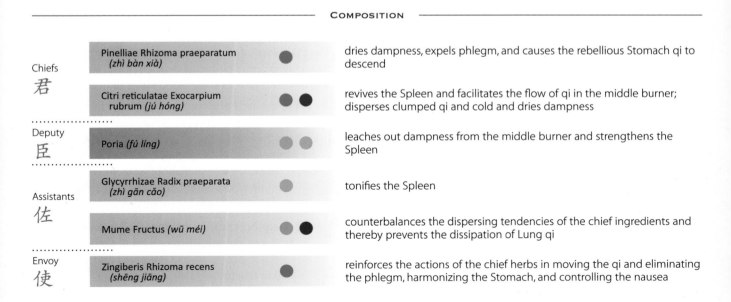

Chiefs 君	Pinelliae Rhizoma praeparatum (*zhì bàn xià*)	dries dampness, expels phlegm, and causes the rebellious Stomach qi to descend
	Citri reticulatae Exocarpium rubrum (*jú hóng*)	revives the Spleen and facilitates the flow of qi in the middle burner; disperses clumped qi and cold and dries dampness
Deputy 臣	Poria (*fú líng*)	leaches out dampness from the middle burner and strengthens the Spleen
Assistants 佐	Glycyrrhizae Radix praeparata (*zhì gān cǎo*)	tonifies the Spleen
	Mume Fructus (*wū méi*)	counterbalances the dispersing tendencies of the chief ingredients and thereby prevents the dissipation of Lung qi
Envoy 使	Zingiberis Rhizoma recens (*shēng jiāng*)	reinforces the actions of the chief herbs in moving the qi and eliminating the phlegm, harmonizing the Stomach, and controlling the nausea

二妙散
Two-Marvel Powder
èr miào săn

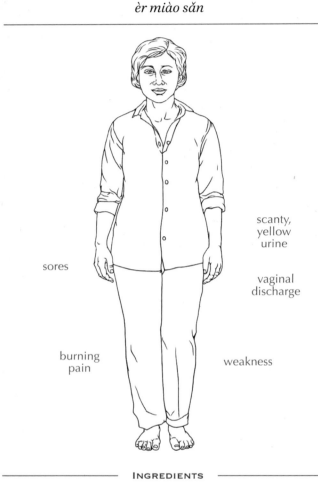

scanty, yellow urine

sores

vaginal discharge

burning pain

weakness

INGREDIENTS

dry-fried Phellodendri Cortex (*chǎo huáng bǎi*)............... 9-12g
Atractylodis Rhizoma (*cāng zhú*)..................................... 6-9g

Preparation notes: When taken in powdered or pill form, equal amounts of the herbs are taken with either warm water or ginger tea.

Actions: clears heat • dries dampness

Main pattern: damp-heat lodged in the lower burner

Key symptoms: scanty, yellow urine in the presence of any of the four secondary symptom patterns

Secondary symptoms: burning pain in the lower back or extremities • red, hot, swollen, and painful feet or knees • weakness or atrophy of the lower extremities • thick, yellow, foul-smelling vaginal discharge • sores or wet, papular rashes on the lower extremities

Tongue: greasy, yellow coating

Pulse: slippery • possibly rapid

Abdomen: no specific signs

▶ CLINICAL NOTES

- This is an important base formula that can be used to treat any pattern of excess damp-heat in the lower body, specifically for symptoms in the skin, flesh, muscles, sinews, and bones. It is not a primary formula for treating damp-heat in the Bladder unless the pattern also includes damp-heat symptoms in these other parts of the body.

- When Coicis Semen (*yì yǐ rén*) is added to enhance the formula's ability to dry dampness, it is called Three-Marvel Pill (*sān miào wán*); when Achyranthis bidentatae Radix (*niú xī*) is also added to help the formula focus on the muscles and sinews and further address the lower body, it is called Four-Marvel Pill (*sì miào wán*).

- The main formula and its variants can all be modified to treat concurrent blood or qi deficiency and stagnation as well as damp-heat causing blood stasis or heat toxin.

  → For damp-heat obstructing the collaterals with burning pain in the back and/or painful red swelling of the joints in the lower extremities, add such herbs as Angelicae sinensis Radix (*dāng guī*), Cyathulae Radix (*chuān niú xī*), Dioscoreae hypoglaucae Rhizoma (*bì xiè*), *fáng jǐ* (Stephaniae/Cocculi/etc. Radix), Erythrinae Cortex (*hǎi tóng pí*), and Trachelospermi Caulis (*luò shí téng*).

  → For damp-heat skin disorders of the lower extremities, add Smilacis glabrae Rhizoma (*tǔ fú líng*), Sophorae flavescentis Radix (*kǔ shēn*), Lonicerae Flos (*jīn yín huā*), or Kochiae Fructus (*dì fū zǐ*).

  → For damp-heat discharge, add Ailanthi Cortex (*chūn pí*), Smilacis glabrae Rhizoma (*tǔ fú líng*), or Sophorae flavescentis Radix (*kǔ shēn*).

→ For signs of blood aspect heat together with any of the above, add Paeoniae Radix rubra (*chì sháo*) and Moutan Cortex (*mǔ dān pí*).

Contraindications: Lung heat • Liver and Kidney deficiency

► FORMULAS WITH SIMILAR INDICATIONS

Polyporus Decoction (*zhū líng tāng*): For dampness and heat in the lower burner in the context of damage to the yin and fluids. This is indicated by reduced urination, incomplete voiding or painful urinary difficulty and/or lower body edema as well as signs of irritability, insomnia, or a darkish, red tongue.

Open the Gate Pill (*tōng guān wán*): For excess fire at the gate of vitality causing damp-heat that obstructs the qi dynamic of the Bladder. This manifests with urinary obstruction or difficulty accompanied by symptoms of upward flaring of yin fire such as tinnitus or irritability.

COMPOSITION

Chief
君 dry-fried Phellodendri Cortex (*chǎo huáng bǎi*) — eliminates heat from the yin aspects of the body, drains lower burner heat, and dries dampness

Deputy
臣 Atractylodis Rhizoma (*zhì cāng zhú*) — dries dampness, promotes the transformation and transportation functions of the Spleen

二仙湯（二仙汤）
Two-Immortal Decoction
èr xiān tāng

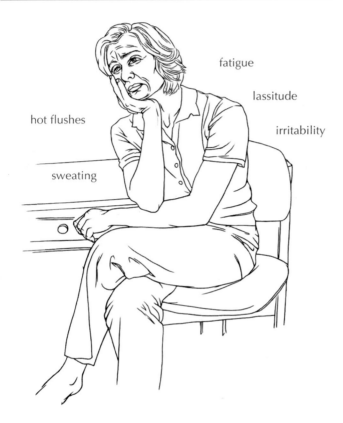

hot flushes

fatigue

lassitude

irritability

sweating

INGREDIENTS

Curculiginis Rhizoma (*xiān máo*)...................................... 6-15g
Epimedii Herba (*yín yáng huò*)... 9-15g
Morindae officinalis Radix (*bā jǐ tiān*)............................. 6-9g
Phellodendri Cortex (*huáng bǎi*)..................................... 6-9g
Anemarrhenae Rhizoma (*zhī mǔ*)................................... 6-9g
Angelicae sinensis Radix (*dāng guī*) 9g

Actions: warms Kidney yang • tonifies Kidney essence • drains fire from the Kidneys • regulates the Penetrating and Conception vessels

Main pattern: deficiency of Kidney yin and yang accompanied by flaring of fire at the gate of vitality

Key symptoms: hot flushes • sweating • fatigue • lassitude • irritability

Secondary symptoms: menstrual irregularity • insomnia • palpitations • nervousness • urinary frequency

Tongue: pale body • red spots or yellow coating

Pulse: deep • rapid

Abdomen: no specific signs

▶ CLINICAL NOTES

- This is a modern formula designed to treat hypertension in menopausal women. It is specifically indicated for patterns manifesting with excess heat (such as hot flushes, sweating, irritability, restlessness, and insomnia) occurring against a background of blood and Kidney yang deficiency (lassitude, fatigue, urinary frequency, and sweating).

- The formula's range of indications has been extended to treat depression and other essence-spirit disorders provided that they manifest with the combined excess/ deficiency pattern for which it is designed.

Contraindications: yin deficiency • fire excess

▶ FORMULAS WITH SIMILAR INDICATIONS

*Anemarrhena, Phellodendron, and Rehmannia Pill (*zhī bǎi dì huáng wán*): For Kidney yin deficiency with flaring of the fire at the gate of vitality (hot flushes, irritability, flooding pulse in the distal positions) as a key symptom.

Kidney Qi Pill (*shèn qì wán*): For Kidney yang and qi deficiency that may manifest with floating fire. Yang and qi deficiency symptoms such as fatigue, feeling cold, increased urination, and backache will be pronounced. Floating yang may manifest as headaches or hot flushes that improve with rest and warmth.

Flow-Warming Decoction (*wēn jīng tāng*): For menstrual irregularities due to internal cold and stagnation in the uterus accompanied by rebellious ascent of yang qi manifesting as hot flushes that are more pronounced in the afternoon or evening, sweating, headaches or nausea.

COMPOSITION

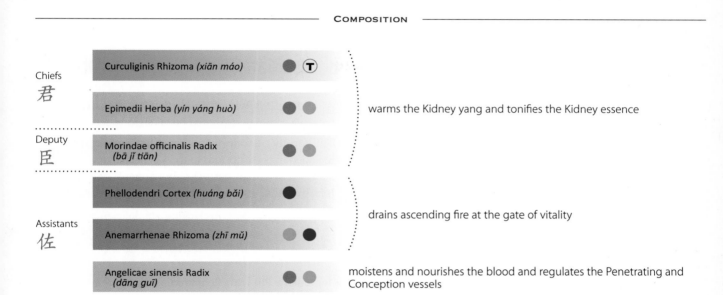

Chiefs
君

Curculiginis Rhizoma *(xiān máo)*

Epimedii Herba *(yín yáng huò)*

warms the Kidney yang and tonifies the Kidney essence

Deputy
臣

Morindae officinalis Radix
(bā jǐ tiān)

Phellodendri Cortex *(huáng bǎi)*

Assistants
佐

Anemarrhenae Rhizoma *(zhī mǔ)*

drains ascending fire at the gate of vitality

Angelicae sinensis Radix
(dāng guī)

moistens and nourishes the blood and regulates the Penetrating and Conception vessels

二至丸
Two-Solstice Pill
èr zhì wán

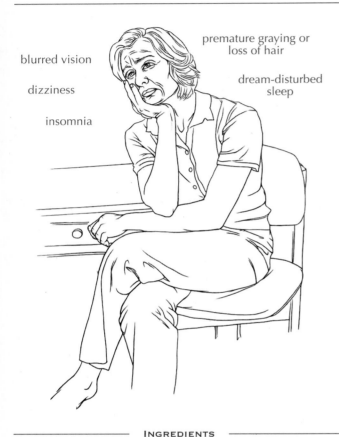

blurred vision

dizziness

insomnia

premature graying or
loss of hair

dream-disturbed
sleep

Pulse: thin or deep and weak

Abdomen: no specific signs

▶ CLINICAL NOTES

- A mild yin-tonifying formula that has the advantage of being easy to digest. Should be taken long-term.
- This formula, or one or another of its ingredients, is often included in prescriptions to treat gynecological problems such as irregular periods, short menstrual cycle, or infertility that involve Liver and Kidney deficiency heat.

Contraindications: patterns lacking yin deficiency or heat

▶ FORMULAS WITH SIMILAR INDICATIONS

Six-Ingredient Pill with Rehmannia (*liù wèi dì huáng wán*): This formula is more nourishing for yin deficiency, but more difficult to digest. More appropriate when there are also signs of water metabolism issues, such as edema or phlegm.

──── INGREDIENTS ────

Ligustri lucidi Fructus (*nū zhēn zǐ*) 15g
Ecliptae Herba (*mò hàn lián*) 15g

Actions: tonifies and benefits the Liver and Kidneys

Main pattern: Liver and Kidney yin deficiency

Key symptoms: premature graying or loss of hair • dizziness • blurred vision • insomnia • dream-disturbed sleep

Secondary symptoms: weakness, soreness, or atrophy of the lower back and knees • dry mouth and throat • spontaneous emissions

Tongue: red and dry body or sides

COMPOSITION

Chiefs
君

Ligustri lucidi Fructus *(nū zhēn zǐ)*	● ●	enriches the Kidneys and nourishes the Liver
Ecliptae Herba *(mò hàn lián)*	● ●	nourishes the yin, benefits the essence, and cools the blood to stop bleeding

防風通聖散（防风通圣散）
Saposhnikovia Powder that Sagely Unblocks
fáng fēng tōng shèng sǎn

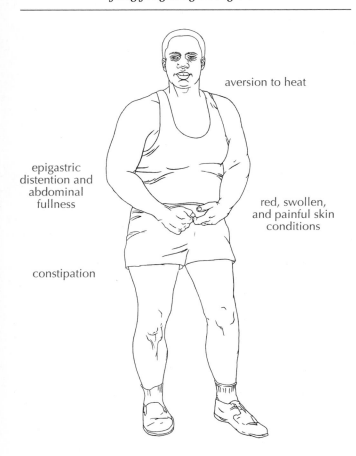

aversion to heat

epigastric distention and abdominal fullness

red, swollen, and painful skin conditions

constipation

—— INGREDIENTS ——

Saposhnikoviae Radix (*fáng fēng*) 6g
Chuanxiong Rhizoma (*chuān xiōng*) 6g
Angelicae sinensis Radix (*dāng guī*) 6g
Paeoniae Radix alba (*bái sháo*) 6g
Rhei Radix et Rhizoma (*dà huáng*) 6g
Menthae haplocalycis Herba (*bò hé*) 6g
[1]Ephedrae Herba (*má huáng*) 6g

1. This herb can be difficult to obtain because of legal issues. Notopterygii Rhizoma seu Radix *(qiāng huó)* may be substituted.

Forsythiae Fructus (*lián qiào*) 6g
Natrii Sulfas (*máng xiāo*) 6g
Gypsum fibrosum (*shí gāo*) 12g
Scutellariae Radix (*huáng qín*) 12g
Platycodi Radix (*jié gěng*) 6g
Talcum (*huá shí*) 15g
Glycyrrhizae Radix (*gān cǎo*) 6g
Gardeniae Fructus (*zhī zǐ*) 6g
Schizonepetae Herba (*jīng jiè*) 6g
Atractylodis macrocephalae Rhizoma (*bái zhú*) 6g
Zingiberis Rhizoma recens (*shēng jiāng*) 6g

Actions: disperses wind • releases the exterior • drains heat • unblocks the bowels

Main pattern: heat excess in both the exterior and interior

Key symptoms: aversion to heat • epigastric distention and abdominal fullness • constipation • furuncles, carbuncles, acne or similar skin conditions involving localized swelling, redness, and pain

Secondary symptoms: strong fever and chills • upward flushing of heat • lightheadedness • dizziness • neck pain and tension • red and sore eyes • difficulty swallowing • nasal congestion with thick and sticky discharge • bitter taste • dry mouth • acid regurgitation • belching • dark urine

Tongue: greasy and white or yellow coating

Pulse: flooding and rapid • wiry and slippery

Abdomen: distended abdomen • aversion to pressure or palpation

▶ CLINICAL NOTES

• The formula treats patterns with heat excess in the interior that accumulates in both the chest and abdomen. This can occur in the course of either acute or chronic disorders. In both cases, effective venting of the heat is constrained by wind-cold fettering the exterior, while in the interior the heat is clumping in the intestines and flooding the Triple Burner. In acute cases, the patient will experience high fever, chest tightness, constipation, and thick nasal discharge. In chronic cases, accumulation of heat is most likely due to dietary irregularity in patients who are already predisposed to excess heat.

- The formula is widely used in Japan to stimulate the elimination of toxins from the body in patients with a strong constitution and signs of heat excess.
- While sometimes promoted as a formula to promote weight loss, this usage should be avoided, especially because long-term use presents a danger to the body's qi and fluids.

Contraindications: deficiency patterns • pregnancy • long-term use

► **FORMULAS WITH SIMILAR INDICATIONS**

*Cool the Diaphragm Powder (*liáng gé săn*): This formula vents wind-heat (rather than wind-cold) from the upper burner and drains clumped heat from the interior. The pattern is marked by sensations of heat and irritability in the chest and abdomen, thirst, flushed face, sore throat, constipation, dark, scanty urine, and a red tongue.

Major Bupleurum Decoction (*dà chái hú tāng*): For a dual lesser yang and yang brightness warp disorder manifesting with alternating chills and fevers rather than simultaneous chills and fevers, as in the main pattern.

COMPOSITION

Chiefs 君			
Saposhnikoviae Radix (*fáng fēng*)	● ●		disperses wind and releases the exterior by inducing sweating
Ephedrae Herba (*má huáng*)	● ●		
Rhei Radix et Rhizoma (*dà huáng*)	●		expels heat through the stool
Natrii Sulfas (*máng xiāo*)	● ● ●		

Deputies 臣			
Schizonepetae Herba (*jīng jiè*)	●		assists in releasing the exterior
Menthae haplocalycis Herba (*bò hé*)	● ●		
Gardeniae Fructus (*zhī zǐ*)	●		drains heat through the urine
Talcum (*huá shí*)	● ●		
Gypsum fibrosum (*shí gāo*)	● ●		
Forsythiae Fructus (*lián qiào*)	● ●		clears heat from the Lungs and Stomach
Scutellariae Radix (*huáng qín*)	●		
Platycodi Radix (*jié gěng*)	● ●		

Assistants 佐			
Chuanxiong Rhizoma (*chuān xiōng*)	●		harmonizes the blood, which helps to disperse wind
Angelicae sinensis Radix (*dāng guī*)	● ●		
Paeoniae Radix alba (*bái sháo*)	● ●		
Atractylodis macrocephalae Rhizoma (*bái zhú*)	● ●		protects the Spleen from the action of the wind-heat clearing herbs

Envoys 使			
Glycyrrhizae Radix (*gān cǎo*)	●		indirectly protects the Spleen by harmonizing the actions of the other ingredients
Zingiberis Rhizoma recens (*shēng jiāng*)	●		strengthens the Stomach to prevent the ingredients from causing upset stomach

[This page intentionally left blank]

防己黃耆湯（防己黃芪汤）
Stephania and Astragalus Decoction
fáng jǐ huáng qí tāng

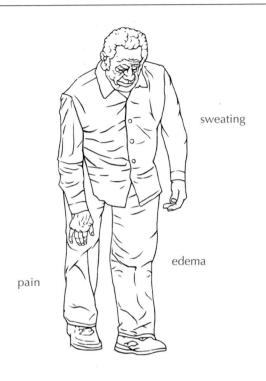

sweating

edema

pain

INGREDIENTS

Astragali Radix (*huáng qí*) 9-15g

Stephaniae tetrandrae Radix (*hàn fáng jǐ*) 6-12g

Atractylodis macrocephalae Rhizoma (*bái zhú*) 4.5-9g

Glycyrrhizae Radix praeparata (*zhì gān cǎo*) 4.5-6g

Zingiberis Rhizoma recens (*shēng jiāng*)........................ 3-4.5g

Jujubae Fructus (*dà zǎo*).. 1-2 pieces

Actions: augments the qi • dispels wind • strengthens the Spleen • promotes urination • reduces edema

Main pattern: wind-dampness or wind edema due to an invasion of wind and dampness in a patient with a deficient exterior

Key symptoms: sweating • superficial edema • pain, swelling, or stiffness in the joints

Secondary symptoms: pale complexion • fatigue on slight exertion • aversion to drafts • heavy sensation in the body • urinary difficulty • slight thirst

Tongue: pale body • white coating

Pulse: floating

Abdomen: weak abdominal wall • increased abdominal fat

▶ CLINICAL NOTES

• This formula treats patients with qi deficiency who present with edema or damp accumulation in the exterior or the joints. This type of patient will often be overweight, sweat easily, have poor muscle tone, and cold, moist skin. The edema is typically more pronounced in the lower body. Swollen and painful knees are also a specific focus.

• The formula's composition helps the body naturally dispel wind-dampness by firming up the protective qi in order to stop the sweating and promote healthy water metabolism.

Contraindications: excess-type edema • water-dampness constraint of the protective yang

▶ FORMULAS WITH SIMILAR INDICATIONS

Jade Windscreen Powder (*yù píng fēng sǎn*): For qi deficiency of the Lungs and Spleen without dampness. This manifests with sweating, aversion to drafts, fatigue, or frequent infections when these symptoms occur without signs of dampness such as edema or swelling.

Five-Peel Powder (*wǔ pí sǎn*): For superficial edema due to excess dampness and stagnation in the greater yin (Lung and Spleen) channels. This manifests as a sensation of heaviness, distention, and fullness in the epigastrium and abdomen, labored, heavy breathing, urinary difficulty, a white, greasy tongue coating, and a submerged, moderate pulse.

─────────────────────────────── COMPOSITION ───────────────────────────────

Chiefs
君

Astragali Radix *(huáng qí)* ● — stabilizes the protective qi

Stephaniae tetrandrae Radix *(hàn fáng jǐ)* ● ● — releases the exterior, unblocks the channels, promotes urination, expels dampness, and relieves pain

Deputy
臣

Atractylodis macrocephalae Rhizoma *(bái zhú)* ● ● — strengthens the Spleen and resolves dampness; assists the chief herbs in stabilizing the exterior and resolving the dampness

Assistant
佐

Glycyrrhizae Radix praeparata *(zhì gān cǎo)* ● — helps tonify the Spleen

Envoys
使

Zingiberis Rhizoma recens *(shēng jiāng)* ●

Jujubae Fructus *(dà zǎo)* ● — regulates and harmonizes the nutritive and protective qi to assist in the stabilization of the exterior and the strengthening of the qi and blood

茯苓丸
Poria Pill
fú líng wán

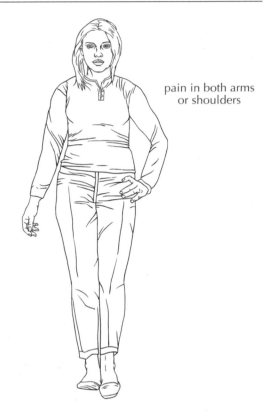

pain in both arms
or shoulders

INGREDIENTS

Poria (*fú líng*) 6-15g
Aurantii Fructus (*zhǐ ké*) 3-12g
Pinelliae Rhizoma praeparatum (*zhì bàn xià*) 9-12g
Natrii Sulfas (*máng xiāo*) 3-9g
Zingiberis Rhizoma recens (*sheng jiāng*) 3-6g

Actions: dries dampness • moves the qi • softens hardness • transforms phlegm

Main pattern: phlegm tarrying in the middle burner from which it overflows into the channels and collaterals

Key symptoms: pain in both arms or shoulders

Secondary symptoms: numbness in both hands • superficial edema in all four extremities

Tongue: white, greasy coating

Pulse: submerged and thin • wiry and slippery

Abdomen: no specific signs

▶ CLINICAL NOTES

- This formula treats shoulder pain with inability to lift the hands. This is often more pronounced on one side than the other. Where phlegm has also led to blood stasis it is useful to add herbs such as Pheretima (*dì lóng*), Mori Ramulus (*sāng zhī*), or Cinnamomi Ramulus (*guì zhī*) to invigorate the blood and unblock the collaterals.

- Treatment with this formula should be discontinued as soon as the symptoms have eased to avoid drying out the body fluids.

- The formula can also be used for other patterns characterized by excess phlegm in the upper burner such as cough, plum-pit qi, or insomnia.

Contraindications: patients with weak constitutions • shoulder pain due to blood deficiency and wind

▶ FORMULAS WITH SIMILAR INDICATIONS

Tonify the Middle to Augment the Qi Decoction (*bǔ zhōng yì qì tāng*): For shoulder pain from qi deficiency and invasion of wind-dampness into the channels. This pattern is recognized by the presence of a deficient pulse and by pain that is significantly ameliorated by rest. When the formula is used to treat shoulder pain, herbs such as Gentianae macrophyllae Radix (*qín jiāo*) and Gastrodiae Rhizoma (*tiān má*) with Mori Ramulus (*sāng zhī*) or Cinnamomi Ramulus (*guì zhī*) are usually added to focus the formula on the shoulder or upper arm.

Notopterygium Decoction to Overcome Dampness (*qiāng huó shèng shī tāng*): For shoulder pain from wind-dampness against a background of blood deficiency. This type of pain is usually sudden in onset and is accompanied by stiffness. For this purpose the original formula is modified by adding herbs like Angelicae sinensis Radix (*dāng guī*) to tonify blood in the channels, while replacing Ligustici Rhizoma (*gǎo běn*) and Saposhnikoviae Radix (*fáng fēng*), which are more specific for the neck, with those that focus on the upper extremities, such as Gentianae macrophyllae Radix (*qín jiāo*) and Mori Ramulus (*sāng zhī*).

*Two Atractylodes Decoction** (*èr zhú tāng*): For shoulder pain owing to dampness, phlegm, or thin mucus in the upper burner. This formula contains herbs to directly address wind-dampness in the channels as well as heat-clearing herbs for any resultant heat from constraint.

COMPOSITION

Chief 君	Pinelliae Rhizoma praeparatum (*zhì bàn xià*)	●	transforms phlegm and facilitates the downward directing of the qi dynamic
Deputy 臣	Poria (*fú líng*)	● ●	strengthens the Spleen, leaches out dampness, and transforms phlegm
Assistants 佐	Aurantii Fructus (*zhǐ ké*)	● ●	moves the qi and eases the middle, smooths the qi dynamic to facilitate the elimination of phlegm
	Natrii Sulfas (*máng xiāo*)	● ● ●	softens hardness and moistens dryness, reduces and guides out lurking phlegm via the bowels
Envoy 使	Zingiberis Rhizoma recens (*shēng jiāng*)	●	counteracts the toxicity of the chief herb, supports the chief and deputy herbs in transforming phlegm and dispersing thin mucus

甘草乾薑茯苓白朮湯
（甘草干姜茯苓白术汤）
Licorice, Ginger, Poria, and White Atractylodes Decoction
gān cǎo gān jiāng fú líng bái zhú tāng

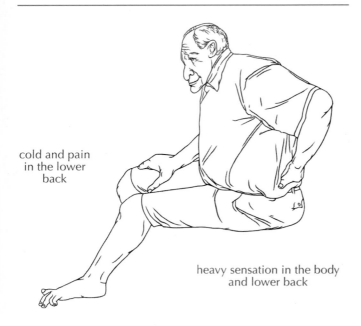

cold and pain in the lower back

heavy sensation in the body and lower back

INGREDIENTS

Glycyrrhizae Radix (*gān cǎo*) 6g
Zingiberis Rhizoma (*gān jiāng*) 12g
Poria (*fú líng*) 12g
Atractylodis macrocephalae Rhizoma (*bái zhú*) 6g

Actions: warms the Spleen • overcomes dampness

Main patterns: painful obstruction of the back and waist • fixed Kidney disorder (腎著 *shèn zhuó*)

Key symptoms: heavy sensation in the body and lower back (as if carrying a heavy weight) • cold and pain in the lower back • difficulty bending

Secondary symptoms: diarrhea • soft stools • increased saliva • sweating • free-flowing urine

Tongue: pale • moist coating that may be thick and greasy at the root

Pulse: submerged • thin • moderate

Abdomen: splashing sounds • soft fullness in lower abdomen

▶ CLINICAL NOTES

- This formula treats damp-cold obstructing the flow of qi in the exterior of the body. This is usually due to an external factor like exposure to rain or cold weather or swimming in cold water. It can also arise from middle-burner yang deficiency.

- The key clinical markers are a sensation of heaviness, cold, or pain in the abdomen or back. The sensation of cold can be subjective, or may be palpable. Heaviness may manifest as a sensation of numbness or insensitivity. The patient may also experience difficulty bending from the waist. The body's effort to shed excess fluids may present as diarrhea or soft stools, copious urination, sweating, profuse saliva, phlegm, or increased skin secretions. Because they are due to underlying cold, they will usually not be malodorous.

- This formula is also used for Girdle vessel disorders that are characterized by cold and dampness.

- Incontinence and edema can be effectively treated with this formula if due to damp-cold lodged in the lower burner.

Contraindications: damp-heat

▶ FORMULAS WITH SIMILAR INDICATIONS

True Warrior Decoction (*zhēn wǔ tāng*): For heaviness in the body and urinary frequency from more severe yang deficiency and water excess. This pattern is sometimes accompanied by signs of floating yang such as fever or palpitations.

Poria, Cinnamon Twig, Atractylodes, and Licorice Decoction (*líng guì zhú gān tāng*): For thin mucus in the abdomen and epigastrium manifesting with dizziness, palpitations, and a wet tongue. These are signs of water excess in the interior along with an upward surge of qi. This latter aspect affects the water pathways, which interferes with free-flowing urination.

Kidney Qi Pill (*shèn qì wán*): For backache and difficulty bending due to Kidney yang deficiency with some accumulation of water-dampness. This formula warms the Kidneys whereas

Licorice, Ginger, Poria, and White Atractylodes Decoction (*gān cǎo gān jiāng fú líng bái zhú tāng*) warms the Spleen.

--- COMPOSITION ---

Chief 君	Zingiberis Rhizoma (*gān jiāng*)	warms the middle and drives out wind-damp painful obstruction
Deputy 臣	Poria (*fú líng*)	strengthens the Spleen and promotes urination to eliminate dampness via the urine
Assistants 佐	Atractylodis macrocephalae Rhizoma (*bái zhú*)	tonifies the Spleen qi even as it dries dampness
	Glycyrrhizae Radix (*gān cǎo*)	harmonizes the function of the other herbs and strengthens the Spleen

甘露消毒丹
Sweet Dew Special Pill to Eliminate Toxin
gān lù xiāo dú dān

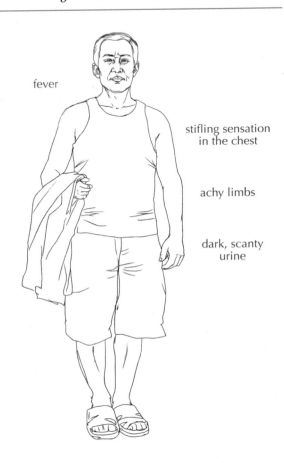

fever

stifling sensation in the chest

achy limbs

dark, scanty urine

Amomi Fructus rotundus (*bái dòu kòu*) 6-9g

Actions: resolves dampness • transforms turbidity • clears heat • resolves toxicity

Main pattern: early stage of a damp-warmth epidemic disorder flooding all three burners and presenting with equally pronounced heat and dampness

Key symptoms: fever • achy limbs • stifling sensation in the chest • abdominal distention • lethargy • dark, scanty urine

Secondary symptoms: swollen and painful throat • swollen lymph nodes • vomiting and diarrhea • jaundice • cloudy, painful urinary dribbling • stiffness and pain in the lower back • sweating

Tongue: red body • white or yellow, greasy coating

Pulse: soggy and rapid • slippery and rapid

Abdomen: focal distention in the epigastrium • distention and fullness in the area between CV-8 and CV-12

▶ CLINICAL NOTES

• This is a main formula for acute and sub-acute damp-heat disorders at the qi level. Key clinical markers are a sensation of fullness in the chest or upper abdomen (indicating dampness obstructing the qi dynamic) along with signs of excess heat such as fever or dark, scanty urine.

• While less well known than formulas such as Honeysuckle and Forsythia Powder (*yín qiáo săn*) or Ephedra Decoction (*má huáng tāng*), this is a key formula for treating flu-type infections and was used as such by the famous Qing dynasty physician Ye Tian-Shi. It is especially useful in regions where dampness is prevalent.

• Because this formula treats damp-heat at the qi aspect of all three burners, it can be used for a very wide range of disorders, most of which are infectious. These include maculopapular rashes, influenza, tonsillitis, mumps, and damp-heat-phlegm cough (disorders of the upper burner and the exterior); hepatitis, jaundice, cholecystitis, and other gastrointestinal disorders (middle burner); and urinary tract infections (lower burner).

INGREDIENTS

Forsythiae Fructus (*lián qiào*) 6-9g
Scutellariae Radix (*huáng qín*) 9-21g
Menthae haplocalycis Herba (*bò hé*) 6-9g
Belamcandae Rhizoma (*shè gān*) 6-9g
Fritillariae cirrhosae Bulbus (*chuān bèi mŭ*) 6-9g
Talcum (*huá shí*) 15-30g
Akebiae Caulis (*mù tōng*) 6-9g
Artemisiae scopariae Herba (*yīn chén*) 9-24g
Pogostemonis/Agastaches Herba (*huò xiāng*) 6-9g
Acori tatarinowii Rhizoma (*shí chāng pŭ*) 9-12g

Contraindications: significant yin deficiency

▶ FORMULAS WITH SIMILAR INDICATIONS

Universal Benefit Drink to Eliminate Toxin (*pǔ jì xiāo dú yǐn*): For wind-heat seasonal epidemic disorders. These manifest with a painful and swollen throat along with thirst and a strong fever. These disorders also present with a powdery, white, or yellow tongue coating that reflects damage to the fluids from massive heat toxin.

Three-Seed Decoction (*sān rén tāng*): For qi aspect damp-warmth with dampness that is more pronounced than heat. This is characterized by a mild fever that worsens in the afternoon, white tongue coating, and a pulse that is soggy but not rapid.

Coptis and Magnolia Bark Drink (*lián pò yǐn*): For qi aspect damp-warmth where dampness and heat are equally strong. Rather than focusing on treating all three burners, this formula focuses on treating diarrhea and vomiting due to obstruction of the middle burner qi dynamic.

COMPOSITION

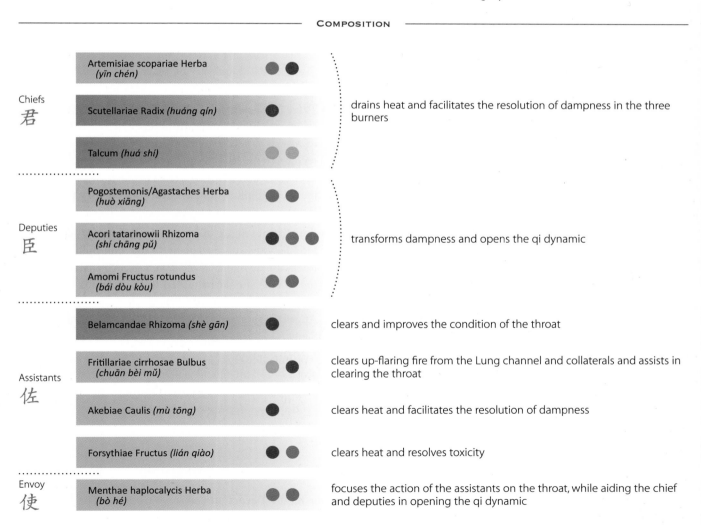

Chiefs 君	Artemisiae scopariae Herba (*yīn chén*)	
	Scutellariae Radix (*huáng qín*)	drains heat and facilitates the resolution of dampness in the three burners
	Talcum (*huá shí*)	
Deputies 臣	Pogostemonis/Agastaches Herba (*huò xiāng*)	
	Acori tatarinowii Rhizoma (*shí chāng pú*)	transforms dampness and opens the qi dynamic
	Amomi Fructus rotundus (*bái dòu kòu*)	
Assistants 佐	Belamcandae Rhizoma (*shè gān*)	clears and improves the condition of the throat
	Fritillariae cirrhosae Bulbus (*chuān bèi mǔ*)	clears up-flaring fire from the Lung channel and collaterals and assists in clearing the throat
	Akebiae Caulis (*mù tōng*)	clears heat and facilitates the resolution of dampness
	Forsythiae Fructus (*lián qiào*)	clears heat and resolves toxicity
Envoy 使	Menthae haplocalycis Herba (*bò hé*)	focuses the action of the assistants on the throat, while aiding the chief and deputies in opening the qi dynamic

甘麥大棗湯 （甘麦大枣汤）
Licorice, Wheat, and Jujube Decoction
gān mài dà zǎo tāng

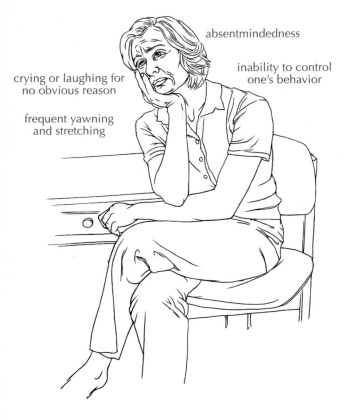

absentmindedness

inability to control one's behavior

crying or laughing for no obvious reason

frequent yawning and stretching

INGREDIENTS

Glycyrrhizae Radix (*gān cǎo*).. 9g
Tritici Fructus (*xiǎo mài*).. 9-30g
Jujubae Fructus (*dà zǎo*)..................................... 5-10 pieces

Actions: nourishes the Heart • calms the spirit • harmonizes the middle burner • relaxes hypertonicity

Main pattern: restless organ disorder

Key symptoms: absentmindedness • inability to control one's behavior • crying or laughing for no obvious reason • frequent yawning and stretching

Secondary symptoms: agitation • mental exhaustion • restless sleep (sometimes with night sweats) • dry mouth • little interest in food • dry stool

Tongue: pale red body • scanty coating

Pulse: thin • frail • rapid

Abdomen: tightness of rectus abdominis muscle specifically on the left side, but otherwise a generally flaccid abdomen • palpitations above the umbilicus

▶ CLINICAL NOTES

- Restless organ disorder is a condition in which patients find it difficult to control their emotions. They feel sad for no reason, yet also agitated and confused. They overreact to emotional stimuli, crying, laughing, or becoming angry with little provocation.

- There is considerable debate as to the precise pathophysiology of this disorder. In practice, it is less important to attach a precise diagnostic label than to learn to recognize the key clinical markers: inability to control one's emotions, desire to stretch or yawn, or tension in the rectus abdominis muscle but without a wiry pulse. Also lacking are clear signs of excess or deficiency heat or cold.

- For distinct signs of Heart yin deficiency with a red tongue body, appropriate herbs like Lilii Bulbus (*bǎi hé*), Rehmanniae Radix (*shēng dì huáng*), or Platycladi Semen (*bǎi zǐ rén*) should be added to the formula to address this issue. For blood deficiency, one may add herbs like Angelicae sinensis Radix (*dāng guī*) and Ziziphi spinosae Semen (*suān zǎo rén*).

- In contemporary practice, this formula has a very wide scope of treatment and is indicated for disorders ranging from childhood nighttime tremors to menopausal syndrome or depression.

Contraindications: none noted

▶ FORMULAS WITH SIMILAR INDICATIONS

Sour Jujube Decoction (*suān zǎo rén tāng*): For Liver deficiency patterns, specifically Liver blood deficiency, characterized by insomnia, fatigue, and anxiety.

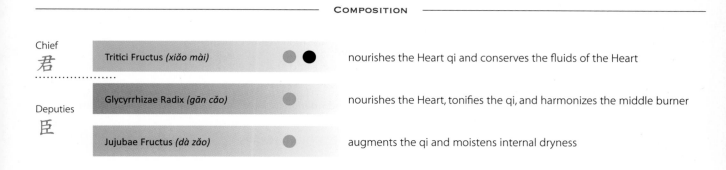

COMPOSITION

Chief
君
Tritici Fructus *(xiǎo mài)*   nourishes the Heart qi and conserves the fluids of the Heart

Deputies
臣
Glycyrrhizae Radix *(gān cǎo)*   nourishes the Heart, tonifies the qi, and harmonizes the middle burner

Jujubae Fructus *(dà zǎo)*   augments the qi and moistens internal dryness

葛根黃芩黃連湯（葛根黄芩黄连汤）
Kudzu, Scutellaria, and Coptis Decoction
gé gēn huáng qín huáng lián tāng

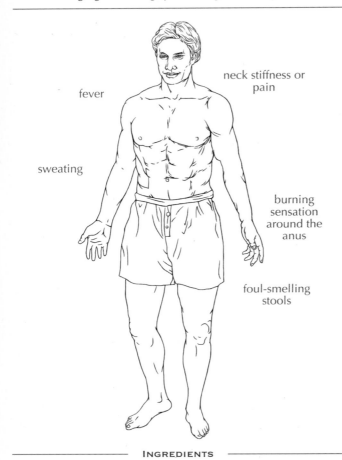

fever

neck stiffness or pain

sweating

burning sensation around the anus

foul-smelling stools

INGREDIENTS

Puerariae Radix (*gé gēn*).. 15g
Scutellariae Radix (*huáng qín*) 9g
Coptidis Rhizoma (*huáng lián*) 9g
Glycyrrhizae Radix praeparata (*zhì gān cǎo*) 6g

Actions: releases the exterior • drains heat

Main patterns: heat excess in both the exterior and interior (yang brightness warp disorder) • heat-type dysenteric disorders

Key symptoms: fever • sweating • foul-smelling stools • burning sensation around the anus • neck stiffness or pain

Secondary symptoms: facial flushing • headache • wheezing • thirst • irritability • insomnia

Tongue: red • yellow coating

Pulse: rapid and slippery • flooding, large, and forceful • rapid-irregular

Abdomen: may have focal distention in epigastrium

▶ CLINICAL NOTES

• A major formula for heat-type dysenteric disorders due to excess heat in the yang brightness warp, where the body simultaneously seeks to vent heat via the exterior and drain it via the Intestines. This includes any disorder characterized by loose or unformed, foul-smelling stools that is accompanied by upward flushing of heat with such signs as a body that is sweaty and hot to the touch, facial flushing, irritability, thirst, insomnia, or a pulse that is rapid-irregular, flooding, large and forceful, or rapid and slippery. While the upward flushing of heat may also manifest as wheezing, dizziness, headache and stiff neck, the source of these signs needs to be carefully differentiated.

Contraindications: dysenteric disorders without fever or with a submerged and slow pulse

▶ FORMULAS WITH SIMILAR INDICATIONS

Scutellaria Decoction (*huáng qín tāng*): For dysenteric disorders that occur in the course of a simultaneous greater yang and lesser yang warp disorder. This is characterized by more severe abdominal pain.

*Peony Decoction (*sháo yào tāng*): For dysenteric disorders with abdominal pain and stools that contain both blood and pus or phlegm and signs of blood deficiency.

Pulsatilla Decoction (*bái tóu wēng tāng*): For dysenteric disorders due to damp-heat excess that has penetrated into the blood aspect. This pattern is characterized by more blood than pus in the stools.

Major Order the Qi Decoction (*dà chéng qì tāng*): Yang

brightness interior excess patterns can also manifest with foul-smelling diarrhea but the abdomen will be distended and painful to the touch. There may be hard bits of stool within the watery evacuation.

COMPOSITION

Chief
君

Puerariae Radix *(gé gēn)* — releases the exterior, clears heat, and treats dysenteric diarrhea by raising the clear yang of the Spleen and Stomach

Deputies
臣

Coptidis Rhizoma *(huáng lián)* — drains heat, dries dampness in the Stomach and Intestines, stops diarrhea

Glycyrrhizae Radix praeparata *(zhì gān cǎo)* — harmonizes the actions of the other herbs and protects the middle burner

Assistant
佐

Scutellariae Radix *(huáng qín)* — enters into the Intestines and is frequently prescribed in the treatment of dysenteric disorders due to damp-heat

葛根湯 （葛根汤）
Kudzu Decoction
gé gēn tāng

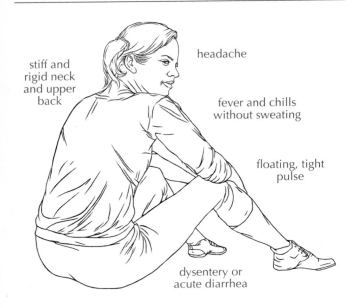

stiff and rigid neck and upper back

headache

fever and chills without sweating

floating, tight pulse

dysentery or acute diarrhea

INGREDIENTS

Puerariae Radix (*gé gēn*) 12g
[1]Ephedrae Herba (*má huáng*) 6g
Cinnamomi Ramulus (*guì zhī*) 6g
Paeoniae Radix alba (*bái sháo*) 6g
Zingiberis Rhizoma recens (*shēng jiāng*) 6g
Jujubae Fructus (*dà zǎo*) .... 3 pieces
Glycyrrhizae Radix praeparata (*zhì gān cǎo*) 5g

Actions: releases pathogens from the exterior and muscle layer • generates fluids

Main pattern: externally-contracted wind-cold penetrating into the greater yang channels of the head and neck

Key symptoms: fever and chills without sweating • stiff and rigid neck and upper back

Secondary symptoms: headache • dry retching • dysentery or acute diarrhea

---

1. This herb can be difficult to obtain because of legal issues. Perillae Folium (*zǐ sū yè*) may be substituted.

Tongue: thin, white coating

Pulse: floating • tight

Abdomen: no specific signs

▶ CLINICAL NOTES

- Indicated for wind-cold yang brightness exterior disorders with symptoms of dryness and heat along the course of the yang brightness channel (neck stiffness, headache, neuralgia, etc.)
- Also for patterns whose major symptoms involve mucous membranes (inflammation of the eyes, nose, bowels, etc.) because the yang brightness is regarded as the "interior of the exterior."

Contraindications: wind-heat disorders with similar symptoms

▶ FORMULAS WITH SIMILAR INDICATIONS

Ephedra Decoction (*má huáng tāng*): For greater yang stage disorders with cold fettering the exterior characterized by fever and chills without sweating and a pulse that is floating and tight.

Cinnamon Twig Decoction (*guì zhī tāng*):For greater yang stage wind attack characterized by chills and fever with sweating and a pulse that is floating and lax.

COMPOSITION

Chief
君

Puerariae Radix *(gé gēn)* — releases the exterior, soothes the muscles (especially of upper back and neck), generates fluids, clears heat

Deputies
臣

Ephedrae Herba *(má huáng)*

Cinnamomi Ramulus *(guì zhī)*

induces sweating, resolves the exterior, disperses cold, and unblocks the collaterals

Paeoniae Radix *(bái sháo)* — preserves the yin by preventing the exterior-releasing herbs from causing excessive sweating

Assistants
佐

Zingiberis Rhizoma recens *(shēng jiāng)*

Jujubae Fructus *(dà zǎo)*

regulates the protective and nutritive qi, harmonizes the Stomach

Envoy
使

Glycyrrhizae Radix praeparata *(zhì gān cǎo)* — harmonizes the actions of the other herbs

葛花解醒散
Kudzu Flower Powder to Relieve Hangovers
gé huā jiě chéng săn

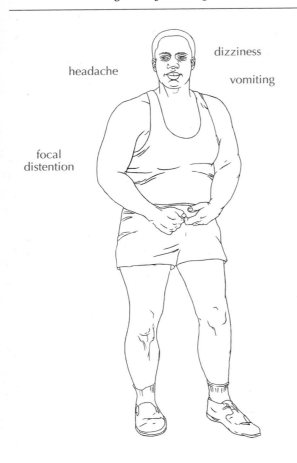

headache • dizziness • vomiting • focal distention

INGREDIENTS

Amomi Fructus rotundus (*bái dòu kòu*) 15g

Amomi Fructus (*shā rén*).. 15g

Puerariae Flos (*gé huā*) 15g

Zingiberis Rhizoma (*gān jiāng*)... 6g

dry-fried Massa medicata fermentata (*chǎo shén qū*) 6g

Alismatis Rhizoma (*zé xiè*) 6g

Atractylodis macrocephalae Rhizoma (*bái zhú*) 6g

Citri reticulatae Pericarpium (*chén pí*)............................ 4.5g

Ginseng Radix (*rén shēn*).. 4.5g

Polyporus (*zhū líng*) 4.5g

Poria (*fú líng*) 4.5g

Aucklandiae Radix (*mù xiāng*) 3g

Citri reticulatae viride Pericarpium (*qīng pí*)..................... 1g

Preparation notes: Grind into a fine powder and take 9g as a draft with water. This will produce a mild sweat after which the hangover should improve.

Actions: separates and reduces alcohol-dampness • warms the middle • strengthens the Spleen

Main pattern: accumulation of damp-heat in the yang brightness channels (Stomach and Large Intestines) due to alcohol consumption and Spleen deficiency

Key symptoms: vomiting • dizziness • headache • focal distention in the chest and diaphragm • reduced appetite • fatigue • inhibited urination

Secondary symptoms: irritability • trembling of the hands and feet • diarrhea

Tongue: greasy coating

Pulse: possibly slippery

Abdomen: discomfort in epigastrium • splashing sounds in upper abdomen

▶ CLINICAL NOTES

• This formula is indicated for acute hangovers as well as stagnation arising from habitual consumption of alcohol. However, due to its warming nature, it must be modified for patients with heat excess. For example, for more signs of damp-heat, Coptidis Rhizoma (*huáng lián*) and Scutellariae Radix (*huáng qín*) can be added.

Contraindications: yin deficiency heat • thirst indicating damage to fluids

──────────────────── COMPOSITION ────────────────────

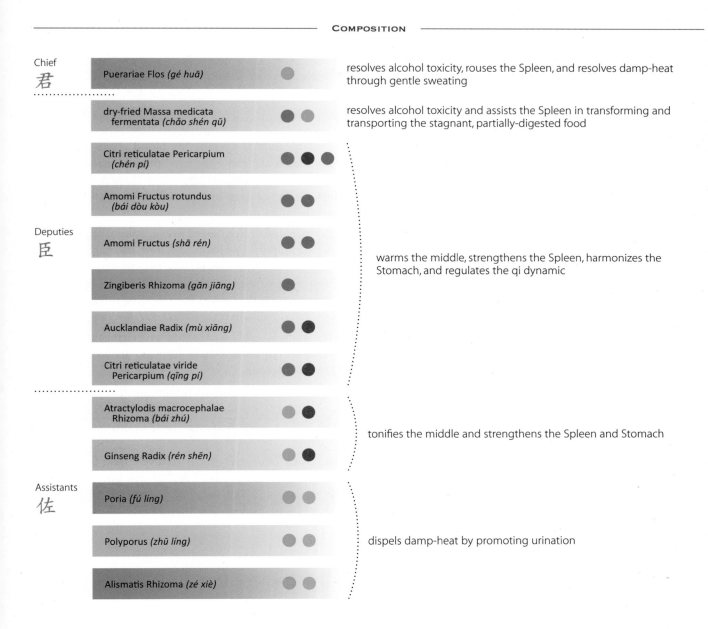

Chief
君

Puerariae Flos (gé huā) — resolves alcohol toxicity, rouses the Spleen, and resolves damp-heat through gentle sweating

dry-fried Massa medicata fermentata (chǎo shén qū) — resolves alcohol toxicity and assists the Spleen in transforming and transporting the stagnant, partially-digested food

Citri reticulatae Pericarpium (chén pí)

Amomi Fructus rotundus (bái dòu kòu)

Deputies
臣

Amomi Fructus (shā rén)

Zingiberis Rhizoma (gān jiāng)

Aucklandiae Radix (mù xiāng)

Citri reticulatae viride Pericarpium (qīng pí)

warms the middle, strengthens the Spleen, harmonizes the Stomach, and regulates the qi dynamic

Atractylodis macrocephalae Rhizoma (bái zhú)

Ginseng Radix (rén shēn)

tonifies the middle and strengthens the Spleen and Stomach

Assistants
佐

Poria (fú líng)

Polyporus (zhū líng)

Alismatis Rhizoma (zé xiè)

dispels damp-heat by promoting urination

膈下逐瘀湯（膈下逐瘀汤）
Drive Out Stasis Below the Diaphragm Decoction
gé xià zhú yū tāng

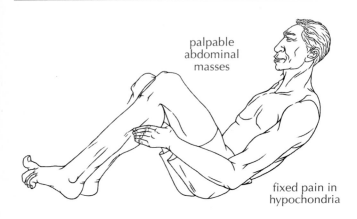

palpable abdominal masses

fixed pain in hypochondria

--- INGREDIENTS ---

dry-fried Trogopterori Faeces (*chǎo wǔ líng zhī*) 6-9g
Angelicae sinensis Radix (*dāng guī*) 9g
Chuanxiong Rhizoma (*chuān xiōng*) 6g
Persicae Semen (*táo rén*).. 9g
Moutan Cortex (*mǔ dān pí*) 6g
Paeoniae Radix rubra (*chì sháo*)................................... 6g
Linderae Radix (*wū yào*)... 6-12g
Corydalis Rhizoma (*yán hú suǒ*) 3g
Glycyrrhizae Radix (*gān cǎo*).. 9g
Cyperi Rhizoma (*xiāng fù*)... 4.5g
Carthami Flos (*hóng huā*)... 9g
Aurantii Fructus (*zhǐ ké*)... 4.5g

Actions: invigorates the blood • dispels blood stasis • promotes the movement of qi • alleviates pain

Main pattern: blood stasis in the area below the diaphragm

Key symptoms: fixed pain in hypochondria • palpable abdominal masses

Secondary symptoms: chronic diarrhea • daybreak diarrhea • amenorrhea • painful periods

Tongue: dark body • stasis spots • distended sublingual veins • white coating

Pulse: wiry and rough, particularly in the middle positions

Abdomen: tenderness below the ribs • palpable masses • abdominal masses visible when lying down • spider nevi or visible arterioles on the chest or abdominal wall

► **CLINICAL NOTES**

• This formula is specific for blood stasis below the diaphragm and above the navel that can manifest either with fixed pain or masses that are visible or palpable. Such masses do not come and go as do accumulations due to qi stagnation.

• For pain due to an enlarged liver or spleen, herbs such as Salviae miltiorrhizae Radix (*dān shēn*) and Bupleuri Radix (*chái hú*) are often added. These patients also commonly have signs of blood deficiency. When this is the case, appropriate herbs such as Paeoniae Radix alba (*bái sháo*) and Salviae miltiorrhizae Radix (*dān shēn*) are added.

• The formula is also used to treat amenorrhea and painful periods even though these disorders are located in the lower abdomen.

Contraindications: deficiency conditions

► **FORMULAS WITH SIMILAR INDICATIONS**

Salvia Drink (*dān shēn yǐn*): A relatively mild formula for epigastric pain due to blood and qi stagnation. Does not treat masses.

COMPOSITION

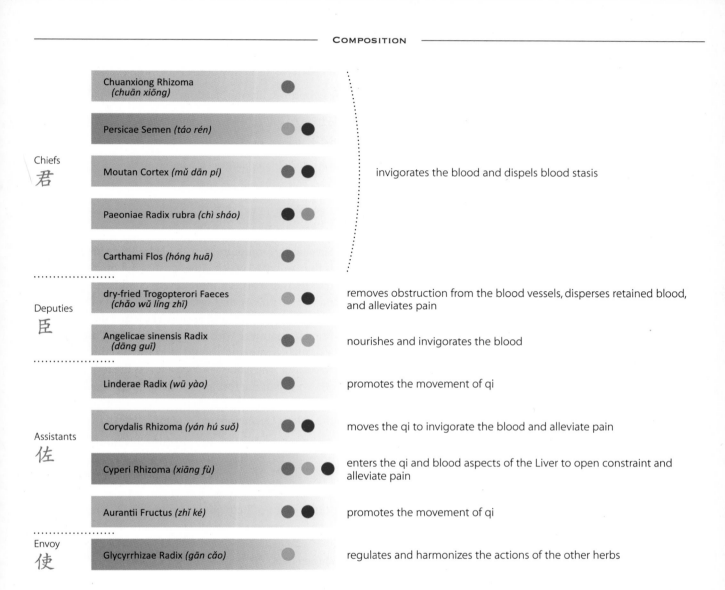

Chiefs
君

Chuanxiong Rhizoma (chuān xiōng)

Persicae Semen (táo rén)

Moutan Cortex (mǔ dān pí)

Paeoniae Radix rubra (chì sháo)

Carthami Flos (hóng huā)

invigorates the blood and dispels blood stasis

Deputies
臣

dry-fried Trogopterori Faeces (chǎo wǔ líng zhī)

removes obstruction from the blood vessels, disperses retained blood, and alleviates pain

Angelicae sinensis Radix (dāng guī)

nourishes and invigorates the blood

Assistants
佐

Linderae Radix (wū yào)

promotes the movement of qi

Corydalis Rhizoma (yán hú suǒ)

moves the qi to invigorate the blood and alleviate pain

Cyperi Rhizoma (xiāng fù)

enters the qi and blood aspects of the Liver to open constraint and alleviate pain

Aurantii Fructus (zhǐ ké)

promotes the movement of qi

Envoy
使

Glycyrrhizae Radix (gān cǎo)

regulates and harmonizes the actions of the other herbs

固衝湯（固冲汤）
Stabilize Gushing Decoction
gù chòng tāng

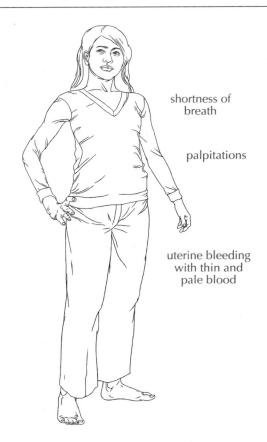

shortness of
breath

palpitations

uterine bleeding
with thin and
pale blood

INGREDIENTS

dry-fried Atractylodis macrocephalae Rhizoma
   (*chǎo bái zhú*).. 30g
Astragali Radix (*huáng qí*)...................................... 18g
Corni Fructus (*shān zhū yú*)................................... 24g
Paeoniae Radix alba (*bái sháo*)............................. 12g
calcined Fossilia Ossis Mastodi (*duàn lóng gǔ*).......... 24g
calcined Ostreae Concha (*duàn mǔ lì*) 24g
Sepiae Endoconcha (*hǎi piāo xiāo*) 12g
charred Trachycarpi Petiolus (*zōng lǘ tàn*) 6g
Galla chinensis (*wǔ bèi zǐ*)..................................... 1.5g
Rubiae Radix (*qiàn cǎo gēn*).................................. 9g

Actions: augments the qi • strengthens the Spleen • stabilizes the Penetrating vessel • stops bleeding

Main pattern: instability of the Penetrating vessel

Key symptoms: uterine bleeding with thin and pale blood

Secondary symptoms: palpitations • shortness of breath

Tongue: pale

Pulse: deficient and large • thin and frail

Abdomen: no specific signs

▶ CLINICAL NOTES

• Specifically for profuse menstrual bleeding with blood that is thin and pale, which either gushes out or continuously trickles out. This is a more severe condition than heavy menstrual flow or mid-cycle bleeding, both of which can be treated by addressing the root cause and do not require branch treatment with astringent agents. This formula, a branch treatment, should stop the bleeding within a week after which one can then address the root deficiency with qi-tonifying formulas such as Tonify the Middle to Augment the Qi Decoction (*bǔ zhōng yì qì tāng*) or Restore the Spleen Decoction (*guī pí tāng*).

• Although indicated for profuse bleeding, it is inappropriate for cases in which the bleeding is so severe that it leads to an abandoned disorder characterized by profuse sweating, cold limbs, and a pulse that is faint to the point of being imperceptible. While traditionally Unaccompanied Ginseng Decoction (*dú shēn tāng*) was the indicated treatment for these patients, at present they should be rushed to an emergency room.

Contraindications: bleeding due to either blood stasis or heat • bleeding that is so severe that it results in qi abandonment

▶ FORMULAS WITH SIMILAR INDICATIONS

Restore the Spleen Decoction (*guī pí tāng*): Tonifies the qi and nourishes the Heart blood to treat chronic but less severe bleeding with signs of Heart blood deficiency.

Tonify the Middle to Augment the Qi Decoction (*bǔ zhōng*

yì qì tāng): For less severe cases of uterine bleeding due qi deficiency leading to sinking qi in the lower abdomen that does not require the use of astringent agents.

Stabilize the Menses Pill (*gù jīng wán*): For severe uterine bleeding due to Liver qi constraint fire in an environment of yin deficiency.

─── COMPOSITION ───

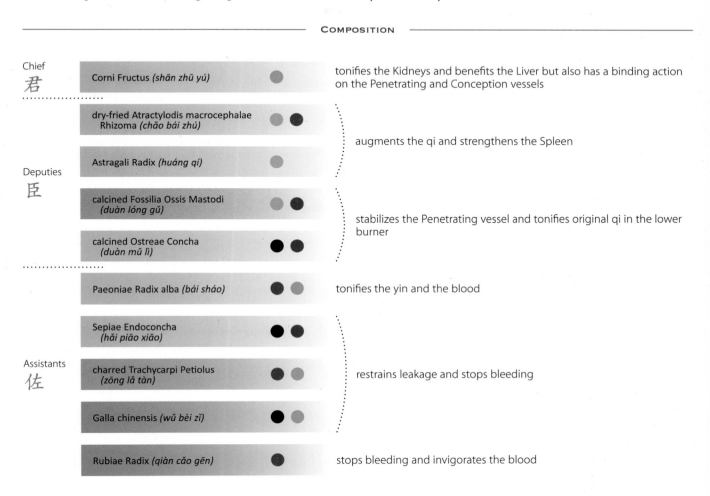

Chief 君	Corni Fructus *(shān zhū yú)*		tonifies the Kidneys and benefits the Liver but also has a binding action on the Penetrating and Conception vessels
Deputies 臣	dry-fried Atractylodis macrocephalae Rhizoma *(chǎo bái zhú)*		augments the qi and strengthens the Spleen
	Astragali Radix *(huáng qí)*		
	calcined Fossilia Ossis Mastodi *(duàn lóng gǔ)*		stabilizes the Penetrating vessel and tonifies original qi in the lower burner
	calcined Ostreae Concha *(duàn mǔ lì)*		
Assistants 佐	Paeoniae Radix alba *(bái sháo)*		tonifies the yin and the blood
	Sepiae Endoconcha *(hǎi piāo xiāo)*		restrains leakage and stops bleeding
	charred Trachycarpi Petiolus *(zōng lǘ tàn)*		
	Galla chinensis *(wǔ bèi zǐ)*		
	Rubiae Radix *(qiàn cǎo gēn)*		stops bleeding and invigorates the blood

固經丸（固经丸）
Stabilize the Menses Pill
gù jīng wán

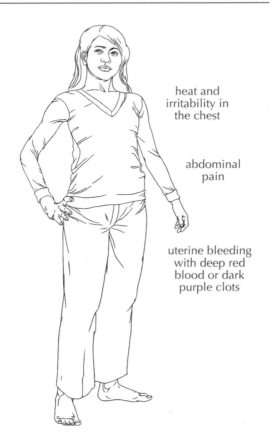

heat and irritability in the chest

abdominal pain

uterine bleeding with deep red blood or dark purple clots

Key symptoms: uterine bleeding with deep red blood or dark purple clots

Secondary symptoms: heat and irritability in the chest • abdominal pain • dark urine • constipation

Tongue: red

Pulse: rapid • wiry

Abdomen: no specific signs

► CLINICAL NOTES

- For severe uterine bleeding that is either continuous or alternates between trickling and gushing of blood. The presence of dark purple clots is a key marker.
- The formula can also be used to treat vaginal discharge, dysenteric disorders, seminal emissions, and heat in the five centers due to yang excess and yin deficiency.

Contraindications: bleeding due to heat from blood stasis

► FORMULAS WITH SIMILAR INDICATIONS

Stabilize Gushing Decoction (*gù chōng tāng*): For sudden and profuse uterine bleeding precipitated by deficiency of qi and blood.

━━━━━━━━━━ INGREDIENTS ━━━━━━━━━━

Testudinis Plastrum (*guī bǎn*) 15-30g
Paeoniae Radix alba (*bái sháo*) 15-30g
Scutellariae Radix (*huáng qín*) 15-30g
Ailanthi Cortex (*chūn pí*) 12-21g
Phellodendri Cortex (*huáng bái*) 6-9g
Cyperi Rhizoma (*xiāng fù*) 6-7.5g

Actions: enriches the yin • clears heat • stops bleeding • stabilizes the menses

Main pattern: heat in the Penetrating and Conception vessels due to Liver qi constraint in the context of yin deficiency

─────────────────── COMPOSITION ───────────────────

Chiefs
君

Testudinis Plastrum *(guī bǎn)*   ● ●   tonifies the yin essence and directs the fire downward

Paeoniae Radix alba *(bái sháo)*   ● ●   preserves the yin and nourishes the blood

Deputies
臣

Scutellariae Radix *(huáng qín)*   ●   drains heat from the upper burner and blood to stop the bleeding

Phellodendri Cortex *(huáng bái)*   ●   drains damp-heat from the lower burner

Assistants
佐

Ailanthi Cortex *(chūn pí)*   ● ●   binds up the blood and prevents an abandoned disorder from developing

Cyperi Rhizoma *(xiāng fù)*   ● ● ●   regulates the qi and relieves Liver constraint

歸脾湯（归脾汤）
Restore the Spleen Decoction
guī pí tāng

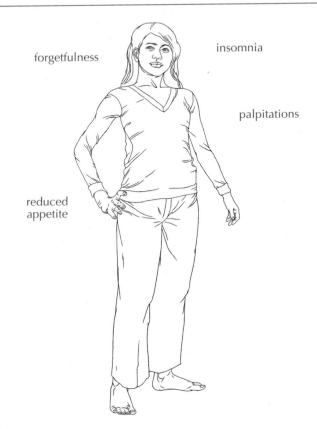

forgetfulness

insomnia

palpitations

reduced appetite

INGREDIENTS

Ginseng Radix (*rén shēn*)... 3-6g
Astragali Radix (*huáng qí*)... 3-12g
Atractylodis macrocephalae Rhizoma (*bái zhú*) 3-9g
Poria (*fú líng*).. 3-9g
Ziziphi spinosae Semen (*suān zǎo rén*)............................ 3-12g
Longan Arillus (*lóng yǎn ròu*).. 3-12g
Aucklandiae Radix (*mù xiāng*)... 3-6g
Glycyrrhizae Radix praeparata (*zhì gān cǎo*) 1-3
Angelicae sinensis Radix (*dāng guī*) 30g 3-9g
processed Polygalae Radix (*zhì yuǎn zhì*) 3-6g
Zingiberis Rhizoma recens (*shēng jiāng*)...................... 3 slices
Jujubae Fructus (*dà zǎo*).. 4 pieces

Actions: augments the qi • tonifies the blood • strengthens the Spleen • nourishes the Heart

Main patterns: Spleen and Heart qi and blood deficiency • Spleen unable to govern the blood • Heart failing to nourish the spirit

Key symptoms: forgetfulness • palpitations • unwarranted worrying • insomnia • reduced appetite • chronic bleeding • pallid and wan complexion

Secondary symptoms: anxiety and phobia • insomnia • panic • dream-disturbed sleep • feverishness • night sweats • withdrawal • dizziness • headaches • heavy and tired limbs • reduced vitality

Tongue: pale body • thin coating

Pulse: thin • frail

Abdomen: weak abdomen • tenderness on pressure in epigastrium • palpable pulsations

▶ CLINICAL NOTES

- There are many formulas that treat blood deficiency. This one is specific for deficiency of Spleen qi and Heart blood that causes the unnourished spirit to lose the comfort of its abode. This gives rise to symptoms such as insomnia, palpitations, and anxiety. Because the Spleen qi is weak, the patient affected by this pattern also presents with impaired digestion.

- In addition, this formula treats bleeding due to the Spleen losing its ability to control the blood. In women this may present as mid-cycle bleeding, menorrhagia, frequent or prolonged periods with copious, pale blood, or scanty blood flow.

Contraindications: none noted

▶ FORMULAS WITH SIMILAR INDICATIONS

Prepared Licorice Decoction (*zhì gān cǎo tāng*): Harmonizes the nutritive and protective qi in a patient whose qi and blood are both deficient. Treats irregular pulse, insomnia, dryness, and deficiency-type wind patterns.

Four-Substance Decoction (*sì wù tāng*): For Liver blood deficiency with stronger signs of dryness and no signs of Spleen deficiency.

Stabilize Gushing Decoction (*gù chōng tāng*): For severe uterine bleeding where the Spleen's ability to control blood is being overwhelmed.

Sour Jujube Decoction (*suān zǎo rén tāng*): Harmonizes the Liver qi and blood in patterns where Liver-Heart deficiency leads to the blood failing to nourish the Heart. This formula is much less tonifying than Restore the Spleen Decoction (*guī pí tāng*).

*Yellow Earth Decoction (*huáng tǔ tāng*): For patterns of yang deficiency bleeding.

COMPOSITION

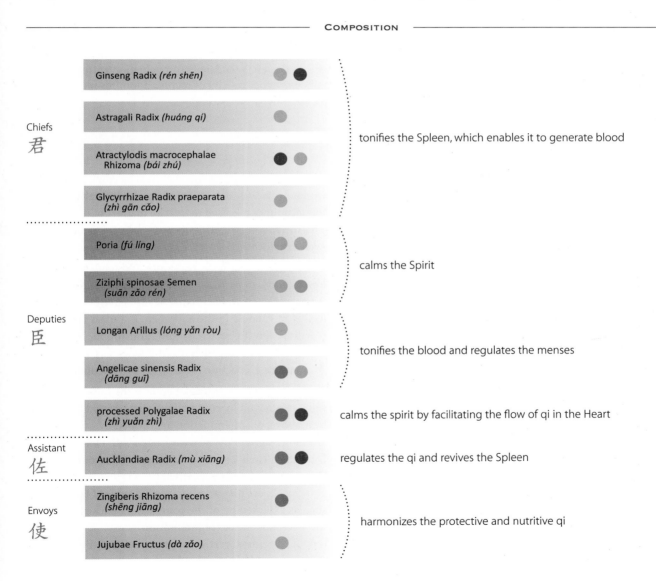

Chiefs
君

- Ginseng Radix (*rén shēn*)
- Astragali Radix (*huáng qí*)
- Atractylodis macrocephalae Rhizoma (*bái zhú*)
- Glycyrrhizae Radix praeparata (*zhì gān cǎo*)

tonifies the Spleen, which enables it to generate blood

Deputies
臣

- Poria (*fú líng*)
- Ziziphi spinosae Semen (*suān zǎo rén*)

calms the Spirit

- Longan Arillus (*lóng yǎn ròu*)
- Angelicae sinensis Radix (*dāng guī*)

tonifies the blood and regulates the menses

- processed Polygalae Radix (*zhì yuǎn zhì*)

calms the spirit by facilitating the flow of qi in the Heart

Assistant
佐

- Aucklandiae Radix (*mù xiāng*)

regulates the qi and revives the Spleen

Envoys
使

- Zingiberis Rhizoma recens (*shēng jiāng*)
- Jujubae Fructus (*dà zǎo*)

harmonizes the protective and nutritive qi

桂枝茯苓丸
Cinnamon Twig and Poria Pill
guì zhī fú líng wán

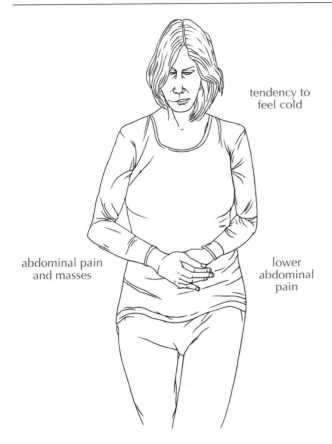

tendency to feel cold

abdominal pain and masses

lower abdominal pain

INGREDIENTS

Cinnamomi Ramulus (*guì zhī*) 9g
Poria (*fú líng*) 9g
[1]Paeoniae Radix (*sháo yào*) 9g
Moutan Cortex (*mǔ dān pí*) 9g
Persicae Semen (*táo rén*) 9g

Actions: invigorates the blood • transforms blood stasis • reduces fixed abdominal masses

Main pattern: blood stasis in the lower abdomen

---

1. As the primary function here is to invigorate the blood, expel stagnation, and stop pain, Paeoniae Radix rubra *(chì sháo)* is preferred.

Key symptoms: lower abdominal pain • pain and masses associated with a variety of gynecological disorders • tendency to feel cold

Secondary symptoms: headaches • dizziness • neck tension or stiffness • hot flushes with cold feet • bruising

Tongue: dark body • stasis spots • distended sublingual veins

Pulse: wiry or rough and deep

Abdomen: pain on palpation in the lower abdomen (more severe on the left) • tenderness on palpation around the umbilicus • hypertonicity of rectus abdominis muscle in the lower abdomen

▶ CLINICAL NOTES

• Although originally intended to treat bleeding in pregnant women that was accompanied by abdominal masses, in modern times it is used to treat all manner of blood stasis. This includes menstrual disorders, abdominal masses, and even extends to systemic circulatory disorders.

• A key clinical marker is resistance and tenderness in the lower abdomen on palpation, most commonly on the left. Alternatively, patients themselves may have a subjective feeling of fullness in the abdomen. If a mass is palpated, it will be tender, relatively soft, and mobile versus the very hard and completely fixed masses that occur in an Appropriate Decoction (*dǐ dàng tāng*) presentation.

• Another important clinical marker is the presence of heat signs in a generally cold patient, such as cold below and heat above, or inflammation aggravated by cold without any of the signs of dryness associated with Flow-Warming Decoction (*wēn jīng tāng*) or dampness associated with Tangkuei and Peony Powder (*dāng guī sháo yào sǎn*) patterns. There may also be systemic signs of blood stasis such as a darkening of the complexion, dark rings under the eyes, increased pigmentation, stasis spots on the tongue, dizziness, vertigo, spots in front of the eyes, and stiffness or pain in the shoulder.

Contraindications: use with caution during pregnancy or postpartum

► FORMULAS WITH SIMILAR INDICATIONS

Peach Pit Decoction to Order the Qi (*táo hé chéng qì tāng*): For blood stasis in the lower abdomen with yang excess, as reflected in signs of dryness and heat and a forceful pulse.

Tangkuei and Peony Powder (*dāng guī sháo yào sǎn*): For blood stasis in the lower abdomen in the context of blood deficiency and water buildup.

Flow-Warming Decoction (*wēn jīng tāng*): For blood stasis in the lower abdomen due to cold in patients who show signs of dryness and upward flushing of heat.

───────────── COMPOSITION ─────────────

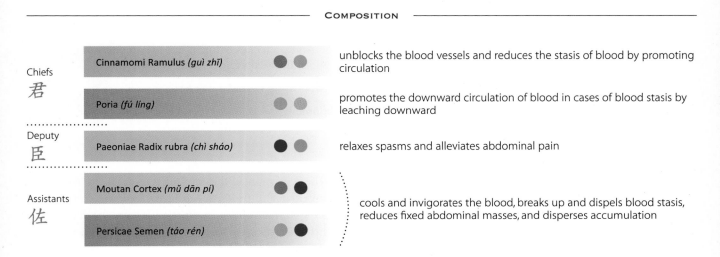

Chiefs
君

Cinnamomi Ramulus *(guì zhī)* — unblocks the blood vessels and reduces the stasis of blood by promoting circulation

Poria *(fú líng)* — promotes the downward circulation of blood in cases of blood stasis by leaching downward

Deputy
臣

Paeoniae Radix rubra *(chì sháo)* — relaxes spasms and alleviates abdominal pain

Assistants
佐

Moutan Cortex *(mǔ dān pí)*

Persicae Semen *(táo rén)*

cools and invigorates the blood, breaks up and dispels blood stasis, reduces fixed abdominal masses, and disperses accumulation

桂枝湯（桂枝汤）
Cinnamon Twig Decoction
guì zhī tang

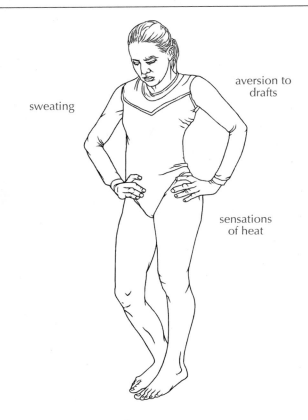

sweating

aversion to drafts

sensations of heat

INGREDIENTS

Cinnamomi Ramulus (*guì zhī*)... 9g
Paeoniae Radix alba (*bái sháo*)... 9g
Zingiberis Rhizoma recens (*shēng jiāng*)............................ 9g
Jujubae Fructus (*dà zǎo*).. 3-4 pieces
Glycyrrhizae Radix praeparata (*zhì gān cǎo*)........................ 6g

Actions: releases pathogens from the muscle layer and regulates the nutritive and protective qi

Main patterns: externally-contracted wind-cold or wind attack (中風 *zhòng fēng*) at the greater yang stage • imbalance of nutritive and protective qi or of yin and yang, qi and blood

Key symptoms: aversion to drafts (including intolerance of drafts or open windows and needing to wear a scarf or other protective clothing) • daytime or nighttime sweating (usually spontaneous or triggered by activity, stress, or wind) • fever or other heat symptoms (triggered by wind-cold)

Secondary symptoms: headache • stiff neck • nasal congestion • aching and pain in the extremities (especially arms and shoulders) • dry heaves • flushing • constipation

Tongue: While many modern textbooks state that the patient will have a white coating, this is not necessarily the case. And if a white coating is due to dampness or phlegm, this formula is contraindicated.

Pulse: floating • either lax or frail

Abdomen: tension in the rectus abdominis muscle

► CLINICAL NOTES

- The key feature of this formula is its ability to harmonize nutritive and protective qi in the exterior, and yin and yang in the interior, in situations where the yang qi has become relatively hyperactive and the yin qi relatively deficient and blocked.

- Hyperactivity of protective qi (yang) manifests as heat in the form of fever, rashes, allergic reactions, muscle tension, etc., or as rebellious qi or qi that cannot be contained manifesting in sweating, dry retching, flushes, and a floating pulse.

- Deficiency of nutritive qi (yin) refers to an inhibition of the normal movement of the nutritive aspect within the vessels. This may imply some true deficiency, but also may be due to obstruction by cold inhibiting physiological movement and manifesting in headache, body aches, a stiff neck, or the aggravation of symptoms by cold. In some cases it may even present as constipation.

- Cinnamon Twig Decoction (*guì zhī tāng*) patients are typically thin, hypersensitive, overexcitable, and averse to wind-cold.

Contraindications: cases with exterior cold and interior heat • significant internal dampness

Note: If mistakenly prescribed, nosebleed, profuse sweating, high fever, severe thirst, palpitations, and irritability may result. In such cases, White Tiger plus Ginseng Decoction (*bái hǔ jiā rén shēn tāng*) is an appropriate follow-up formula.

▶ FORMULAS WITH SIMILAR INDICATIONS

Ephedra Decotion (*má huáng tāng*): For greater yang cold-damage disorder with fever and chills in the absence of sweating and with a floating, tight pulse.

Kudzu Decoction (*gé gēn tāng*): For a yang brightness channel disorder with pronounced head/neck symptoms and a floating, excessive pulse.

Augmented Cyperus and Perilla Leaf Powder (*jiā wei xiāng sū sǎn*): For common cold in children or weak patients or where diagnosis is not clear; usually presents with some digestive discomfort.

──────────── COMPOSITION ────────────

Chief 君	Cinnamomi Ramulus (*guì zhī*)	promotes sweating, resolves the muscle layer, warms and unblocks the nutritive qi and the vessels
Deputy 臣	Paeoniae Radix alba (*bái sháo*)	augments the function of the nutritive qi
Assistants 佐	Zingiberis Rhizoma recens (*shēng jiāng*)	releases the exterior, disperses cold, warms the yang
	Jujubae Fructus (*dà zǎo*)	augments the qi, generates fluids
Envoy 使	Glycyrrhizae Radix praeparata (*zhì gān cǎo*)	harmonizes the effects of the other ingredients

滾痰丸
Flushing Away Roiling Phlegm Pill
gǔn tán wán

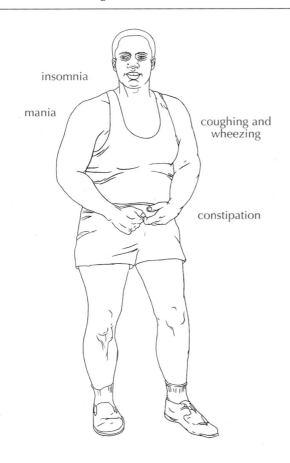

insomnia

mania

coughing and wheezing

constipation

INGREDIENTS

calcined Chloriti Lapis/Micae Lapis aureus (*duàn méng shí*) 30g
wine-washed Rhei Radix et Rhizoma (*jiǔ xǐ dà huáng*) 240g
wine-washed Scutellariae Radix (*jiǔ xǐ huáng qín*) 240g
Aquilariae Lignum resinatum (*chén xiāng*) 5g

Preparation notes: Powder the ingredients and make into pills with water. The normal dosage is 6-9g taken 1-2 times a day with warm water.

Actions: drains fire • drives out phlegm

Main pattern: excess fire with chronic phlegm

Key symptoms: constipation • mania or confusion • insomnia • strange dreams • palpitations • coughing and wheezing with thick, viscous sputum • vertigo • tinnitus

Secondary symptoms: focal distention • stifling sensation in the chest and epigastrium • facial tics • deep pain in the joints • nodules in the neck

Tongue: old, yellow, thick coating

Pulse: slippery • rapid • forceful

Abdomen: discomfort in epigastrium • palpable accumulations around the umbilicus but no pain on pressure

▶ CLINICAL NOTES

- This formula was composed to treat phlegm patterns that mutate to produce a large range of strange symptoms. In modern terms these might be labeled epilepsy, schizophrenia, bipolar disorder, depression, anxiety, or sleep-walking. However, the formula can also be used for more commonly seen disorders such as migraines, dizziness, or chronic cough. The key clinical markers are constipation and a yellow, old-looking tongue coating.

Contraindications: pregnancy and postpartum • deficiency conditions

▶ FORMULAS WITH SIMILAR INDICATIONS

Warm Gallbladder Decoction (*wēn dǎn tāng*): For phlegm causing constraint in the middle burner and flanks (Stomach and Gallbladder). This may manifest with similar symptoms but without constipation and with a slippery, white or slightly yellow tongue coating.

Major Order the Qi Decoction (*dà chéng qì tāng*): For yang brightness interior, excess-heat patterns that manifest with constipation, mania, or agitation. The pulse in this pattern is deep and excessive, the tongue coating is dry, and the abdomen is distended and painful when pressed.

--- COMPOSITION ---

Chief 君	calcined Chloriti Lapis/Micae Lapis aureus *(duàn méng shí)*	● ●	strongly drives phlegm retained in the Stomach and Intestines downward and out of the body; directs the qi downward to calm wheezing, arrests palpitations, pacifies the Liver, and suppresses jitteriness and convulsions
Deputy 臣	wine-washed Rhei Radix et Rhizoma *(jiǔ xǐ dà huáng)*	●	cleanses fire from the upper burner by directing it downward through the Large Intestine in the lower burner, unblocks the obstruction of the yang organs
Assistants 佐	wine-washed Scutellariae Radix *(jiǔ xǐ huáng qín)*	●	clears fire from the upper burner to prevent it from scorching the fluids and thereby generating more phlegm
	Aquilariae Lignum resinatum *(chén xiāng)*	● ● ●	regulates the qi and opens constraint, rapidly directing the rebellious qi downward in order to eliminate the phlegm; its warming nature slightly buffers the cooling action of the three other ingredients in order to protect the normal qi

蒿芩清膽湯（蒿芩清胆汤）
Sweet Wormwood and Scutellaria Decoction to Clear the Gallbladder
hāo qín qīng dǎn tāng

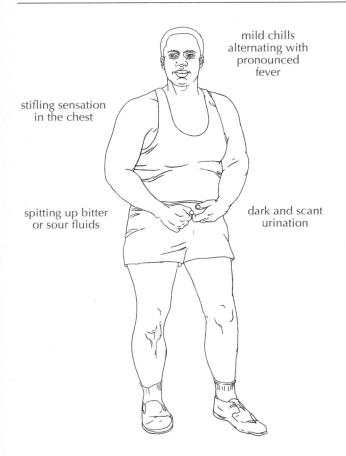

mild chills alternating with pronounced fever

stifling sensation in the chest

spitting up bitter or sour fluids

dark and scant urination

INGREDIENTS

Artemisiae annuae Herba (*qīng hāo*) 4.5-6g
Scutellariae Radix (*huáng qín*) 4.5-9g
Bambusae Caulis in taeniam (*zhú rú*) 9g
Aurantii Fructus (*zhǐ ké*) 4.5g
Citri reticulatae Pericarpium (*chén pí*) 4.5g
Pinelliae Rhizoma praeparatum (*zhì bàn xià*) 4.5g
Poria rubra (*chì fú líng*) 9g
Talcum (*huá shí*) 6g
Glycyrrhizae Radix (*gān cǎo*) 1g

Indigo naturalis (*qīng dài*) 2g

Preparation notes: The last three of these ingredients, also known as Jasper Powder (*bì yù sǎn*), should be ground into a powder, placed in a cheesecloth bag, and cooked with the other ingredients.

Actions: clears Gallbladder heat • harmonizes the Stomach qi • resolves dampness • transforms phlegm

Main pattern: damp-heat and phlegm turbidity in the lesser yang channels constraining the qi dynamic

Key symptoms: mild chills alternating with pronounced fever • stifling sensation in the chest • spitting up bitter or sour fluids • focal distention and pain in the chest and hypochondrium • dark and scant urination

Secondary symptoms: bitter taste in the mouth • thirst, with or without a desire to drink • vomiting yellow, brackish fluids • dry heaves

Tongue: red body with a thick, greasy coating • coating is usually white but may be yellow or a mixture of both colors

Pulse: rapid • slippery on the right and wiry on the left

Abdomen: focal distention in the chest and epigastrium

► CLINICAL NOTES

• Originally used for malarial disorders, this formula is now prescribed for a wide range of acute and chronic inflammatory disorders presenting with symptoms of heat, phlegm, and dampness including cholecystitis, icteric hepatitis, pyelonephritis, malaria, typhoid, pelvic inflammatory disease, and pneumonia.

• Clears phlegm, heat, and dampness from the lesser yang channels in connection with symptoms such as tinnitus, deafness, dizziness, jaundice, hemorrhoids, or urinary obstruction.

• Can also be used to treat systemic manifestations of damp-heat such as night sweats, hot flushes, palpitations, or sleep disorders.

Contraindications: phlegm-dampness due to yang deficiency

▶ FORMULAS WITH SIMILAR INDICATIONS

Minor Bupleurum Decoction (*xiǎo chái hú tāng*): For cold invading the lesser yang with pronounced chills in addition to feverishness, vomiting of acidic fluids or expectoration of white or clear rather than yellow and sticky sputum, and a wiry rather than slippery and rapid pulse.

COMPOSITION

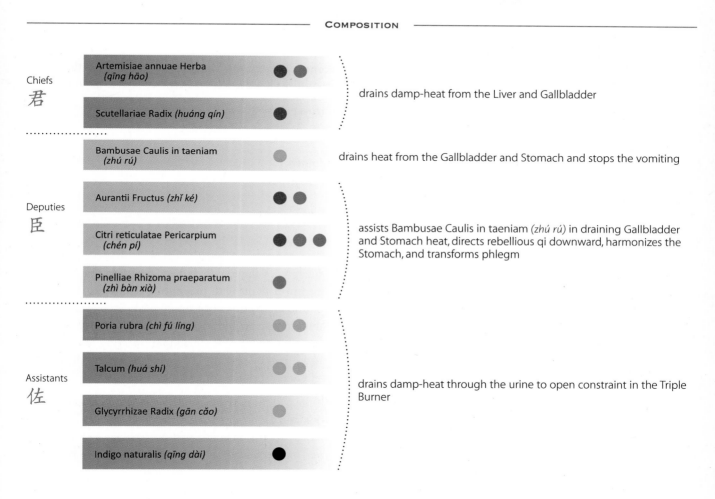

Chiefs
君

Artemisiae annuae Herba
(*qīng hāo*)

Scutellariae Radix (*huáng qín*)

drains damp-heat from the Liver and Gallbladder

Bambusae Caulis in taeniam
(*zhú rú*)

drains heat from the Gallbladder and Stomach and stops the vomiting

Deputies
臣

Aurantii Fructus (*zhǐ ké*)

Citri reticulatae Pericarpium
(*chén pí*)

Pinelliae Rhizoma praeparatum
(*zhì bàn xià*)

assists Bambusae Caulis in taeniam (*zhú rú*) in draining Gallbladder and Stomach heat, directs rebellious qi downward, harmonizes the Stomach, and transforms phlegm

Assistants
佐

Poria rubra (*chì fú líng*)

Talcum (*huá shí*)

Glycyrrhizae Radix (*gān cǎo*)

Indigo naturalis (*qīng dài*)

drains damp-heat through the urine to open constraint in the Triple Burner

厚樸溫中湯（厚朴温中汤）
Magnolia Bark Decoction for Warming the Middle
hòu pò wēn zhōng tāng

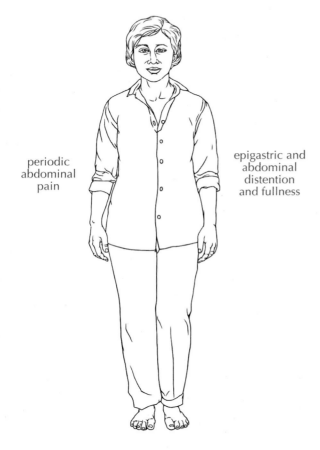

periodic abdominal pain

epigastric and abdominal distention and fullness

INGREDIENTS

Ginger-fried Magnoliae officinalis Cortex (*jiāng hòu pò*) . 9-15g

Alpiniae katsumadai Semen (*cǎo dòu kòu*) 6-9g

Citri reticulatae Pericarpium (*chén pí*)............................. 9-15g

Aucklandiae Radix (*mù xiāng*)... 6-9g

Zingiberis Rhizoma (*gān jiāng*)..................................... 1.5-6g

Poria (*fú líng*)... 9-12g

Glycyrrhizae Radix praeparata (*zhì gān cǎo*) 3-9g

Zingiberis Rhizoma recens (*shēng jiāng*).......................... 6-9g

Actions: promotes the movement of qi • eliminates fullness • dries dampness • warms the middle burner

Main pattern: dampness obstructing the middle burner with Spleen and Stomach excess cold

Key symptoms: epigastric and abdominal distention and fullness • periodic abdominal pain • vomiting of clear liquid

Secondary symptoms: loss of appetite • fatigue in the extremities • loose stools or diarrhea • cold extremities

Tongue: pale body • white, slippery coating

Pulse: slow

Abdomen: focal distention in the epigastrium • abdominal distention but soft abdomen

► CLINICAL NOTES

• This formula is specific for cold obstructing the qi dynamic of the middle burner, a pattern that is usually seen in patients with preexisting dampness who ingest cold food or drink. The key clinical markers are sudden abdominal pain and a feeling of distention that responds favorably to warmth (including warming foods) but is aggravated by pressure. The pain and distention are also relieved by belching or passing of gas.

• If the pattern is accompanied by long-term food stagnation and even more severe pain, one can add herbs that reduce food stagnation such as Crataegi Fructus (*shān zhā*) or Massa medicata fermentata (*shén qū*), or herbs that warm the Stomach such as Alpiniae officinarum Rhizoma (*gāo liáng jiāng*).

• If there is concomitant Liver qi stagnation with Liver qi invading the Stomach, one may add such herbs as Cyperi Rhizoma (*xiāng fù*), Evodiae Fructus (*wú zhū yú*), or Sepiae Endoconcha (*hǎi piāo xiāo*). For severe rebelliousness with vomiting of clear fluid, one may add herbs like Pinelliae Rhizoma praeparatum (*zhì bàn xià*) or Bambusae Caulis in taeniam (*zhú rú*).

Contraindications: qi deficiency • yin deficiency

▶ FORMULAS WITH SIMILAR INDICATIONS

*Galangal and Cyperus Pill (*liáng fù wán*): Focuses on abdominal pain and distention in patterns that involve stagnation and disharmony of Liver and Stomach qi.

Regulate the Middle Pill (*lǐ zhōng wán*): For abdominal distention due to dampness and deficiency cold of the middle burner.

Six-Gentlemen Decoction (*liù jūn zǐ tāng*): For deficiency cold of the Spleen and Stomach accompanied by symptoms of phlegm and dampness. This formula emphasizes treatment of the root deficiency and is therefore generally used for chronic conditions. By contrast, Magnolia Bark Decoction for Warming the Middle (*hòu pò wēn zhōng tāng*) focusses more on treating the branches of cold, dampness, and stagnation, and is used for more acute cases.

─────── COMPOSITION ───────

Chiefs 君	Ginger-fried Magnoliae officinalis Cortex (*jiāng hòu pò*)	● ●	warms the middle burner, dries dampness, promotes the descent of qi, and expands the chest
	Citri reticulatae Pericarpium (*chén pí*)	● ● ●	moves the qi, particularly in the upper and middle burners, dries dampness, and harmonizes the middle burner
Deputy 臣	Alpiniae katsumadai Semen (*cǎo dòu kòu*)	● ●	disperses cold and dries dampness
	Aucklandiae Radix (*mù xiāng*)	● ●	promotes the movement of qi, expands the chest, and stops the pain
Assistants 佐	Zingiberis Rhizoma (*gān jiāng*)	●	warms the Spleen, harmonizes the Stomach, and disperses cold
	Zingiberis Rhizoma recens (*shēng jiāng*)	●	
	Poria (*fú líng*)	● ●	strengthens the Spleen, leaches out dampness, and harmonizes the functions of the middle burner
	Glycyrrhizae Radix praeparata (*zhì gān cǎo*)	●	

虎潛丸 (虎潜丸)
Hidden Tiger Pill
hŭ qían wán

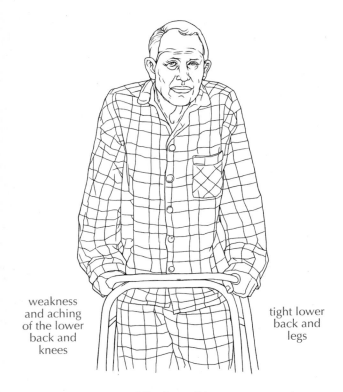

weakness
and aching
of the lower
back and
knees

tight lower
back and
legs

difficulty walking

the original formulation. Note that some pills with this name contain Canis Os (*gŏu gŭ*) as a substitute and that commercial powders substitute Cyathulae Radix (*chuān niú xī*) and Angelicae sinensis Radix (*dāng guī*) instead.

Actions: enriches the yin • directs fire downward • strengthens the sinews and bones

Main pattern: atrophy disorder due to Liver and Kidney deficiency

Key symptoms: weakness and aching of the lower back and knees • tight lower back and legs • difficulty walking

Secondary symptoms: wasting of the muscles of the legs and feet • dizziness • tinnitus • spontaneous emissions • urinary incontinence

Tongue: red body • scanty or no yellow coating

Pulse: thin • frail

Abdomen: no specific signs

▶ CLINICAL NOTES

- This formula primarily treats tightness and contraction of the sinews in the lower back and legs caused by fire from Kidney deficiency. The fire consumes the essence and marrow and causes the sinews to contract.
- Can also be used for other manifestations of Kidney deficiency fire such as dizziness, tinnitus, spontaneous emissions, and urinary incontinence.

Contraindications: damp-heat patterns

▶ FORMULAS WITH SIMILAR INDICATIONS

Two-Marvel Powder (*èr miào săn*): For damp-heat patterns leading to wasting of the muscles in the lower extremities.

Great Tonify the Yin Pill (*dà bŭ yīn wán*): For yin deficiency fire where the fire flares upward harassing the Heart with such symptoms as night sweats, tinnitus, or irritability.

INGREDIENTS

wine-fried Phellodendri Cortex (*jiŭ chăo huáng băi*) 9g
wine-fried Anemarrhenae Rhizoma (*jiŭ chăo zhī mŭ*).......... 9g
Rehmanniae Radix praeparata (*shú dì huáng*) 12g
wine-fried Testudinis Plastrum (*jiŭ chăo guī băn*).............. 12g
Paeoniae Radix alba (*bái sháo*)... 6g
Cynomorii Herba (*suŏ yáng*) 6g
Cervi Cornus Colla (*lù jiǎo jiāo*)... 6g
Zingiberis Rhizoma (*gān jiāng*)... 1.5g
Citri reticulatae Pericarpium (*chén pí*)................................. 6g

Preparation notes: Cervi Cornus Colla (*lù jiǎo jiāo*) is a commonly-used substitute for Tigris Os (*hŭ gŭ*) that was used in

COMPOSITION

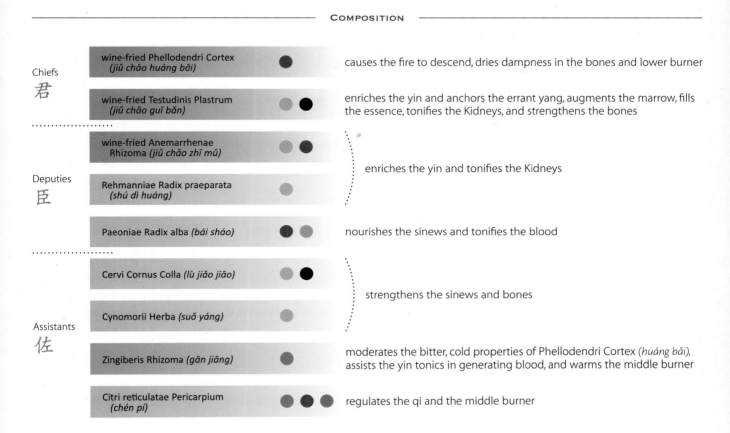

Chiefs
君

wine-fried Phellodendri Cortex
(jiŭ chăo huáng băi)
causes the fire to descend, dries dampness in the bones and lower burner

wine-fried Testudinis Plastrum
(jiŭ chăo guī băn)
enriches the yin and anchors the errant yang, augments the marrow, fills the essence, tonifies the Kidneys, and strengthens the bones

Deputies
臣

wine-fried Anemarrhenae Rhizoma *(jiŭ chăo zhī mŭ)*

Rehmanniae Radix praeparata
(shú dì huáng)
enriches the yin and tonifies the Kidneys

Paeoniae Radix alba *(bái sháo)*
nourishes the sinews and tonifies the blood

Assistants
佐

Cervi Cornus Colla *(lù jiăo jiāo)*

Cynomorii Herba *(suŏ yáng)*
strengthens the sinews and bones

Zingiberis Rhizoma *(gān jiāng)*
moderates the bitter, cold properties of Phellodendri Cortex *(huáng băi)*, assists the yin tonics in generating blood, and warms the middle burner

Citri reticulatae Pericarpium
(chén pí)
regulates the qi and the middle burner

黄連解毒湯（黄连解毒汤）
Coptis Decoction to Resolve Toxicity
huáng lián jiě dú tāng

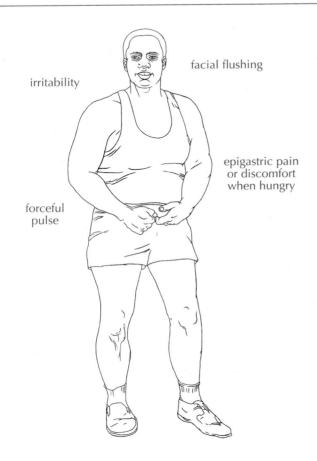

irritability

facial flushing

epigastric pain or discomfort when hungry

forceful pulse

--- INGREDIENTS ---

Coptidis Rhizoma (*huáng lián*) 9g
Scutellariae Radix (*huáng qín*) 6g
Phellodendri Cortex (*huáng bǎi*)... 6g
Gardeniae Fructus (*zhī zǐ*)... 6-12g

Actions: drains fire • resolves toxicity

Main patterns: fire toxin or overwhelming excess heat in any or all of the three burners

Key symptoms: fever • irritability • facial flushing • epigastric pain or discomfort when hungry

Secondary symptoms: insomnia • nosebleed, vomiting of blood, blood in the stools, or increased menstrual bleeding due to qi aspect heat excess • bad breath • carbuncles and furuncles • itching • toxic swellings • diarrhea or constipation • dark urine

Tongue: tip and sides very red • may have a yellow coating

Pulse: forceful and rapid • flooding and large

Abdomen: discomfort and pain on palpation in the epigastrium • hypertonicity of rectus abdominis muscle in the upper abdomen

▶ CLINICAL NOTES

- The name of the formula points toward its main function, namely, to rid the body of toxic heat. The herbs in the formula act on all three burners and can therefore be used to eliminate qi aspect excess heat, qi aspect heat causing the blood to move chaotically, or damp-heat in the Heart, Liver-Gallbladder, Stomach-Spleen, or Bladder. A forceful and rapid pulse is a key sign in all of these patterns.

- This is an important formula for draining excess heat that pushes blood toward the exterior where it stagnates, manifesting in itching and inflammation in both the skin and mucous membranes, and eventually bleeding.

- The formula can be used to treat acute fevers as well as flare-ups of chronic conditions characterized by excess heat such as hypertension, insomnia, psychiatric disorders, or menopausal hot flushes.

- The formula is extremely bitter and cooling. Some physicians advise to take the decocted formula only after it has cooled down to room temperature to increase its ability to clear heat.

Contraindications: yin deficiency heat • excess cold in the middle burner • qi deficiency

▶ FORMULAS WITH SIMILAR INDICATIONS

White Tiger Decoction (*bái hǔ tāng*): For qi-aspect heat damaging the fluids and leading to dryness. By contrast, the present formula is indicated for damp-heat and for qi-aspect heat entering the blood.

*Drain the Epigastrium Decoction (*xiè xīn tāng*): For a similar pattern with very pronounced upward flushing of heat leading to bleeding from the orifices of the upper body.

Major Order the Qi Decoction (*dà chéng qì tāng*): For upward flushing of heat due to heat clumping in the interior as reflected in constipation and abdominal fullness.

COMPOSITION

Chief
君

Coptidis Rhizoma *(huáng lián)* ● drains fire from the middle burner

Deputy
臣

Scutellariae Radix *(huáng qín)* ● clears heat from the upper burner

Assistants
佐

Phellodendri Cortex *(huáng bǎi)* ● clears heat from the lower burner

Gardeniae Fructus *(zhī zǐ)* ● drains heat from the three burners via the urine, relieves irritability

黃耆桂枝五物湯（黄芪桂枝五物汤）
Astragalus and Cinnamon Twig Five-Substance Decoction
huáng qí guì zhī wǔ wù tāng

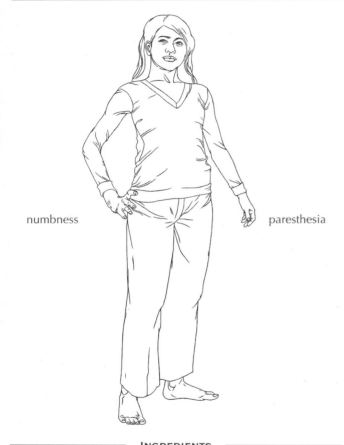

numbness   paresthesia

Main patterns: blood painful obstruction

Key symptoms: numbness • paresthesia (especially in extremities)

Secondary symptoms: aversion to drafts • sweating • mild paralysis • pain in the extremities

Tongue: pale with a white coating

Pulse: faint in the distal and mid positions • choppy and tight in the proximal positions

Abdomen: hypertonicity of the rectus abdominis muscle

▶ CLINICAL NOTES

• In modern times, with appropriate modifications, this formula is used to treat chronic painful obstruction patterns presenting with pain as a main symptom. For example, Curcumae longae Rhizoma (*jiāng huáng*) and Notopterygii Rhizoma seu Radix (*qiāng huó*) can be added to treat chronic shoulder pain. Typically the pain in these patterns will come and go and is aggravated by cold. There will also be signs of qi deficiency in the exterior such as aversion to drafts.

• Treats impairment of circulation in the periphery due to penetration of wind, cold, and dampness at a superficial level. It is thus primarily indicated for numbness and paresthesia such as that occurring suddenly in the course of transient ischemic attacks, or chronically in conditions such as diabetes, chilblains, peripheral neuropathy, or multiple sclerosis.

Contraindications: any condition involving internal Liver wind

▶ FORMULAS WITH SIMILAR INDICATIONS

Tangkuei Decoction for Frigid Extremities (*dāng guī sì nì tāng*): For more pronounced cold, reflected in long-standing cold in the extremities, with blood rather than qi deficiency, reflected in a submerged and thin or imperceptible pulse.

INGREDIENTS

Astragali Radix (*huáng qí*) 9-12g

[1]Paeoniae Radix (*sháo yào*) 9g

Cinnamomi Ramulus (*guì zhī*) 9g

Zingiberis Rhizoma recens (*shēng jiāng*)...................... 12-18g

Jujubae Fructus (*dà zǎo*).. 4 pieces

Actions: augments the qi • warms and harmonizes the channels • unblocks painful obstruction

---

1. As the primary function here is to restrain, tonify, or soften, Paeoniae Radix alba (*bái sháo*) is preferred.

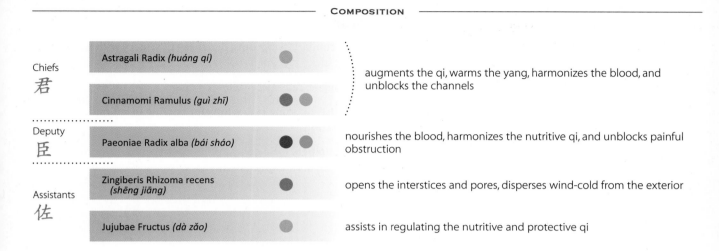

COMPOSITION

Chiefs
君

Astragali Radix *(huáng qí)*

augments the qi, warms the yang, harmonizes the blood, and unblocks the channels

Cinnamomi Ramulus *(guì zhī)*

Deputy
臣

Paeoniae Radix alba *(bái sháo)*

nourishes the blood, harmonizes the nutritive qi, and unblocks painful obstruction

Assistants
佐

Zingiberis Rhizoma recens *(shēng jiāng)*

opens the interstices and pores, disperses wind-cold from the exterior

Jujubae Fructus *(dà zǎo)*

assists in regulating the nutritive and protective qi

黃芩湯（黄芩汤）
Scutellaria Decoction
huáng qín tāng

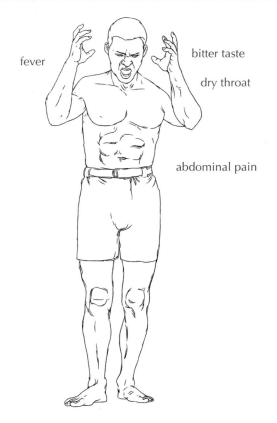

fever

bitter taste

dry throat

abdominal pain

INGREDIENTS

Scutellariae Radix (*huáng qín*) 9g

¹Paeoniae Radix (*sháo yào*) 9g

Glycyrrhizae Radix praeparata (*zhì gān cǎo*) 3-6g

Jujubae Fructus (*dà zǎo*) .... 4 pieces

Actions: clears heat • alleviates dysenteric disorders • harmonizes the middle burner • stops pain

Main patterns: diarrhea or dysenteric disorder caused by heat constraint in the lesser yang that overcomes the Stomach and Intestines

---

1. As the primary function here is to restrain and contain, Paeoniae Radix alba (*bái sháo*) is preferred.

Key symptoms: fever • bitter taste • dry throat • abdominal pain

Secondary symptoms: diarrhea • dysentery with pus, blood, or sticky phlegm

Tongue: red sides • yellow coating

Pulse: flooding • wiry, forceful, stirring in left middle position

Abdomen: focal distention in epigastrium • hypertonicity of rectus abdominis muscle

▶ CLINICAL NOTES

- This is constrained interior heat excess in the lesser yang warp. To drain heat from the interior, the body forces this heat into the Stomach and Intestines where it causes diarrhea and dysentery. This can occur in the course of feverish disorders or in those unrelated to exterior patterns.

- The formula is also used to treat fevers due to heat at the qi level arising from retained pathogens. Such patterns are characterized by fever, a deep rather than superficial pulse at the onset, and no aversion to cold, differentiating this pattern from greater yang stage fevers as well as newly-contracted warm pathogens at the protective level of the lesser yin.

Contraindications: initial stages of dysenteric or feverish disorders with pronounced exterior symptoms • cold or deficiency patterns

▶ FORMULAS WITH SIMILAR INDICATIONS

Kudzu, Scutellaria, and Coptis Decoction (*gé gēn huáng qín huáng lián tang*): For hot dysenteric disorders arising from heat in the greater yang channel (as reflected in such symptoms as neck stiffness or headache accompanying the diarrhea) that attacks the interior.

*Peony Decoction (*sháo yào tāng*): For conditions with less heat but more pronounced qi stagnation as reflected in abdominal pain and tenesmus.

COMPOSITION

| Chief 君 | Scutellariae Radix *(huáng qín)* | ● | drains heat from the lesser yang and yang brightness, resolves toxicity, and stops dysentery and diarrhea |

| Deputy 臣 | Paeoniae Radix alba *(bái sháo)* | ● ● | drains heat from the middle burner, astringes and contains the yin |

| Assis/Env 佐/使 | Glycyrrhizae Radix praeparata *(zhì gān căo)* | ● | harmonizes the middle burner, augments the qi, and enriches the yin |
| | Jujubae Fructus *(dà zăo)* | ● | |

藿香正氣散 （藿香正气散）
Patchouli/Agastache Powder to Rectify the Qi
huò xiāng zhèng qì sǎn

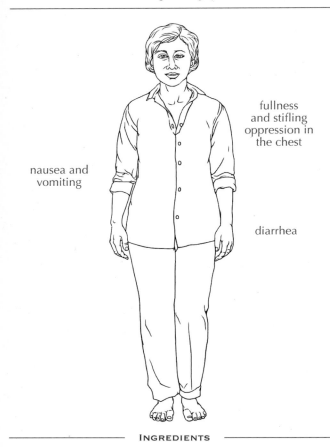

fullness and stifling oppression in the chest

nausea and vomiting

diarrhea

INGREDIENTS

Pogostemonis/Agastaches Herba (*huò xiāng*)....................... 9g
ginger-fried Magnoliae officinalis Cortex (*jiāng chǎo hòu pò*) 9g
Citri reticulatae Pericarpium (*chén pí*)................................. 9g
Perillae Folium (*zǐ sū yè*)... 9g
Angelicae dahuricae Radix (*bái zhǐ*) 9g
Pinelliae Rhizoma praeparatum (*zhì bàn xià*)..................... 12g
Arecae Pericarpium (*dà fù pí*) 15g
Atractylodis macrocephalae Rhizoma (*bái zhú*) 9g
Poria (*fú líng*) 15g
Platycodi Radix (*jié gěng*)... 9g
Glycyrrhizae Radix praeparata (*zhì gān cǎo*) 3g
Zingiberis Rhizoma recens (*shēng jiāng*)............................. 3g

Jujubae Fructus (*dà zǎo*)... 1 piece

Preparation notes: Decoct for just 10-20 minutes.

Actions: releases the exterior • transforms dampness • regulates the qi • harmonizes the middle burner

Main pattern: externally-contracted wind-cold with concurrent dampness and stagnation in the middle burner

Key symptoms: fullness and stifling oppression in the chest • nausea and vomiting • diarrhea

Secondary symptoms: fever and chills • headache • pain in the epigastrium and abdomen • loss of taste • borborygmus

Tongue: white, greasy coating

Pulse: moderate • slippery

Abdomen: distention and discomfort in epigastrium and abdomen

▶ CLINICAL NOTES

• Because the formula simultaneously resolves the exterior and harmonizes the middle burner, it is useful when a person with damp obstruction in the middle burner suffers an attack of wind-cold leading to acute gastrointestinal symptoms such as vomiting and/or diarrhea; or when middle burner dampness is accompanied by pronounced symptoms in the exterior such as headaches and nasal discharge.

• This formula is widely used as a patent medicine for motion sickness.

Contraindications: should not be used without significant modification for disorders due to wind-heat or fire from deficiency

▶ FORMULAS WITH SIMILAR INDICATIONS

Calm the Stomach Powder (*píng wèi sǎn*): For damp obstruction of the qi dynamic of the Spleen and Stomach in the absence of exterior symptoms.

Coptis and Magnolia Bark Drink (*lián pò yǐn*): For acute vomiting and diarrhea due to damp-heat in the middle burner.

COMPOSITION

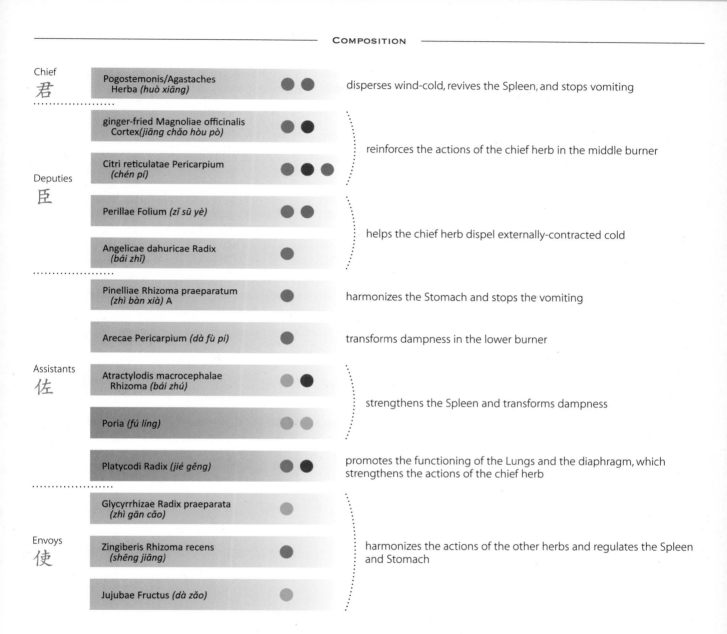

Chief
君

Pogostemonis/Agastaches Herba (huò xiāng) — disperses wind-cold, revives the Spleen, and stops vomiting

Deputies
臣

ginger-fried Magnoliae officinalis Cortex(jiāng chǎo hòu pò)

Citri reticulatae Pericarpium (chén pí) — reinforces the actions of the chief herb in the middle burner

Perillae Folium (zǐ sū yè)

Angelicae dahuricae Radix (bái zhǐ) — helps the chief herb dispel externally-contracted cold

Assistants
佐

Pinelliae Rhizoma praeparatum (zhì bàn xià) A — harmonizes the Stomach and stops the vomiting

Arecae Pericarpium (dà fù pí) — transforms dampness in the lower burner

Atractylodis macrocephalae Rhizoma (bái zhú)

Poria (fú líng) — strengthens the Spleen and transforms dampness

Platycodi Radix (jié gěng) — promotes the functioning of the Lungs and the diaphragm, which strengthens the actions of the chief herb

Envoys
使

Glycyrrhizae Radix praeparata (zhì gān cǎo)

Zingiberis Rhizoma recens (shēng jiāng) — harmonizes the actions of the other herbs and regulates the Spleen and Stomach

Jujubae Fructus (dà zǎo)

濟川煎（济川煎）
Benefit the River [Flow] Decoction
jì chuān jiān

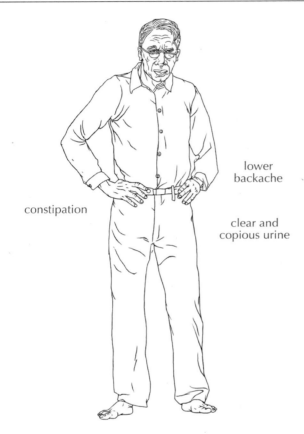

constipation

lower backache

clear and copious urine

Key symptoms: constipation • clear and copious urine • lower backache

Secondary symptoms: generalized weakness and fatigue • cold sensation, especially in back

Tongue: pale body • thin, white coating

Pulse: deep and slow or deep and rough

Abdomen: weak and cold lower abdomen

► CLINICAL NOTES

• Indicated for patients with habitual constipation due to long-term deficiency of the original qi. For severe Kidney deficiency, add Rehmanniae Radix praeparata (*shú dì huáng*); for severe lower back pain, replace Alismatis Rhizoma (*zé xiè*) with Lycii Fructus (*gǒu qǐ zǐ*) and Eucommiae Cortex (*dù zhòng*).

• Also used for post-partum constipation.

Contraindications: constipation due to heat in the Intestines

► FORMULAS WITH SIMILAR INDICATIONS

Hemp Seed Pill (*má zǐ rén wán*): Constipation with increased urination but with heat in the Intestines and an absence of cold signs.

INGREDIENTS

Cistanches Herba (*ròu cōng róng*)......................................6-9g
Angelicae sinensis Radix (*dāng guī*) 9-15g
Achyranthis bidentatae Radix (*niú xī*)................................6g
Alismatis Rhizoma (*zé xiè*) 4.5g
Aurantii Fructus (*zhǐ ké*)..3g
Cimicifugae Rhizoma (*shēng má*)...............................1.5-3g

Actions: warms the Kidneys • nourishes blood • augments essence • moistens the Intestines • unblocks the bowels

Main pattern: constipation due to Kidney deficiency where the Kidneys are unable to transform fluids leading to dryness in the Intestines

COMPOSITION

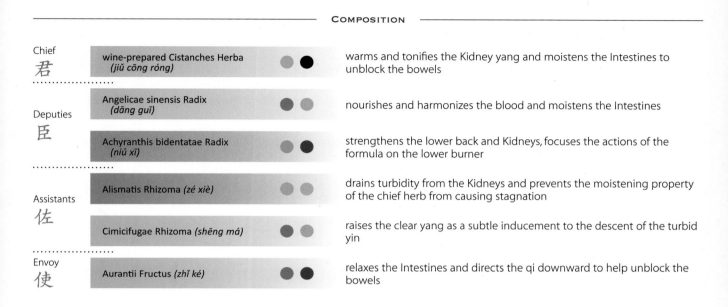

Chief 君	wine-prepared Cistanches Herba (jiǔ cōng róng)		warms and tonifies the Kidney yang and moistens the Intestines to unblock the bowels
Deputies 臣	Angelicae sinensis Radix (dāng guī)		nourishes and harmonizes the blood and moistens the Intestines
	Achyranthis bidentatae Radix (niú xī)		strengthens the lower back and Kidneys, focuses the actions of the formula on the lower burner
Assistants 佐	Alismatis Rhizoma (zé xiè)		drains turbidity from the Kidneys and prevents the moistening property of the chief herb from causing stagnation
	Cimicifugae Rhizoma (shēng má)		raises the clear yang as a subtle inducement to the descent of the turbid yin
Envoy 使	Aurantii Fructus (zhǐ ké)		relaxes the Intestines and directs the qi downward to help unblock the bowels

雞鳴散 （鸡鸣散）
Powder to Take at Cock's Crow
jī míng săn

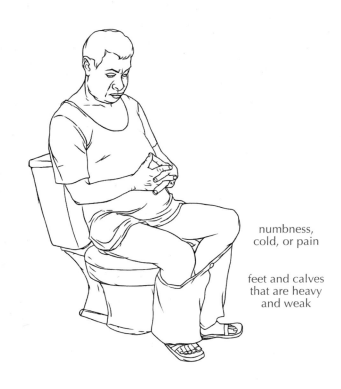

numbness, cold, or pain

feet and calves that are heavy and weak

INGREDIENTS

Arecae Semen (*bīng láng*) 12g

Chaenomelis Fructus (*mù guā*) 15g

Evodiae Fructus (*wú zhū yú*) 6g

Citri reticulatae Pericarpium (*chén pí*) 15g

Perillae Folium (*zǐ sū yè*) 9g

Platycodi Radix (*jié gěng*) 9g

Zingiberis Rhizoma recens (*shēng jiāng*) 9g

Preparation notes: Best taken divided into two doses before breakfast. Some sources recommend making the decoction the night before and then taking it cold the following morning.

Actions: promotes the movement of qi • directs turbidity downward • dissipates and transforms damp-cold

Main pattern: damp leg qi from damp-cold settling in the legs and feet where it clogs the channels and interrupts the smooth flow of qi and blood

Key symptoms: feet and calves that are heavy and weak resulting in difficulty walking • numbness, cold, or pain in the feet or calves • stifling sensation in the chest or upper abdomen

Secondary symptoms: spasms • up-surging of qi from the abdomen to the chest • stifling sensation in the chest • nausea • oozing skin lesions in the lower extremities

Tongue: white, moist coating

Pulse: deep and soft • deep and tense

Abdomen: no specific signs

▶ CLINICAL NOTES

- This formula is specific for damp-cold settling in the lower extremities. Key markers are stiffness, pain, swelling, or cold in the feet and calves as in arthritic conditions, restless leg syndrome, gout, or edema. The pathogen is strong and requires a fierce response. The formula should be taken early in the morning and induce a dark, soft stool. It is not indicated for long-term use.

- Also indicated for damp-cold skin disorders in the lower extremities characterized by oozing, but lacking acute inflammation. If one alters the formula by combining it with such formulas as Two-Marvel Powder (*èr miào săn*) or Coptis Decoction to Resolve Toxicity (*huáng lián jiě dú tāng*), the modification can treat red, hot, itching, or painful damp-heat sores.

Contraindications: leg qi due to dryness • long-term use • pregnancy

▶ FORMULAS WITH SIMILAR INDICATIONS

Licorice, Ginger, Poria, and White Atractylodes Decoction (*gān căo gān jiāng fú líng bái zhú tāng*): Treats damp-cold that affects the lower back and legs. More strongly supplements the Spleen to rid the body of dampness but is less adept at attacking the damp-cold pathogen.

COMPOSITION

Chief
君

Arecae Semen *(bīng láng)* ● ●
breaks up stagnation, directs rebellious qi downward, and eliminates lurking pathogens

Deputies
臣

Chaenomelis Fructus *(mù guā)* ●
transforms dampness, relaxes the sinews, and invigorates the collaterals

Citri reticulatae Pericarpium *(chén pí)* ● ● ●
regulates the qi and strengthens the Spleen, indirectly resolving the dampness

Assistants
佐

Perillae Folium *(zǐ sū yè)* ● ●
disperses wind-cold

Platycodi Radix *(jié gěng)* ● ●
unblocks and disseminates the Lung qi

Envoys
使

Zingiberis Rhizoma recens *(shēng jiāng)* ●
warms and disperses cold and thereby helps treat the leg qi

Evodiae Fructus *(wú zhū yú)* ● ●
disperses cold and causes the turbidity to descend

加味香穌散 （加味香苏散）
Augmented Cyperus and Perilla Leaf Powder
jiā wèi xiāng sū sǎn

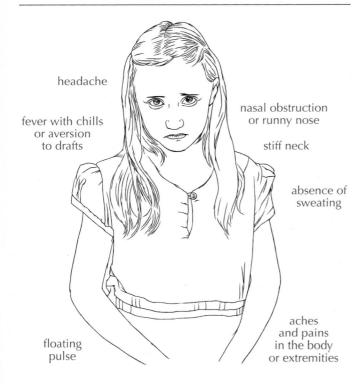

headache

fever with chills
or aversion
to drafts

nasal obstruction
or runny nose

stiff neck

absence of
sweating

floating
pulse

aches
and pains
in the body
or extremities

INGREDIENTS

Perillae Folium (*zǐ sū yè*) 5g
Cyperi Rhizoma (*xiāng fù*) 4g
Citri reticulatae Pericarpium (*chén pí*) 4g
Glycyrrhizae Radix praeparata (*zhì gān cǎo*) 2.5g
Schizonepetae Herba (*jīng jiè*) 3g
Saposhnikoviae Radix (*fáng fēng*) 3g
Gentianae macrophyllae Radix (*qín jiāo*) 3g
Viticis Fructus (*màn jīng zǐ*) 3g
Chuanxiong Rhizoma (*chuān xiōng*) 1.5g
Zingiberis Rhizoma recens (*shēng jiāng*) .... 3 slices

Preparation notes: Do not cook for more than 20 minutes.

Actions: promotes sweating and releases the exterior

Main pattern: common cold in any season

Key symptoms: headache, nasal obstruction, or runny nose • fever with chills or aversion to drafts • absence of sweating

Secondary symptoms: aches and pains in the body or extremities • stiff neck • focal distention • nausea

Tongue: thin, white coating

Pulse: floating

Abdomen: no specific signs

▶ CLINICAL NOTES

• For wind-cold "common cold" (感冒 *gǎn mào*) rather than the more severe cold damage disorders. Can be used in any season.

• Regulates qi dynamic in the interior and is thus suitable where exterior wind-cold patterns that are accompanied by signs of qi constraint such as nausea or other symptoms of digestive upset.

• Suitable for weak patients, children, the elderly, and pregnant women.

Contraindications: deficiency patterns

▶ FORMULAS WITH SIMILAR INDICATIONS

Ephedra Decoction (*má huáng tāng*): For greater yang stage disorders with cold fettering the exterior characterized by fever and chills, absence of sweating, and a pulse that is floating and tight.

Cinnamon Twig Decoction (*guì zhī tāng*): For greater yang stage wind attack disorders characterized by chills and fever with sweating and a pulse that is floating and lax.

*Cyperus and Perilla Leaf Powder (*xiāng sū sǎn*): This formula is less able to release pathogens from the exterior. It is indicated for cases with more pronounced digestive symptoms.

*Ten Divine Decoction (*shí shén tāng*): For patients with a stronger constitution or with more severe external symptoms.

COMPOSITION

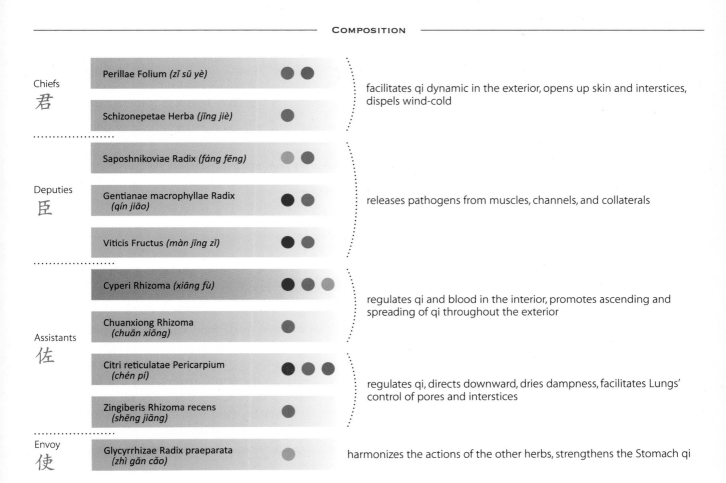

Chiefs
君

Perillae Folium *(zǐ sū yè)*

Schizonepetae Herba *(jīng jiè)*

facilitates qi dynamic in the exterior, opens up skin and interstices, dispels wind-cold

Deputies
臣

Saposhnikoviae Radix *(fáng fēng)*

Gentianae macrophyllae Radix *(qín jiāo)*

Viticis Fructus *(màn jīng zǐ)*

releases pathogens from muscles, channels, and collaterals

Assistants
佐

Cyperi Rhizoma *(xiāng fù)*

Chuanxiong Rhizoma *(chuān xiōng)*

regulates qi and blood in the interior, promotes ascending and spreading of qi throughout the exterior

Citri reticulatae Pericarpium *(chén pí)*

Zingiberis Rhizoma recens *(shēng jiāng)*

regulates qi, directs downward, dries dampness, facilitates Lungs' control of pores and interstices

Envoy
使

Glycyrrhizae Radix praeparata *(zhì gān cǎo)*

harmonizes the actions of the other herbs, strengthens the Stomach qi

健脾丸
Strengthen the Spleen Pill
jiàn pí wán

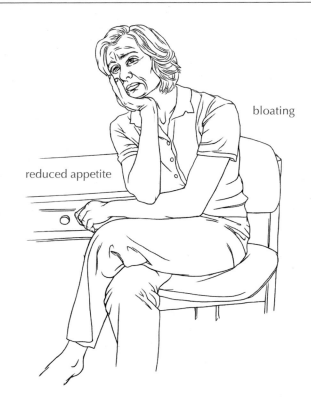

reduced appetite

bloating

INGREDIENTS

dry-fried Atractylodis macrocephalae Rhizoma
(*chǎo bái zhú*) 15g
Poria (*fú líng*) 12g
Ginseng Radix (*rén shēn*) 9g
Dioscoreae Rhizoma (*shān yào*) 6g
roasted Myristicae Semen (*wēi ròu dòu kòu*) 6g
Crataegi Fructus (*shān zhā*) 6g
dry-fried Massa medicata fermentata (*chǎo shén qū*) 6g
dry-fried Hordei Fructus germinatus (*chǎo mài yá*) 6g
Aucklandiae Radix (*mù xiāng*) 4g
Citri reticulatae Pericarpium (*chén pí*) 6g
Amomi Fructus (*shā rén*) 6g
wine-fried Coptidis Rhizoma (*jiǔ chǎo huáng lián*) 3g

Glycyrrhizae Radix (*gān cǎo*) 35g

Actions: strengthens the Spleen • reduces food stagnation • stops diarrhea

Main pattern: food stagnation that has begun to transform into heat in the context of Spleen and Stomach deficiency

Key symptoms: reduced appetite with indigestion • bloating • focal distention of the epigastrium and abdomen

Secondary symptoms: loose stools • fatigue

Tongue: greasy, slightly yellow coating

Pulse: deficient • frail

Abdomen: discomfort in epigastrium • weak abdominal wall

▶ CLINICAL NOTES

• This formula treats food stagnation in patients with Spleen deficiency. Abdominal bloating and lack of appetite are the key clinical markers. It should be modified according to the actual presentation. For example, for more pronounced Spleen deficiency, substitute Coptidis Rhizoma (*huáng lián*) with Zingiberis Rhizoma (*gān jiāng*). If symptoms of dampness are pronounced, add Plantaginis Semen (*chē qián zǐ*) and Alismatis Rhizoma (*zé xiè*).

Contraindications: patterns with prominent signs of excess

▶ FORMULAS WITH SIMILAR INDICATIONS

Preserve Harmony Pill (*bǎo hé wán*): For acute food stagnation in the Stomach in both adults and children.

Unripe Bitter Orange Pill to Reduce Focal Distention (*zhǐ shí xiāo pí wán*): For mixed excess and deficiency patterns where food stagnation arises in the context of Spleen deficiency. However, this formula focuses more strongly on eliminating stagnation and only secondarily on tonifying deficiency. Accordingly, constipation or alternating diarrhea and constipation are typical. For habitually loose stools, Strengthen the Spleen Pill (*jiàn pí wán*) is a better base formula.

COMPOSITION

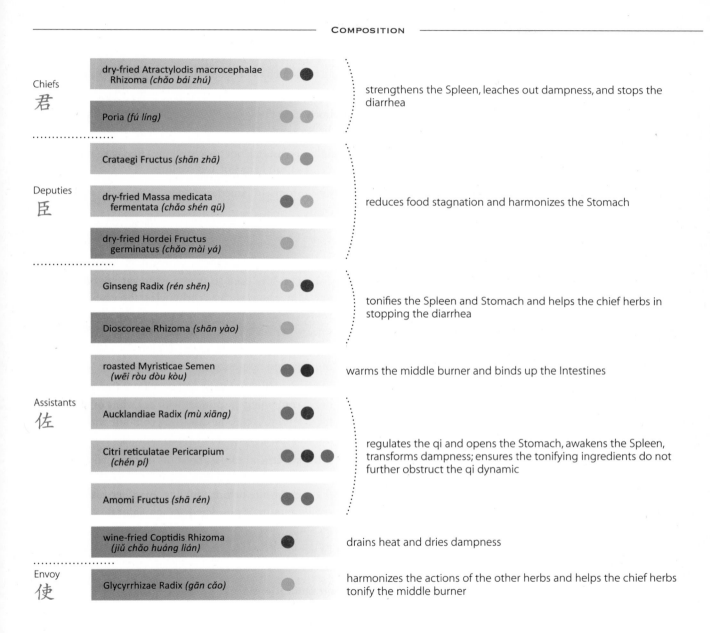

Chiefs
君

dry-fried Atractylodis macrocephalae Rhizoma *(chǎo bái zhú)*

Poria *(fú líng)*

strengthens the Spleen, leaches out dampness, and stops the diarrhea

Deputies
臣

Crataegi Fructus *(shān zhā)*

dry-fried Massa medicata fermentata *(chǎo shén qū)*

dry-fried Hordei Fructus germinatus *(chǎo mài yá)*

reduces food stagnation and harmonizes the Stomach

Assistants
佐

Ginseng Radix *(rén shēn)*

Dioscoreae Rhizoma *(shān yào)*

tonifies the Spleen and Stomach and helps the chief herbs in stopping the diarrhea

roasted Myristicae Semen *(wēi ròu dòu kòu)*

warms the middle burner and binds up the Intestines

Aucklandiae Radix *(mù xiāng)*

Citri reticulatae Pericarpium *(chén pí)*

Amomi Fructus *(shā rén)*

regulates the qi and opens the Stomach, awakens the Spleen, transforms dampness; ensures the tonifying ingredients do not further obstruct the qi dynamic

wine-fried Coptidis Rhizoma *(jiǔ chǎo huáng lián)*

drains heat and dries dampness

Envoy
使

Glycyrrhizae Radix *(gān cǎo)*

harmonizes the actions of the other herbs and helps the chief herbs tonify the middle burner

金黃散/金黃膏
Golden-Yellow Plaster
jīn huáng săn/jīn huáng gāo

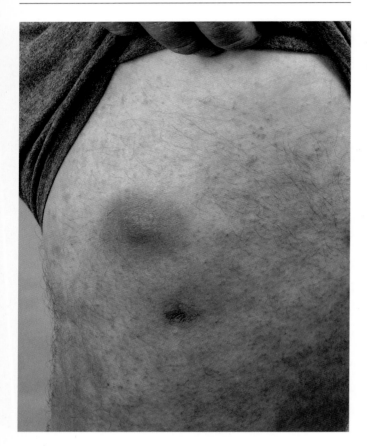

---------- INGREDIENTS ----------

Trichosanthis Radix (*tiān huā fěn*).....................................50g

Phellodendri Cortex (*huáng băi*)......................................25g

Rhei Radix et Rhizoma (*dà huáng*)...................................25g

Curcumae longae Rhizoma (*jiāng huáng*).........................25g

Angelicae dahuricae Radix (*bái zhĭ*) 25g

Magnoliae officinalis Cortex (*hòu pò*)..............................10g

Citri reticulatae Pericarpium (*chén pí*)............................10g

Glycyrrhizae Radix (*gān căo*)...10g

Atractylodis Rhizoma (*cāng zhú*).....................................10g

Arisaematis Rhizoma praeparatum (*zhì tiān nán xīng*)........10g

Preparation notes: Grind the herbs to a fine powder, sift in an 80*mu* (80 openings per inch) sieve, and make into a paste with petroleum jelly, vegetable oil, tea water, or a decoction of an herb such as Taraxaci Herba (*pú gōng yīng*), as noted below.

Actions: clears heat • resolves toxicity • disperses swelling • relieves pain

Main patterns: red, hot toxic swellings that have not yet come to a head • any hot, red swelling

Key symptoms: inflamed swellings

▶ CLINICAL NOTES

• This is the classic external formula for hot, red, toxic swellings. It is used to treat a wide variety of swellings and skin lesions such as carbuncles, abscesses, furuncles, rooted sores, burns, acute mastitis, infected lymph nodes, infected or toxic insect bites, infections of the fleshy area surrounding the toenails or fingernails, cellulitis, styes, mumps, and herpes zoster and simplex.

• For hot swellings or yang toxic swellings that have not yet burst, combining the powder with egg white or tea water is ideal. For more chronic disorders, combine with vegetable oil (sesame oil is used in China) or honey.

• If the superficial sore is moist (as in impetigo or herpes), one can apply the powder directly or mix with sesame oil or egg white before applying. In either case, adding a small amount of powdered Indigo naturalis (*qīng dài*) is recommended.

• Generally, if applied as a plaster, the dressing is changed once every 24 hours.

Contraindications: Do not apply to open sores unless the preparation has been appropriately sterilized. Applying to the area surrounding the sore is permissible.

▶ FORMULAS WITH SIMILAR INDICATIONS

Indigo Powder (*qīng dài săn*): Best for hot and damp skin rashes. By contrast, Golden-Yellow Powder (*jīn huáng săn*) is ideal for toxic swellings.

COMPOSITION

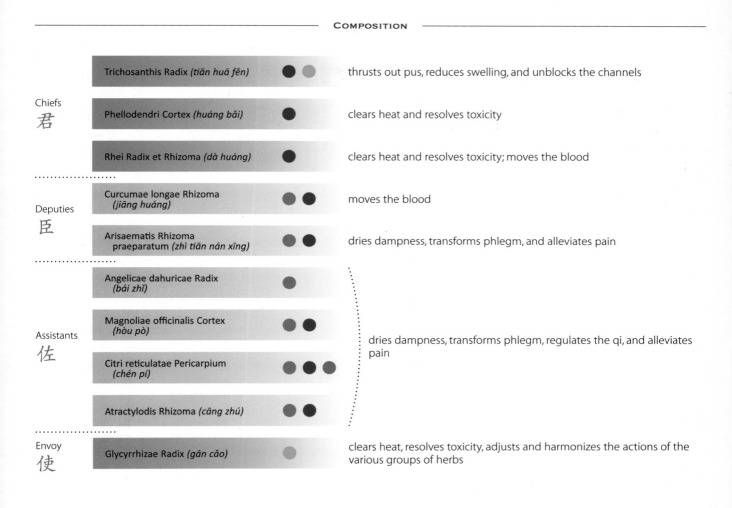

Chiefs 君	Trichosanthis Radix *(tiān huā fěn)*	thrusts out pus, reduces swelling, and unblocks the channels
	Phellodendri Cortex *(huáng bǎi)*	clears heat and resolves toxicity
	Rhei Radix et Rhizoma *(dà huáng)*	clears heat and resolves toxicity; moves the blood
Deputies 臣	Curcumae longae Rhizoma *(jiāng huáng)*	moves the blood
	Arisaematis Rhizoma praeparatum *(zhì tiān nán xīng)*	dries dampness, transforms phlegm, and alleviates pain
Assistants 佐	Angelicae dahuricae Radix *(bái zhǐ)*	dries dampness, transforms phlegm, regulates the qi, and alleviates pain
	Magnoliae officinalis Cortex *(hòu pò)*	
	Citri reticulatae Pericarpium *(chén pí)*	
	Atractylodis Rhizoma *(cāng zhú)*	
Envoy 使	Glycyrrhizae Radix *(gān cǎo)*	clears heat, resolves toxicity, adjusts and harmonizes the actions of the various groups of herbs

金铃子散（金铃子散）
Melia Toosendan Powder
jīn líng zǐ sǎn

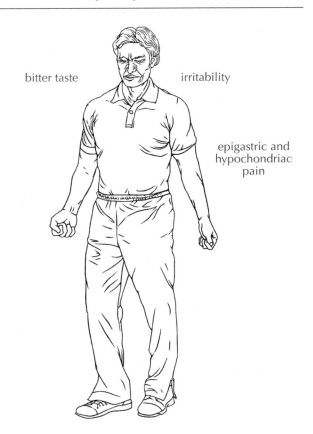

bitter taste

irritability

epigastric and hypochondriac pain

INGREDIENTS

Toosendan Fructus (*chuān liàn zǐ*).....................................30g
Corydalis Rhizoma (*yán hú suǒ*).......................................30g

Preparation notes: Usually ground into a powder with 9g taken each time, chased with either wine or hot water.

Actions: spreads Liver qi • drains heat • invigorates the blood • alleviates pain

Main pattern: Liver constraint transforming into heat

Key symptoms: intermittent epigastric and hypochondriac pain that is aggravated by the ingestion of hot food or beverage • chest pain • hernial pain • menstrual pain

Secondary symptoms: irritability • bitter taste

Tongue: red body

Pulse: wiry • rapid

Abdomen: hypochondrial tenderness • tense rectus abdominis muscle

▶ CLINICAL NOTES

• This is the core formula for Liver constraint transforming into heat, which causes Liver qi to transgress its bounds and also dries up the fluids and causes the blood to stagnate. The formula is therefore indicated for treating pain anywhere, not just along the course of the Liver channel. Key clinical markers are a wiry pulse that may be rapid or rough, irritability, and frustration.

• If the yin fluids or blood have been damaged, this formula should be combined with appropriate tonifying herbs such as Angelicae sinensis Radix (*dāng guī*), Salviae miltiorrhizae Radix (*dān shēn*), Paeoniae Radix alba (*bái sháo*), Lycii Fructus (*gǒu qǐ zǐ*), Rehmanniae Radix (*shēng dì huáng*), or Ophiopogonis Radix (*mài mén dōng*), or a formula containing these herbs.

Contraindications: use with caution during pregnancy • inappropriate for pain from Liver qi constraint in the context of cold disorders

▶ FORMULAS WITH SIMILAR INDICATIONS

*Left Metal Pill** (*zuǒ jīn wán*): For Liver fire that attacks the Stomach in the absence of deficiency signs and symptoms.

*Augmented Rambling Powder** (*jiā wèi xiāo yáo sǎn*): Treats Liver qi constraint which transforms into fire in the context of qi and blood deficiency. It puts less emphasis on treating the pain and more on addressing the upward flaring of fire.

──────────────── **COMPOSITION** ────────────────

| Chief
君 | Toosendan Fructus *(chuān liàn zǐ)* | ● | clears heat from the chest, hypochondrium, and groin by draining it through the urine |
| Assis/Env
佐/使 | Corydalis Rhizoma *(yán hú suǒ)* | ● ● | invigorates the blood by moving the qi |

金鎖固精丸（金锁固精丸）
Metal Lock Pill to Stabilize the Essence
jīn suǒ gù jīng wán

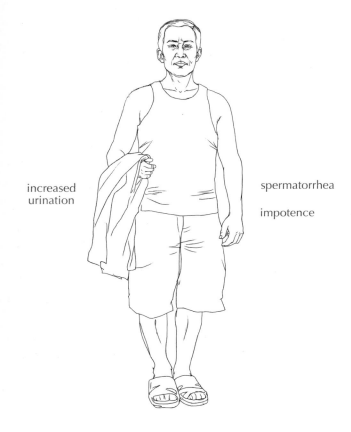

increased urination

spermatorrhea

impotence

INGREDIENTS

Astragali complanati Semen (*shā yuàn zǐ*)..........................60g

Euryales Semen (*qiàn shí*)..60g

Nelumbinis Stamen (*lián xū*)..60g

calcined Fossilia Ossis Mastodi (*duàn lóng gǔ*).................30g

calcined Ostreae Concha (*duàn mǔ lì*).............................30g

Nelumbinis Semen (*lián zǐ*)...120g

Preparation notes: This formula is usually taken in pill form, 6-9g twice daily, with slightly salty water.

Actions: tonifies and stabilizes the Kidneys • binds essence • secures emissions

---

Main pattern: Kidney deficiency leading to instability of the gate of essence

Key symptoms: chronic spermatorrhea • impotence • increased urination

Secondary symptoms: fatigue and weakness • sore and weak limbs • lower back pain • tinnitus

Tongue: pale body • white coating

Pulse: thin • frail

Abdomen: no specific signs

▶ CLINICAL NOTES

• This formula focuses on securing the leakage of essence due to Kidney deficiency. Key indicators for this formula are seminal emissions that do not occur during dreams and the absence of heat signs such as night sweats and heat in the five centers.

• Although spontaneous emissions are the classic indication for this formula, it can also be used to treat excessive sweating, diarrhea (especially if it occurs when walking or running), urinary incontinence, profuse uterine bleeding, or postpartum disorders associated with weak Kidneys that are unable to contain the essence.

• Sexual intercourse and ingestion of acrid, spicy-hot foods should be avoided while taking this formula. Due to its astringent nature, the formula should be discontinued if the patient contracts an external pathogen during the course of treatment.

Contraindications: damp-heat • blazing fire from deficiency

▶ FORMULAS WITH SIMILAR INDICATIONS

*Mantis Egg-Case Powder (*sāng piāo xiāo sǎn*): Focuses on tonifying the Heart while securing the essence in patients with a pattern of Heart and Kidney failing to communicate. Symptoms of this pattern include dark urine, heightened sexual arousal, and nocturnal emissions during dreams.

—————————————— COMPOSITION ——————————————

Chief 君	Astragali complanati Semen (*shā yuàn zǐ*)	● ●	tonifies the Kidneys and benefits the essence, and stops the leakage of semen by stabilizing the gate of essence
Deputies 臣	Euryales Semen (*qiàn shí*)	● ●	assists the chief ingredient in stabilizing the gate of essence and stopping the leakage of semen
	Nelumbinis Stamen (*lián xū*)	● ●	
	Nelumbinis Semen (*lián zǐ*)	● ●	
Assistants 佐	calcined Fossilia Ossis Mastodi (*duàn lóng gǔ*)	● ●	binds the semen and prevents it from leaking
	calcined Ostreae Concha (*duàn mǔ lì*)	● ●	

九味羌活湯（九味羌活汤）
Nine-Herb Decoction with Notopterygium
jiǔ wèi qiāng huó tāng

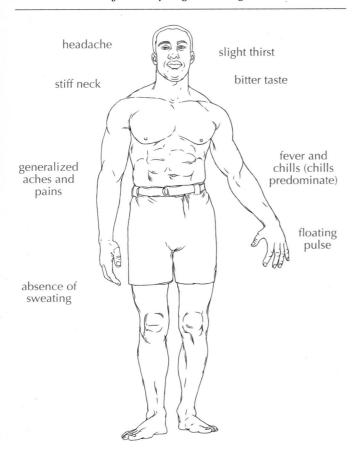

headache
stiff neck
slight thirst
bitter taste
generalized aches and pains
fever and chills (chills predominate)
floating pulse
absence of sweating

INGREDIENTS

Notopterygii Rhizoma seu Radix (*qiāng huó*) 5-9g

Saposhnikoviae Radix (*fáng fēng*) 5-9g

Atractylodis Rhizoma (*cāng zhú*) 5-9g

¹Asari Herba (*xì xīn*) 1-3g

Chuanxiong Rhizoma (*chuān xiōng*) 3-6g

Angelicae dahuricae Radix (*bái zhǐ*) 3-6g

Scutellariae Radix (*huáng qín*) 3-6g

1. This herb can be difficult to obtain because of legal issues. Clematidis Radix *(wēi líng xiān)* may be substituted.

Rehmanniae Radix (*shēng dì huáng*)............................ 3-6g
Glycyrrhizae Radix (*gān cǎo*)................................... 3-6g

Actions: induces sweating and dispels dampness while simultaneously draining interior heat

Main patterns: externally-contracted wind-cold-dampness with concurrent internal accumulation of heat

Key symptoms: fever and chills (chills predominate) • absence of sweating • headache • stiff neck • generalized aches and pains

Secondary symptoms: slight thirst • bitter taste

Tongue: white or slightly yellow coating

Pulse: floating

Abdomen: no specific signs

▶ CLINICAL NOTES

• For wind-cold-dampness in the exterior with accumulation of heat in the interior.

• Should be adjusted to match the precise location of symptoms in particular channels of the head or body, and the severity of the symptoms, by increasing or decreasing the amount of individual constituents. For instance, for greater yang channel symptoms, increase the amount of Notopterygii Rhizoma seu Radix (*qiāng huó*); for lesser yang channel symptoms, increase the amount of Saposhnikoviae Radix (*fáng fēng*); for yang brightness headaches, increase the amount of Angelicae dahuricae Radix (*bái zhǐ*); for greater yin headaches, increase the amount of *Atractylodis Rhizoma* (*cāng zhú*); for lesser yin headaches, increase the amount of Asari Radix et Rhizoma (*xì xīn*); and for terminal yin headaches, increase the amount of Chuanxiong Rhizoma (*chuān xiōng*).

• Less effective in releasing wind-cold from the exterior than Ephedra Decotion (*má huáng tāng*) or Cinnamon Twig Decoction (*guì zhī tāng*), but also less dispersing of the body's qi.

Contraindications: warm pathogen disorders • yin deficiency

► FORMULAS WITH SIMILAR INDICATIONS

Three-Seed Decoction (*sān rén tāng*): For damp-warmth in the exterior where the symptoms are aggravated by heat rather than cold and present without thirst or other signs of damage to the fluids.

──────────────── COMPOSITION ────────────────

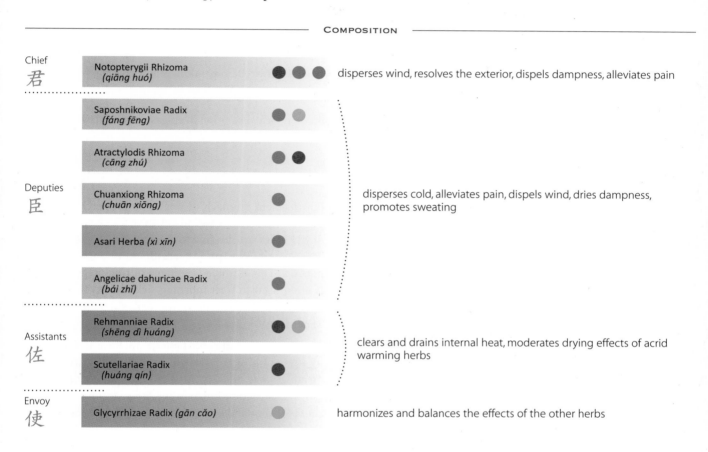

Chief 君	Notopterygii Rhizoma (*qiāng huó*)	disperses wind, resolves the exterior, dispels dampness, alleviates pain
Deputies 臣	Saposhnikoviae Radix (*fáng fēng*)	disperses cold, alleviates pain, dispels wind, dries dampness, promotes sweating
	Atractylodis Rhizoma (*cāng zhú*)	
	Chuanxiong Rhizoma (*chuān xiōng*)	
	Asari Herba (*xì xīn*)	
	Angelicae dahuricae Radix (*bái zhǐ*)	
Assistants 佐	Rehmanniae Radix (*shēng dì huáng*)	clears and drains internal heat, moderates drying effects of acrid warming herbs
	Scutellariae Radix (*huáng qín*)	
Envoy 使	Glycyrrhizae Radix (*gān cǎo*)	harmonizes and balances the effects of the other herbs

橘皮竹茹湯（橘皮竹茹汤）
Tangerine Peel and Bamboo Shavings Decoction
jú pí zhú rú tāng

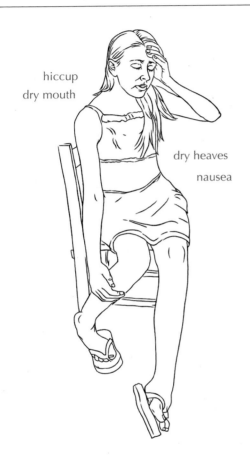

hiccup
dry mouth

dry heaves

nausea

─────────── **INGREDIENTS** ───────────

Citri reticulatae Pericarpium (*chén pí*)............................ 9-12g

Bambusae Caulis in taeniam (*zhú rú*) 9-12g

Ginseng Radix (*rén shēn*)... 3g

Zingiberis Rhizoma recens (*shēng jiāng*)................................. 9g

Glycyrrhizae Radix (*gān cǎo*)... 6g

Jujubae Fructus (*dà zǎo*)... 5 pieces

Actions: directs rebellious Stomach qi downward • stops hiccup • augments the qi • clears heat

Main patterns: qi stagnation and constraint due to long-term Stomach deficiency • injury to the Stomach qi due to vomiting, diarrhea, or other causes

Key symptoms: hiccup • nausea • dry heaves

Secondary symptoms: dry mouth • irritability • breathlessness • vomiting

Tongue: slightly red body • thin, yellow coating

Pulse: deficient • rapid

Abdomen: focal distention in epigastrium • splashing sounds

▶ CLINICAL NOTES

• For deficient Stomach qi unable to properly direct the pure upward and the turbid downward such that Stomach qi rebels upward, leading to hiccup, retching, and nausea. This occurs after prolonged illness or in qi-deficient patients. This formula is suitable during pregnancy and is often used to treat morning sickness. As the relief of nausea is usually temporary, the patient should eat as soon as her nausea subsides.

• The formula is suited for patterns that are accompanied by signs of heat from qi constraint such as irritability, breathlessness, and dry mouth. If the heat is from excess, Pinellia Decoction to Drain the Epigastrium (*bàn xià xiè xīn tāng*) should be used; if it is from yin deficiency, use Ophiopogonis Decoction (*mài mén dōng tāng*) instead.

• If the pattern includes vomiting, it is best to add herbs to enhance the downward-directing action of the formula, such as Kaki Calyx (*shì dì*). If heat is prominent, add Coptidis Rhizoma (*huáng lián*); if phlegm is present, add Pinelliae Rhizoma praeparatum (*zhì bàn xià*) .

Contraindications: hiccup due to cold or excess heat

▶ FORMULAS WITH SIMILAR INDICATIONS

*Clove and Persimmon Calyx Decoction (*dīng xiāng shī dì tāng*): For hiccup due to deficiency cold in the Stomach as reflected in a pale tongue with a white coating and a submerged, slow pulse.

*Inula and Haematite Decoction (*xuán fù dài zhě tāng*): For incessant hiccup, belching, or vomiting due to the presence of phlegm fluids as reflected in hard focal distention in the epigastrium.

COMPOSITION

Chief 君	Citri reticulatae Pericarpium *(chén pí)*	●●●	harmonizes the Stomach and stops the hiccup
	Bambusae Caulis in taeniam *(zhú rú)*	●	clears heat, calms the Stomach, and stops the hiccup
Deputies 臣	Ginseng Radix *(rén shēn)*	●●	tonifies qi
	Zingiberis Rhizoma recens *(shēng jiāng)*	●	harmonizes the Stomach and stops the vomiting
Assis/Env 佐/使	Glycyrrhizae Radix *(gān cǎo)*	●	augments qi
Assistant 佐	Jujubae Fructus *(dà zǎo)*	●	

蠲痹湯 (蠲痹汤)
Remove Painful Obstruction Decoction
juān bì tāng

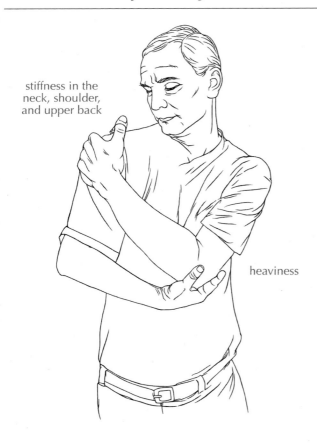

stiffness in the
neck, shoulder,
and upper back

heaviness

Actions: tonifies and harmonizes the protective and nutritive qi • dispels wind • eliminates dampness

Main pattern: painful obstruction in a patient with qi and blood deficiency

Key symptoms: generalized heaviness in the body • stiffness in the neck, shoulder, and upper back • difficulty moving

Secondary symptoms: numbness in the extremities

Tongue: white coating

Pulse: moderate

Abdomen: no specific signs

▶ CLINICAL NOTES

- For painful obstruction pattern, specifically in the upper body and upper extremities, in the context of blood and qi deficiency. Adding Gentianae macrophyllae Radix (*qín jiāo*) can increase the efficacy of this formula.
- The dregs from the decoction can be re-cooked and used externally as a wash, compress, or steam bath. Because these applications open the pores, patients should cover the treated area immediately after treatment in order to avoid contracting a new wind or cold pathogen.

Contraindications: damp-heat painful obstruction patterns

▶ FORMULAS WITH SIMILAR INDICATIONS

Pubescent Angelica and Taxillus Decoction (*dú huó jì shēng tāng*): For wind-cold-damp painful obstruction manifesting with symptoms in the lower extremities and back or at the level of the sinews and bones in patients who present with Kidney and Liver deficiency.

INGREDIENTS

Notopterygii Rhizoma seu Radix (*qiāng huó*)......................9g
Curcumae longae Rhizoma (*jiāng huáng*)..........................9g
wine-washed Angelicae sinensis Radix (*jiǔ xǐ dāng guī*)........9g
honey-prepared Astragali Radix (*mì zhì huáng qí*)..............9g
Paeoniae Radix alba (*bái sháo*)...................................9g
Saposhnikoviae Radix (*fáng fēng*)................................9g
Glycyrrhizae Radix praeparata (*zhì gān cǎo*)....................3g
Zingiberis Rhizoma recens (*shēng jiāng*)........................9g
Jujubae Fructus (*dà zǎo*)...................................2 pieces

Preparation notes: Commonly, the first seven ingredients are powdered and then cooked for 20 minutes with the last two.

COMPOSITION

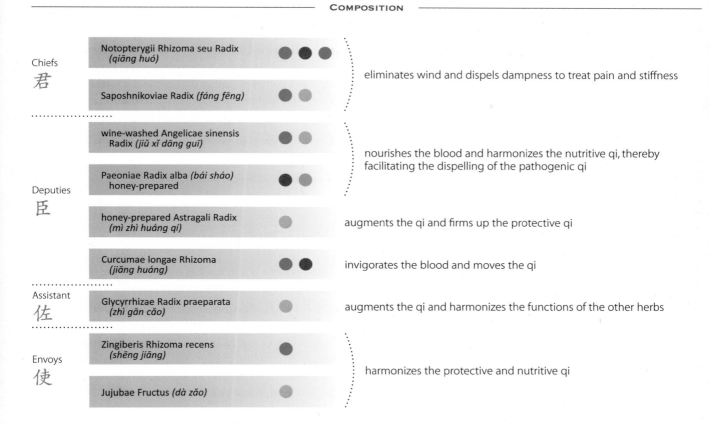

Chiefs
君

Notopterygii Rhizoma seu Radix
(qiāng huó)

Saposhnikoviae Radix (fáng fēng)

eliminates wind and dispels dampness to treat pain and stiffness

Deputies
臣

wine-washed Angelicae sinensis
Radix (jiǔ xǐ dāng guī)

Paeoniae Radix alba (bái sháo)
honey-prepared

nourishes the blood and harmonizes the nutritive qi, thereby
facilitating the dispelling of the pathogenic qi

honey-prepared Astragali Radix
(mì zhì huáng qí)

augments the qi and firms up the protective qi

Curcumae longae Rhizoma
(jiāng huáng)

invigorates the blood and moves the qi

Assistant
佐

Glycyrrhizae Radix praeparata
(zhì gān cǎo)

augments the qi and harmonizes the functions of the other herbs

Envoys
使

Zingiberis Rhizoma recens
(shēng jiāng)

Jujubae Fructus (dà zǎo)

harmonizes the protective and nutritive qi

苦參湯（苦参汤）
Sophora Root Wash
kǔ shēn tāng

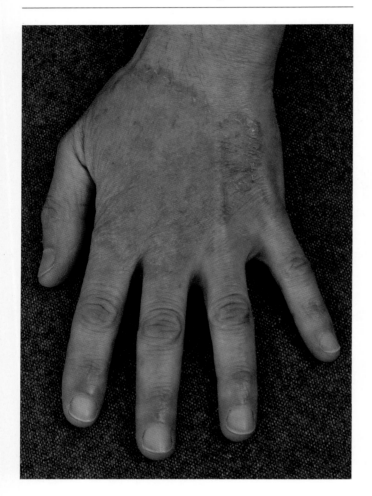

Preparation notes: Soak the ingredients in six cups of water for 30 minutes and bring to a boil. Lower the heat and simmer for 25 minutes. Strain out the liquid, which can be stored and re-used for three days. Re-heat before use. Use as a soak or a compress for 20-30 minutes, 1-2 times per day. If used as a compress, apply the dampened washcloth to the affected area and re-dip into the warm solution every few minutes to keep it warm.

Actions: dispels wind • dries dampness • kills parasites • relieves itching

Main pattern: scabbing skin disorders

Key symptoms: red, itchy swellings • dry, scaly, itchy rashes

▶ CLINICAL NOTES

- This formula is also used as a douche in the treatment of itching and irritation of the female genitals.
- This is a valuable formula for stubborn skin disorders. Most valuable is its use in treating various fungal infections of the skin. For this purpose it should be modified by adding Sulfur (*liú huáng*), Hydnocarpi Semen (*dà fēng zǐ*), and Meliae Cortex (*kǔ liàn gēn pí*) and cooked with rice wine and rice vinegar.

Contraindications: none noted

INGREDIENTS

Sophorae flavescentis Radix (*kǔ shēn*).............................. 60g
Cnidii Fructus (*shé chuáng zǐ*).. 30g
Angelicae dahuricae Radix (*bái zhǐ*) 15g
Lonicerae Flos (*jīn yín huā*) 30g
Chrysanthemi Flos (*jú huā*)... 30g
Phellodendri Cortex (*huáng bǎi*).. 15g
Kochiae Fructus (*dì fū zǐ*).. 15g
Acori tatarinowii Rhizoma (*shí chāng pǔ*) 9g

───── COMPOSITION ─────

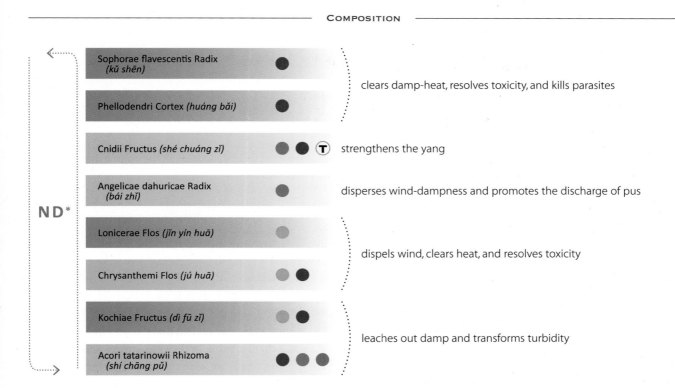

Sophorae flavescentis Radix *(kǔ shēn)*

Phellodendri Cortex *(huáng bǎi)*

clears damp-heat, resolves toxicity, and kills parasites

Cnidii Fructus *(shé chuáng zǐ)* (T) strengthens the yang

Angelicae dahuricae Radix *(bái zhǐ)* disperses wind-dampness and promotes the discharge of pus

Lonicerae Flos *(jīn yín huā)*

Chrysanthemi Flos *(jú huā)*

dispels wind, clears heat, and resolves toxicity

Kochiae Fructus *(dì fū zǐ)*

Acori tatarinowii Rhizoma *(shí chāng pǔ)*

leaches out damp and transforms turbidity

ND*

*herb roles are not differentiated

理中丸
Regulate the Middle Pill
lǐ zhōng wán

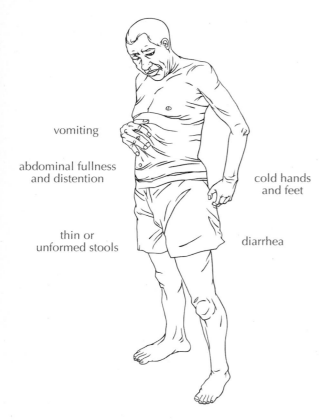

vomiting

abdominal fullness
and distinction

cold hands
and feet

thin or
unformed stools

diarrhea

INGREDIENTS

Zingiberis Rhizoma (*gān jiāng*).. 9g
Ginseng Radix (*rén shēn*)... 9g
Atractylodis macrocephalae Rhizoma (*bái zhú*) 9g
Glycyrrhizae Radix praeparata (*zhì gān cǎo*) 9g

Actions: warms the middle burner • strengthens the Spleen
and Stomach

Main patterns: middle burner deficiency cold • bleeding due to
middle burner yang deficiency

Key symptoms: abdominal fullness and distention • vomiting
• thin or unformed stools • diarrhea with watery stools • cold
hands and feet

Secondary symptoms: emaciation • fatigue • loss of appetite
• excess frothy saliva • cough with thin, watery sputum
• absence of thirst despite diarrhea or thirst with no desire
to drink • various types of bleeding

Tongue: pale red body • white coating that may be thick,
greasy, or wet

Pulse: submerged and thin • frail • thin and forceless • slow
and frail

Abdomen: hard focal distention in the epigastrium • weak
and cold abdomen

▶ CLINICAL NOTES

• In this pattern all of the symptoms are aggravated by eating
raw and cold foods. It is important not to be confused by
symptoms of stagnation, such as focal distention in the
epigastrium, and to mistake these symptoms to mean that
the condition is at root excessive.

• The pattern may present with branch symptoms of excess,
such as focal distention in the epigastrium and vomiting.
These symptoms are associated with stagnation that
results from a cold and deficient middle burner losing its
ability to transport. Treatment is primarily aimed at the
root, supplementing the center and dispersing cold.

• This important formula for treating deficiency cold in
the interior focuses specifically on the greater yin warp.
The manifestations thus involve impaired digestive
functions (nausea, vomiting, abdominal distention and
pain, diarrhea) but can also extend to the respiratory
system (coughing up watery sputum). When treating
acute conditions, such as sudden turmoil disorder, its use
should be discontinued once the vomiting and diarrhea
have stopped, which indicates that the condition has been
resolved or that the pathogen has moved to a different
warp.

• Today this formula is mainly used to treat chronic
deficiency-cold diarrhea or abdominal pain. While dietary
irregularities and the contraction of cold from the exterior
are the traditional causes of this pattern, treatment by
antibiotics and antifungals that damage the interior may
also be contributing factors.

- As the Spleen governs the blood, this formula can be used to treat various types of bleeding due to deficiency cold in the middle burner. This includes nosebleeds, vomiting of blood, excessive menstrual bleeding, bleeding from the rectum, or internal bleeding.

Contraindications: externally-contracted disorders with fever • yin deficiency or excess conditions

▶ FORMULAS WITH SIMILAR INDICATIONS

Magnolia Bark Decoction for Warming the Middle (*hòu pò wēn zhōng tāng*): For invasion of damp-cold into the middle burner marked by epigastric and abdominal distention and fullness, and a white, slippery tongue coating.

Four-Gentlemen Decoction (*sì jūn zǐ tāng*): For qi deficiency leading to impaired movement and transformation but without the prominent presence of cold.

Frigid Extremities Decoction (*sì nì tāng*): For unrelenting diarrhea resulting from the yang of the middle burner having been cut off from its source in the gate of vitality. This is indicated by systemic signs of deficiency cold such as cold extremities and fatigue that are symptomatic of lesser yin warp disorders.

Mume Pill (*wū méi wán*): For patterns characterized by heat above and cold below (terminal yin warp) as reflected in diarrhea accompanied by hunger, thirst, or qi rushing upward toward the chest.

COMPOSITION

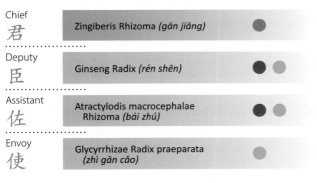

Chief 君	Zingiberis Rhizoma (*gān jiāng*)	●	warms the Spleen and Stomach yang and eliminates interior cold
Deputy 臣	Ginseng Radix (*rén shēn*)	● ●	strongly tonifies the source qi, rectifies the ascending and descending functions of the middle burner
Assistant 佐	Atractylodis macrocephalae Rhizoma (*bái zhú*)	● ●	aids the deputy herb in tonifying the Spleen and Stomach, strengthens the Spleen and dries dampness
Envoy 使	Glycyrrhizae Radix praeparata (*zhì gān cǎo*)	●	augments the qi of the middle burner and harmonizes the actions of the other herbs in the formula

連樸飲 （连朴饮）
Coptis and Magnolia Bark Drink
lián pò yǐn

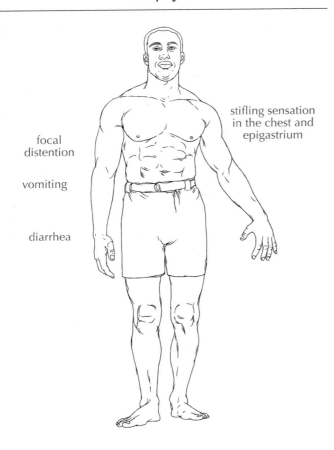

focal
distention

vomiting

diarrhea

stifling sensation
in the chest and
epigastrium

INGREDIENTS

ginger Coptidis Rhizoma (*jiāng huáng lián*)................... 3-12g
prepared Magnoliae officinalis Cortex (*zhì hòu pò*).......... 6-15g
Gardeniae Fructus (*zhī zǐ*)... 9g
dry-fried Sojae Semen praeparatum (*chǎo dòu chǐ*).............. 9g
Acori tatarinowii Rhizoma (*shí chāng pǔ*) 3-6g
Pinelliae Rhizoma praeparatum (*zhì bàn xià*)................. 3-12g
Phragmitis Rhizoma (*lú gēn*) 21-60g

Actions: clears heat • transforms dampness • regulates the qi
• harmonizes the middle burner

Main pattern: damp-heat smoldering in the middle burner,
which disrupts the ascending and descending functions of
the Spleen and Stomach

Key symptoms: stifling sensation in the chest and
epigastrium • focal distention • nausea and vomiting • loose
stools or yellow diarrhea

Secondary symptoms: bitter taste • irritability • dark, scanty
urine • sudden turmoil

Tongue: yellow, greasy coating

Pulse: slippery • rapid

Abdomen: focal distention in chest and upper abdomen

▶ CLINICAL NOTES

• This formula treats damp-heat obstructing the middle
burner qi dynamic in patterns where heat and dampness
are equally strong (reflected in the moist or greasy, yellow
tongue coating) and the heat has already damaged the
fluids (reduced urination). It can be used for acute or
chronic patterns. Such conditions are not limited to
digestive disorders but also include impotence, infertility,
and post-viral fatigue syndrome.

• Originally for sudden turmoil disorder (simultaneous
vomiting and diarrhea) due to an aggregation of damp-
heat smoldering in the body. It is still useful for this
problem, which carries such biomedical diagnoses as
acute gastroenteritis, typhoid, and paratyphoid.

• This formula should be taken cool to increase its efficacy
in relieving nausea and vomiting.

Contraindications: dampness and cold obstructing the
middle burner

▶ FORMULAS WITH SIMILAR INDICATIONS

Patchouli/Agastache Powder to Rectify the Qi (*huò xiāng
zhèng qì sǎn*): For simultaneous vomiting and diarrhea in
patients where wind-cold fetters the protective yang and
dampness obstructs the interior. This is reflected in symptoms like chills and fever and such signs as a white tongue
coating.

Sweet Dew Special Pill to Eliminate Toxin (*gān lù xiāo dú* *dān*): For damp-heat patterns with equally strong dampness and heat, but affecting all three burners rather than just the middle burner. The associated symptoms are primarily seen on the face, head, and exterior.

──────────── **COMPOSITION** ────────────

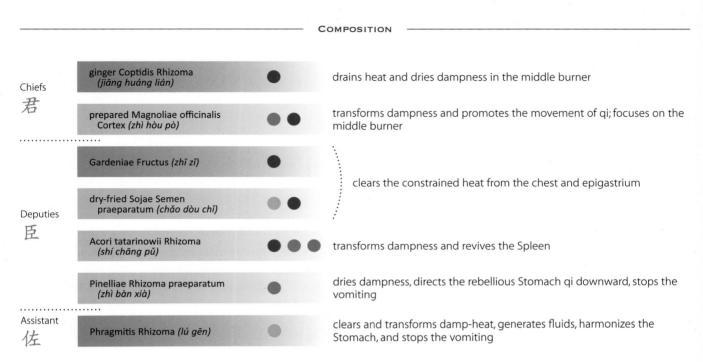

Chiefs
君

ginger Coptidis Rhizoma *(jiāng huáng lián)* — drains heat and dries dampness in the middle burner

prepared Magnoliae officinalis Cortex *(zhì hòu pò)* — transforms dampness and promotes the movement of qi; focuses on the middle burner

Deputies
臣

Gardeniae Fructus *(zhī zǐ)*

dry-fried Sojae Semen praeparatum *(chǎo dòu chǐ)* — clears the constrained heat from the chest and epigastrium

Acori tatarinowii Rhizoma *(shí chāng pǔ)* — transforms dampness and revives the Spleen

Pinelliae Rhizoma praeparatum *(zhì bàn xià)* — dries dampness, directs the rebellious Stomach qi downward, stops the vomiting

Assistant
佐

Phragmitis Rhizoma *(lú gēn)* — clears and transforms damp-heat, generates fluids, harmonizes the Stomach, and stops the vomiting

苓桂朮甘湯（苓桂术甘汤）
Poria, Cinnamon Twig, Atractylodes, and Licorice Decoction
líng guì zhú gān tāng

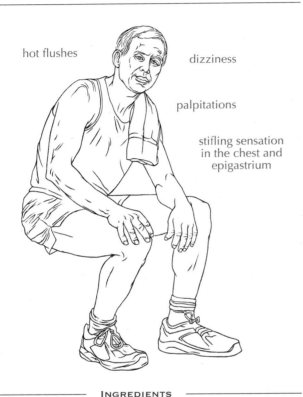

hot flushes

dizziness

palpitations

stifling sensation in the chest and epigastrium

INGREDIENTS

Poria (*fú líng*) 12g
Cinnamomi Ramulus (*guì zhī*) 9g
Atractylodis macrocephalae Rhizoma (*bái zhú*) 6g
Glycyrrhizae Radix praeparata (*zhì gān cǎo*) 6g

Actions: warms and transforms phlegm and thin mucus • strengthens the Spleen • resolves dampness

Main pattern: thin mucus in the epigastrium

Key symptoms: dizziness • stifling sensation in the chest and epigastrium • palpitations or tachycardia • hot flushes

Secondary symptoms: headaches • expectoration of watery sputum • shortness of breath • simultaneous vomiting and diarrhea • focal distention • irritability, restlessness

Tongue: pale, swollen, and wet body • thin, white coating

Pulse: slippery and wiry • slippery and soggy

Abdomen: splashing sounds in upper abdomen • discomfort in epigastrium • pulsations above or around umbilicus

▶ CLINICAL NOTES

- Although originally for thin mucus in the epigastrium, this formula can be prescribed for thin mucus affecting any aspect of the Triple Burner, specifically including heart disease and cardiovascular disorders, eye disorders, digestive and urinary problems. Such conditions are often characterized by periods of acute ill health alternating with times when few or no symptoms are present.

- Specific clinical markers for thin mucus include: (i) dizziness or lightheadedness when rising from a prone or sitting position; (ii) hot flushes, palpitations, tachycardia, or nervousness; (iii) cold abdomen or splashing sounds in the stomach on palpation, or large areas of coldness on the back or along the spine; (iv) pale tongue with a slippery, white coating together with a submerged and wiry pulse; (v) visible signs of excess fluid accumulation such as edema, coughing up of watery sputum, or excess saliva. All symptoms related to thin mucus are aggravated by fatigue, nervous tension, or the contraction of external pathogens.

Contraindications: damp-heat • yin deficiency and hyperactive Liver yang

▶ FORMULAS WITH SIMILAR INDICATIONS

Licorice, Ginger, Poria, and White Atractylodes Decoction (*gān cǎo gān jiāng fú líng bái zhú tāng*): For damp-cold painful obstruction of the back manifesting as a heavy sensation in the body, cold and pain in the lower back, pressure in the lower back as if carrying a heavy weight, normal appetite, absence of thirst, and copious urine.

True Warrior Decoction (*zhēn wǔ tāng*): For Spleen and Kidney yang deficiency (greater yin or lesser yin warps)

with retention of pathogenic water. There may also be loose stools, dizziness, a heavy sensation in the head, palpitations, coughing, or vomiting. The pulse in this pattern is usually submerged, thin, and forceless in contrast to the wiry or slippery pulse associated with a Poria, Cinnamon Twig, Atractylodes, and Licorice Decoction (*líng guì zhú gān tāng*) presentation.

COMPOSITION

Chief 君	Poria *(fú líng)*	● ●	strengthens the Spleen and leaches out dampness
Deputy 臣	Cinnamomi Ramulus *(guì zhī)*	● ●	warms the yang and improves the transforming power of the qi, which resolves the thin mucus
Assistant 佐	Atractylodis macrocephalae Rhizoma *(bái zhú)*	● ●	strengthens the transforming and transportive functions of the Spleen, and dries dampness
Envoy 使	Glycyrrhizae Radix praeparata *(zhì gān cǎo)*	●	augments the qi of the middle burner

羚角鉤藤湯（羚角钩藤汤）
Antelope Horn and Uncaria Decoction
líng jiǎo gōu téng tāng

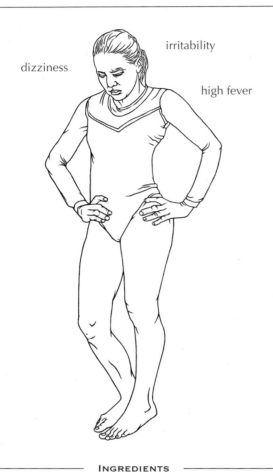

dizziness

irritability

high fever

INGREDIENTS

Saigae tataricae Cornu (*líng yáng jiǎo*) 4.5g
Uncariae Ramulus cum Uncis (*gōu téng*) 9g
Mori Folium (*sāng yè*) 6g
Chrysanthemi Flos (*jú huā*) 9g
Paeoniae Radix alba (*bái sháo*) 9g
Rehmanniae Radix (*shēng dì huáng*) 15g
Fritillariae cirrhosae Bulbus (*chuān bèi mǔ*) 12g
Bambusae Caulis in taeniam (*zhú rú*) 15g
Poriae Sclerotium pararadicis (*fú shén*) 9g
Glycyrrhizae Radix (*gān cǎo*)... 2.4-3g

Preparation & ingredient notes: Traditionally, Saigae tataricae Cornu (*líng yáng jiǎo*) and Bambusae Caulis in taeniam (*zhú rú*) were first decocted together and the remaining ingredients were then cooked in the liquid from that decoction. Because Saigae tataricae Cornu (*líng yáng jiǎo*) is no longer used owing to CITES concerns, a large dose of Haliotidis Concha (*shí jué míng*) or Margaritiferae Concha usta (*zhēn zhū mǔ*) can be substituted. One modern text also mentions Phragmitis Rhizoma (*lú gēn*) as an effective substitute.

Actions: cools the Liver • extinguishes wind • increases the fluids • relaxes the sinews

Main pattern: heat excess in the Liver channel that results in stirring of internal wind

Key symptoms: persistent high fever • dizziness • vertigo • twitching and spasms of the extremities

Secondary symptoms: irritability • restlessness • palpitations • clouded consciousness • tinnitus

Tongue: deep-red and dry • burnt with prickles

Pulse: wiry and rapid • forceful

Abdomen: no specific signs

▶ CLINICAL NOTES

• This formula cools the Liver and extinguishes wind. It can be used when external wind-heat pathogens penetrate into the nutritive and blood aspects, as well as for patterns due to Liver yin deficiency with hyperactivity of Liver yang.

• The ability of this formula to clear heat is relatively mild. If there are signs of strong heat in the qi aspect, one should add herbs that clear heat and resolve toxicity such as Gypsum fibrosum (*shí gāo*) and Anemarrhenae Rhizoma (*zhī mǔ*). If the heat causes blood stasis, it is best to add herbs that cool and move the blood such as Paeoniae Radix rubra (*chì sháo*), Salviae miltiorrhizae Radix (*dān shēn*), and Moutan Cortex (*mǔ dān pí*).

Contraindications: internal wind due to blood or qi deficiency

► FORMULAS WITH SIMILAR INDICATIONS

Sedate the Liver and Extinguish Wind Decoction (*zhèn gān xī fēng tāng*): For internal Liver wind with gushing upward of qi and heat in the Penetrating vessel. This formula focuses on directing the yang and blood downward rather than on venting heat and extinguishing wind.

Gastrodia and Uncaria Drink (*tiān má gōu téng yǐn*): For hyperactivity of Liver yang against a background of yin deficiency.

Specifically designed to treat hypertension with such symptoms as headache, dizziness, and insomnia.

*Major Arrest Wind Pearls (*dà dìng fēng zhū*): For internal stirring of wind due to severe yin deficiency reflected in a deep-red tongue with a scanty or peeled coating.

*Ass-Hide Gelatin and Egg Yolk Decoction (*ē jiāo jī zi huáng tāng*): For the extended presence of a heat pathogen that damages the body's blood and yin and gives rise to wind.

─────────────── COMPOSITION ───────────────

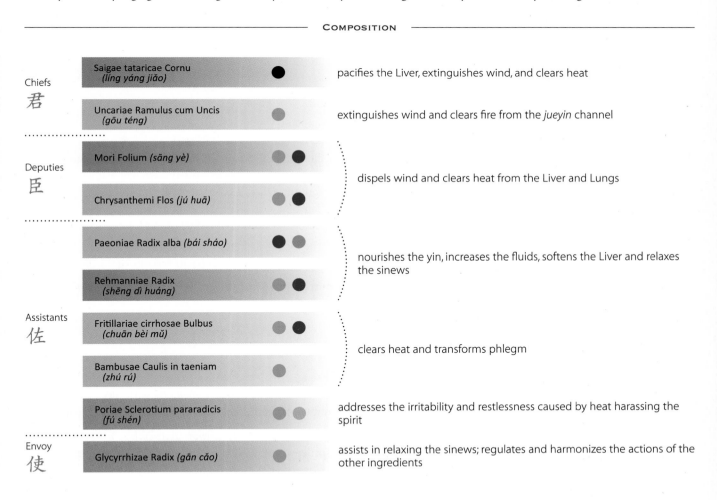

Chiefs 君	Saigae tataricae Cornu (*líng yáng jiǎo*)	pacifies the Liver, extinguishes wind, and clears heat
	Uncariae Ramulus cum Uncis (*gōu téng*)	extinguishes wind and clears fire from the *jueyin* channel
Deputies 臣	Mori Folium (*sāng yè*)	dispels wind and clears heat from the Liver and Lungs
	Chrysanthemi Flos (*jú huā*)	
Assistants 佐	Paeoniae Radix alba (*bái sháo*)	nourishes the yin, increases the fluids, softens the Liver and relaxes the sinews
	Rehmanniae Radix (*shēng dì huáng*)	
	Fritillariae cirrhosae Bulbus (*chuān bèi mǔ*)	clears heat and transforms phlegm
	Bambusae Caulis in taeniam (*zhú rú*)	
	Poriae Sclerotium pararadicis (*fú shén*)	addresses the irritability and restlessness caused by heat harassing the spirit
Envoy 使	Glycyrrhizae Radix (*gān cǎo*)	assists in relaxing the sinews; regulates and harmonizes the actions of the other ingredients

六君子湯（六君子汤）
Six-Gentlemen Decoction
liù jūn zǐ tāng

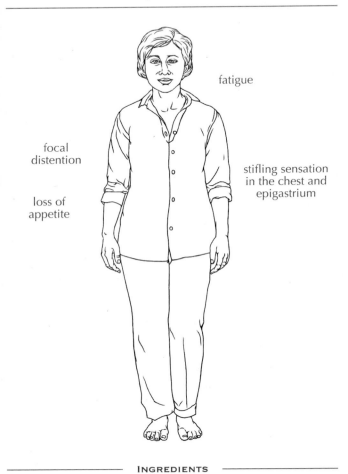

fatigue

focal distention

loss of appetite

stifling sensation in the chest and epigastrium

Key symptoms: fatigue • loss of appetite • focal distention • stifling sensation in the chest and epigastrium

Secondary symptoms: nausea • vomiting • coughing of copious, thin, and white sputum • borborygmus • thin or unformed stools

Tongue: swollen body • tooth-marked • thin, greasy, white coating

Pulse: deep • thin • weak

Abdomen: soft abdomen lacking muscle tone • splashing sounds • epigastric tenderness • pencil-line hardness between the umbilicus and xiphoid process

▶ CLINICAL NOTES

• Similar range of indications to Four-Gentlemen Decoction (*sì jūn zǐ tāng*), but with both qi deficiency and phlegm-dampness. This manifests with a stifling sensation in the epigastrium, nausea, or the presence of visible phlegm or sputum. Often a base formula for asthma due to Spleen deficiency or other patterns manifesting with Spleen qi deficiency accompanied by upward rebellion of qi.

• The formula can also be used to treat bleeding caused by the Spleen losing its capacity to control the blood.

Contraindications: phlegm and dampness without Spleen deficiency

▶ FORMULAS WITH SIMILAR INDICATIONS

Ginseng, Poria, and White Atractylodes Powder (*shēn líng bái zhú sǎn*): For Spleen deficiency with more pronounced dampness manifesting with edema, diarrhea, and soft stools.

Restore the Spleen Decoction (*guī pí tāng*): For spirit-related disorders or for bleeding due to qi deficiency in patients presenting with deficiency of Spleen qi and Heart blood without significant phlegm or dampness.

INGREDIENTS

Ginseng Radix (*rén shēn*)...3g

Atractylodis macrocephalae Rhizoma (*bái zhú*)...............4.5g

Poria (*fú líng*)...3g

Glycyrrhizae Radix praeparata (*zhì gān cǎo*).......................3g

Citri reticulatae Pericarpium (*chén pí*)...............................3g

Pinelliae Rhizoma praeparatum (*zhì bàn xià*)..................4.5g

Actions: strengthens the Spleen • transforms phlegm • stops vomiting

Main pattern: Spleen qi deficiency accompanied by phlegm

COMPOSITION

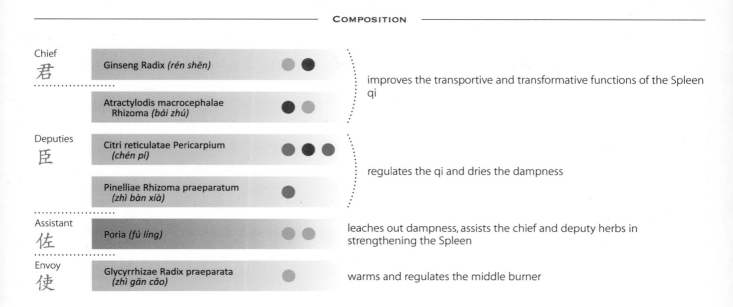

Chief 君	Ginseng Radix (rén shēn)		improves the transportive and transformative functions of the Spleen qi
	Atractylodis macrocephalae Rhizoma (bái zhú)		
Deputies 臣	Citri reticulatae Pericarpium (chén pí)		regulates the qi and dries the dampness
	Pinelliae Rhizoma praeparatum (zhì bàn xià)		
Assistant 佐	Poria (fú líng)		leaches out dampness, assists the chief and deputy herbs in strengthening the Spleen
Envoy 使	Glycyrrhizae Radix praeparata (zhì gān cǎo)		warms and regulates the middle burner

六味地黃丸
Six-Ingredient Pill with Rehmannia
liù wèi dì huáng wán

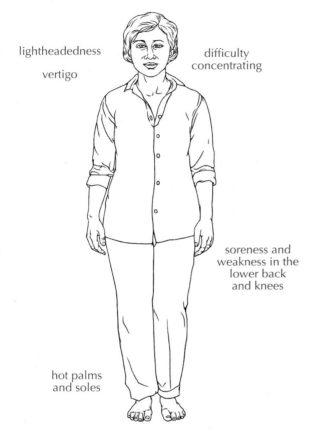

lightheadedness

vertigo

difficulty concentrating

soreness and weakness in the lower back and knees

hot palms and soles

INGREDIENTS

Rehmanniae Radix praeparata (*shú dì huáng*) 24g
Corni Fructus (*shān zhū yú*).. 12g
Dioscoreae Rhizoma (*shān yào*) 12g
Poria (*fú líng*) 9g
Moutan Cortex (*mǔ dān pí*) 9g
Alismatis Rhizoma (*zé xiè*) 9g

Actions: enriches the yin • nourishes the Kidneys

Main pattern: Kidney and Liver yin deficiency

Key symptoms: soreness and weakness in the lower back and knees • hot palms and soles • lightheadedness • vertigo

• difficulty concentrating

Secondary symptoms: impaired hearing • tinnitus • chronic dry and sore throat • toothache • spontaneous or nocturnal emissions • night sweats • nocturia • difficult or excessive urination • hard stools • reduced menstrual flow • loss of libido • impotence • premature ejaculation

Tongue: red with scanty coating • dry • may have cracks

Pulse: rapid • thin

Abdomen: hypertonicity of rectus abdominis muscle below the umbilicus together with weakness or numbness of the center of the lower abdomen • pencil-line tightness of linea alba below the umbilicus • palpable pulsations between umbilicus and pubic bone

▶ CLINICAL NOTES

• The classic formula for Kidney yin deficiency (weak back and legs, hearing loss, nocturnal emissions or urination) that cannot control yang fire (hot soles and palms, dizziness, night sweats, dry throat, or toothache). While all of these symptoms are associated with the lesser yin warp (Heart and Kidneys), the formula also treats problems related to the yin of Liver and Spleen (hunger, inflamed gums, or dryness of the skin or mucous membranes.)

• Manifestations of uncontrolled water often accompany Kidney deficiency. If this water combines with fire, it produces phlegm. This formula is excellent for yin deficiency patterns accompanied by phlegm as well as dryness and heat. This is often seen in illnesses such as diabetes, hypertension, menopausal problems, and other hormonal disorders for which the formula is commonly used.

• Originally a pediatric formula, it can be used to treat patients of any age. In fact, it is often in childhood and during puberty, when the body needs to draw on the Kidneys for growth and development, that Kidney deficiency problems present.

Contraindications: Spleen deficiency accompanied by a white, greasy tongue coating indicating difficulty in digesting rich and cloying herbs • heat patterns due to the presence of external pathogens

▶ FORMULAS WITH SIMILAR INDICATIONS ⇢

Restore the Left [Kidney] Pill (*zǔo guī wán*): Used for treating relatively straight forward conditions of deficiency without fire from deficiency.

COMPOSITION

Chief 君	Rehmanniae Radix praeparata (*shú dì huáng*)	●	strongly enriches the Kidney yin and essence
Deputies 臣	Corni Fructus (*shān zhū yú*)	●	nourishes the Liver and restrains the leakage of essence
	Dioscoreae Rhizoma (*shān yào*)	●	stabilizes the essence by tonifying the Spleen
Assistants 佐	Poria (*fú líng*)	● ●	leaches out dampness from the Spleen
	Moutan Cortex (*mǔ dān pí*)	● ●	clears and drains Liver fire
	Alismatis Rhizoma (*zé xiè*)	● ●	clears and drains the overabundance of Kidney fire

六一散
Six-to-One Powder
liù yī sǎn

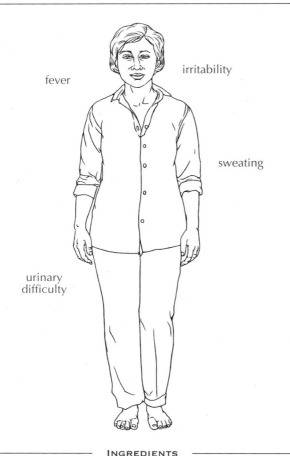

fever

irritability

sweating

urinary difficulty

Tongue: thin body • yellow or white and greasy coating

Pulse: soggy • rapid

Abdomen: slight fullness in lower burner

► CLINICAL NOTES

• Core indications are the combination of fever and irritability (indicating heat) and reduced urination (indicating dampness). The formula effectively unblocks the Triple Burner and drains heat without damaging the qi or engendering more heat.

• In clinical practice the formula is usually combined with other herbs or formulas that focus more specifically on the precise location of the obstruction and/or the relative weighting of heat and dampness.

• Because of its ability to drain heat, the formula can also be effectively used in treating damp-heat obstructing the Triple Burner due to other causes such as painful urinary dribbling or damp-heat skin disorders like papules, sores, and prickly heat.

• Note that while White Tiger Decoction (*bái hǔ tāng*) treats summerheat excess without dampness by clearing heat via the skin and pores, when there is dampness present it would block the pores and thus constrain the heat inside. It must therefore be drained via urination. As a fine powder this formula can be applied externally to treat damp-heat rashes.

Contraindications: yin deficiency • heat excess without dampness

► FORMULAS WITH SIMILAR INDICATIONS

*Cinnamon and Poria Sweet Dew Drink (*guì líng gān lù yǐn*): For more severe presentations where both heat and dampness are pronounced and with symptoms indicating location of the pathology in the Stomach and Intestines.

─────── INGREDIENTS ───────

Talcum (*huá shí*) 6g
Glycyrrhizae Radix (*gān cǎo*).............................. 1g

Preparation notes: Powder and place in a cheesecloth bag for decoctions.

Actions: clears summerheat • resolves dampness • augments the qi

Main pattern: summerheat obstructing the Triple Burner

Key symptoms: fever • sweating • irritability • urinary difficulty

Secondary symptoms: thirst • diarrhea • nausea • vomiting

———————————————————————— COMPOSITION ————————————————————

Chief
君   Talcum *(huá shí)*   ● ●   clears summerheat and resolves dampness through the Triple Burner

Deputy
臣   Glycyrrhizae Radix *(gān cǎo)*   ●   harmonizes the middle and mildly clears heat and resolves toxicity

龍膽瀉肝湯（龙胆泻肝汤）
Gentian Decoction to Drain the Liver
lóng dǎn xiè gān tāng

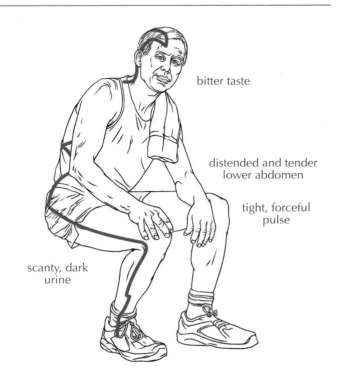

bitter taste

distended and tender lower abdomen

tight, forceful pulse

scanty, dark urine

INGREDIENTS

Gentianae Radix (*lóng dǎn cǎo*) 6g

dry-fried Scutellariae Radix (*chǎo huáng qín*) 9g

Gardeniae Fructus (*zhī zǐ*) 9g

Akebiae Caulis (*mù tōng*) 6-9g

Plantaginis Semen (*chē qián zǐ*) 9g

Alismatis Rhizoma (*zé xiè*) 12g

Bupleuri Radix (*chái hú*) 6g

Rehmanniae Radix (*shēng dì huáng*) 9g

wine-washed Angelicae sinensis Radix (*jiǔ xǐ dāng guī*) 3-6g

Glycyrrhizae Radix (*gān cǎo*) 6g

Actions: drains fire excess from the Liver and Gallbladder • clears and drains damp-heat from the lower burner

Main pattern: damp-heat excess in the Liver and/or Gallbladder channels

Key symptoms: bitter taste • irritability • short temper • scanty, dark urine

Secondary symptoms: headache • dizziness • red and sore eyes • swelling in the ears • hearing loss • difficult and painful urination with a sensation of heat in the urethra • foul-smelling leucorrhea • swollen and pruritic external genitalia • short menstrual cycle • reddish-purple menstrual blood • damp-heat skin problems along the course of the Liver and Gallbladder channels

Tongue: red body • yellow coating

Pulse: tight • forceful

Abdomen: distention of lower abdomen with pain or resistance on pressure • hypertonicity of rectus abdominis muscle • tenderness laterally to the rectus abdominis muscle

▶ CLINICAL NOTES

- This is the main formula for draining damp-heat from the Liver and Gallbladder channels. If one adjusts the composition of the formula to match the degree of heat or dampness present, it has a very wide range of indications extending to any pattern involving the presence of excess heat and dampness along the course of these channels. Typical areas include the ears (otitis, tinnitus, skin rashes); head (headaches, migraines); eyes (acute swellings, herpes zoster, infections); hypochondrium (acute cholecystitis, hepatitis, herpes zoster); the urinary system (cystitis, infections); the external genitals (itching, discharges, foul odor, eczema and other skin rashes in the genital area); and the lower abdomen, specifically involving the male and female reproductive organs (pelvic inflammatory disease, endometriosis, infertility, prostatitis, enlarged prostate).

- The formula can also be used to treat acute episodes of psycho-emotional manifestations of damp-heat excess in the Liver or Gallbladder such as irritability, severe anger, or hypertension.

Contraindications: Spleen deficiency • long-term use

▶ FORMULAS WITH SIMILAR INDICATIONS

*Augmented Rambling Powder (*jiā wèi xiāo yáo sǎn*): For

Liver heat excess patterns involving constraint from qi and blood deficiency; any dampness present will have its root in Spleen deficiency.

Tangkuei, Gentian, and Aloe Pill (*dāng guī lóng huì wán*): For Liver and Gallbladder fire with clumping in the interior. While this formula is stronger at clearing heat, it is less able to drain damp-heat.

Polyporus Decoction (*zhū líng tāng*): For accumulation of water in the lower burner arising from yang brightness

disorders. Patterns are characterized by the simultaneous presence of dampness, heat, and blood deficiency and often involve hematuria.

*Clear the Heart Drink with Lotus Seed (*qīng xīn lián zǐ yǐn*): For Heart and Lung qi deficiency patterns accompanied by damp-heat in the Bladder with painful urinary dribbling.

*Anemarrhena, Phellodendron, and Rehmannia Pill (*zhī bǎi dì huáng wán*): For damp-heat patterns in patients with vulnerable yin involving the Kidney and Bladder channels.

──── COMPOSITION ────

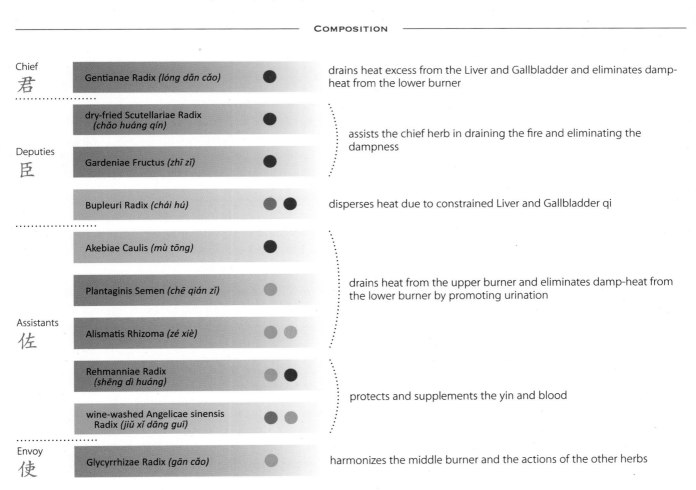

Chief 君
Gentianae Radix (*lóng dǎn cǎo*) — drains heat excess from the Liver and Gallbladder and eliminates damp-heat from the lower burner

Deputies 臣
dry-fried Scutellariae Radix (*chǎo huáng qín*)
Gardeniae Fructus (*zhī zǐ*) — assists the chief herb in draining the fire and eliminating the dampness

Bupleuri Radix (*chái hú*) — disperses heat due to constrained Liver and Gallbladder qi

Assistants 佐
Akebiae Caulis (*mù tōng*)
Plantaginis Semen (*chē qián zǐ*)
Alismatis Rhizoma (*zé xiè*) — drains heat from the upper burner and eliminates damp-heat from the lower burner by promoting urination

Rehmanniae Radix (*shēng dì huáng*)
wine-washed Angelicae sinensis Radix (*jiǔ xǐ dāng guī*) — protects and supplements the yin and blood

Envoy 使
Glycyrrhizae Radix (*gān cǎo*) — harmonizes the middle burner and the actions of the other herbs

麻黃湯 （麻黄汤）
Ephedra Decoction
má huáng tāng

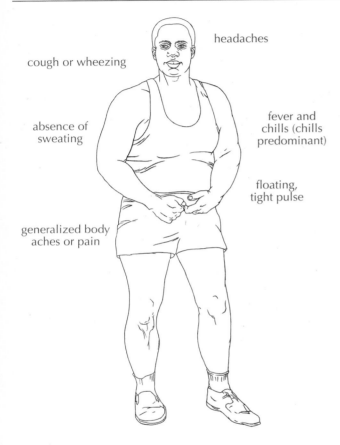

headaches

cough or wheezing

absence of sweating

fever and chills (chills predominant)

floating, tight pulse

generalized body aches or pain

Main patterns: wind-cold attacking the exterior or cold damage at the greater yang stage

Key symptoms: fever and chills (chills predominant) • absence of sweating

Secondary symptoms: cough or wheezing • headaches • generalized body aches or pain • painful obstruction (due to wind-cold-dampness) • runny nose or nasal obstruction

Tongue: thin • white coating

Pulse: floating • tight

Abdomen: no specific signs

▶ CLINICAL NOTES

- Mainly used in the treatment of acute wind-cold disorders in patients with a strong constitution. The high fever is a key clinical pointer and not a contraindication. This is caused by cold constraining yang qi at the surface.

- Used for skin disorders presenting with both redness (heat due to constraint of yang) and dryness (blocked circulation of fluids), especially where such conditions are triggered or aggravated by cold, as in certain types of urticaria or dermatitis.

- Used for asthma only when it is associated with a wind-cold exterior pattern that is not complicated by phlegm, heat, dryness, or deficiency.

- May be considered for use in gynecological disorders characterized by cold obstruction such as amenorrhea or dysmenorrhea.

- Designed for short-term use. Even though this formula is quite strong, it can be used whenever the presenting symptoms match the core pattern, even if the patient is a child or elderly.

Contraindications: weak patients • recent blood loss • patients who are prone to bleeding (especially nosebleed) • hypertension (especially in the elderly) • anxiety and restlessness in patients who tend to be overstimulated

INGREDIENTS

[1]Ephedrae Herba (*má huáng*)... 6-9g
Cinnamomi Ramulus (*guì zhī*)... 4-6g
Armeniacae Semen (*xìng rén*)... 6-9g
Glycyrrhizae Radix praeparata (*zhì gān cǎo*)...................... 3g

Preparation notes: Do not cook for more than 20 minutes.

Actions: releases wind-cold from the exterior and arrests wheezing

1. This herb can be difficult to obtain because of legal issues. Perillae Folium *(zǐ sū yè)* and the combination of Schizonepetae Herba *(jīng jiè)* and Saposhnikoviae Radix *(fáng fēng)* may be substituted.

► FORMULAS WITH SIMILAR INDICATIONS

Kudzu Decoction (*gé gēn tāng*): For wind-cold in the yang brightness channel with pronounced head/neck symptoms and a floating, excessive pulse in addition to chills and fevers.

Augmented Cyperus and Perilla Leaf Powder (*jiā wèi xiāng sū sǎn*): For exterior patterns in children or weak patients who may not be able to tolerate formulas containing Ephedrae Herba (*má huáng*). It is more appropriate for those with digestive tract symptoms. It is also used at present when the ingredients of Ephedra Decoction (*má huáng tāng*) are unavailable.

COMPOSITION

Chief 君	Ephedrae Herba (*má huáng*) ● ●	promotes sweating, resolves the exterior, disperses the Lungs, calms wheezing
Deputy 臣	Cinnamomi Ramulus (*guì zhī*) ● ●	promotes sweating, resolves muscle layer, warms and unblocks the nutritive qi and the vessels
Assistant 佐	Armeniacae Semen (*xìng rén*) ●	directs Lung qi downward, moistens dryness, transforms phlegm, stops coughing
Envoy 使	Glycyrrhizae Radix praeparata (*zhì gān cǎo*) ●	augments the qi, harmonizes the middle, facilitates synergy of the other herbs

麻黃細辛附子湯（麻黄细辛附子汤）
Ephedra, Asarum, and Aconite Accessory Root Decoction
má huáng xì xīn fù zǐ tāng

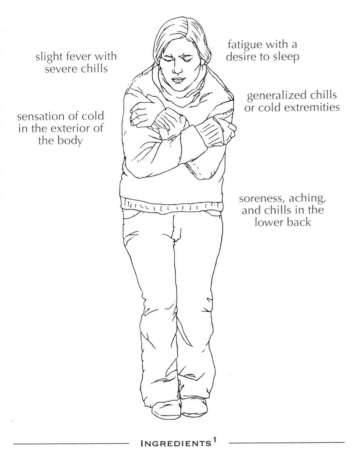

slight fever with severe chills

fatigue with a desire to sleep

sensation of cold in the exterior of the body

generalized chills or cold extremities

soreness, aching, and chills in the lower back

INGREDIENTS[1]

Ephedrae Herba (*má huáng*)..6g
Aconiti Radix lateralis praeparata (*zhì fù zǐ*)....................3-9g
Asari Herba (*xì xīn*)..3g

Actions: assists the yang • releases pathogens from the exterior

Main pattern: exterior wind-cold in patients with preexisting yang deficiency

---

1. All of the ingredients in this formula may be difficult to obtain due to legal restrictions. For this particular combination, there are no substitutes.

Key symptoms: slight fever with severe chills • sensation of cold in the exterior of the body • fatigue with a desire to sleep

Secondary symptoms: generalized chills or cold extremities • soreness, aching, and chills in the lower back • chills are not relieved by wearing more clothing or adding covers

Tongue: pale and swollen body that may have tooth marks • white or moist and greasy coating

Pulse: submerged • perhaps faint

Abdomen: no specific signs

▶ CLINICAL NOTES

- For disorders that simultaneously affect both the greater yang and lesser yin warps, or both the Lungs and Kidneys, such as headache due to cold deficiency with sore throat and a raspy voice, laryngitis, chronic coughing or wheezing, edema, etc.

- Warms the Kidneys and disperses cold to treat deep-seated cold in the lesser yin warp manifesting with headaches, toothache, or pain in the throat.

- Warms and opens the Heart yang and disperses cold and transforms stagnation. It is thus able to treat patterns where Heart and Kidney yang deficiency are accompanied by turbid obstruction such as sick sinus syndrome, cardiac insufficiency, pulmonary heart disease, Keshan disease, etc.

- Warms the channels and disperses cold to alleviate pain aggravated by cold and exhaustion, including trigeminal neuralgia, stubborn headaches, sciatica, rheumatoid arthritis, etc.

Contraindications: unsuitable for cases where symptoms of yang deficiency are dominant, characterized by undigested food in the stool and a faint, almost imperceptible pulse, as its use could lead to devastated yang

▶ FORMULAS WITH SIMILAR INDICATIONS

Renewal Powder (*zài zào sǎn*): For exterior conditions with preexisting qi and yang deficiency marked by a lusterless, somber, pallid complexion, a weak voice, and a large and empty pulse.

Frigid Extremities Decoction (*sì nì tāng*): For lesser yin disorders marked by cold extremities, sense of intense cold, and lethargy without exterior symptoms or signs of obstruction of the lesser yin channel.

COMPOSITION

Chief 君	Ephedrae Herba *(má huáng)*	● ●	promotes sweating, resolves the exterior, disperses cold
Deputy 臣	Aconiti Radix lateralis praeparata *(zhì fù zǐ)*	● Ⓣ	warms the Kidneys and assists the yang
Assis/Env 佐/使	Asari Herba *(xì xīn)*	●	helps chief herb to release the exterior and the deputy to scatter interior cold

麻杏石甘湯(麻杏石甘汤)
Ephedra, Apricot Kernel, Gypsum, and Licorice Decoction
má xìng shí gān tāng

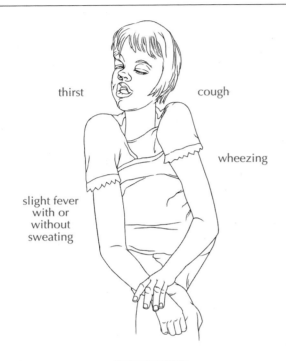

thirst · cough · wheezing · slight fever with or without sweating

INGREDIENTS

[1]Ephedrae Herba (*má huáng*).. 6-9g
Gypsum fibrosum (*shí gāo*).. 18-24g
Armeniacae Semen (*xìng rén*) 9g
Glycyrrhizae Radix praeparata (*zhì gān cǎo*) 3-6g

Actions: facilitates the flow of Lung qi · clears heat · calms wheezing by directing rebellious qi downward

Main pattern: heat lodged in the Lungs where it obstructs the flow of qi

Key symptoms: slight fever with or without sweating · thirst · wheezing · cough

Secondary symptoms: labored breathing · nasal flaring · chest tightness · difficult expectoration of sticky, greenish-yellow phlegm

Tongue: thin coating that tends to be white and dry

Pulse: rapid · floating · slippery

Abdomen: hypertonicity of rectus abdominis muscle in upper abdomen

▶ CLINICAL NOTES

• The main indication for this formula is bronchial spasms due to acute bronchial infections or hypersensitivity.

Contraindications: cough due to cold fettering the exterior · wheezing due to Kidneys unable to grasp qi · strong fever and sweating due to yang brightness heat excess

▶ FORMULAS WITH SIMILAR INDICATIONS

*Cinnamon Twig Decoction plus Magnolia Bark and Apricot Kernel (*guì zhī jiā hòu pò xìng zǐ tāng*): For wheezing and sweating accompanied by an aversion to drafts and/or subjective sensations of qi gushing upward.

Drain the White Powder from *Craft of Medicinal Treatment for Childhood Disease Patterns* (*xiè bái sǎn*): For Lung fire from constraint against a background of yin deficiency. This pattern is characterized by a sensation of steaming heat in the afternoons and skin that is warm to the touch but dry.

Minor Bluegreen Dragon Decoction (*xiǎo qīng lóng tāng*): For coughing and wheezing with thin fluids accumulating in the chest and Lungs and cold in the exterior. The pattern is confirmed by a wet tongue with white coating, nasal discharge, and thin, clear expectorate that may contain bubbles.

Ophiopogonis Decoction (*mài mén dōng tāng*): Treats yin deficiency in the Lungs and Stomach giving rise to a pattern that includes coughing and phlegm that is difficult to expectorate.

---

1. This herb can be difficult to obtain because of legal issues. Perillae Folium (*zǐ sū yè*) may be used as a substitute.

COMPOSITION

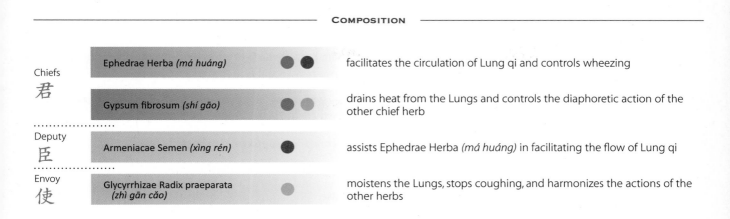

Chiefs
君

Ephedrae Herba (*má huáng*) — facilitates the circulation of Lung qi and controls wheezing

Gypsum fibrosum (*shí gāo*) — drains heat from the Lungs and controls the diaphoretic action of the other chief herb

Deputy
臣

Armeniacae Semen (*xìng rén*) — assists Ephedrae Herba (*má huáng*) in facilitating the flow of Lung qi

Envoy
使

Glycyrrhizae Radix praeparata (*zhì gān cǎo*) — moistens the Lungs, stops coughing, and harmonizes the actions of the other herbs

麻子仁丸
Hemp Seed Pill
má zǐ rén wán

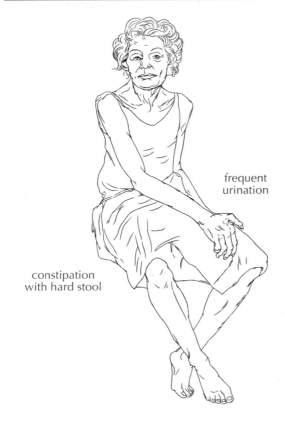

frequent urination

constipation with hard stool

INGREDIENTS

Cannabis Semen (*huǒ má rén*)..................................... 30g
Armeniacae Semen (*xìng rén*)..................................... 15g
¹Paeoniae Radix (*sháo yào*).. 15g
Aurantii Fructus immaturus (*zhǐ shí*)........................ 10g
Magnoliae officinalis Cortex (*hòu pó*)........................ 15g
Rhei Radix et Rhizoma (*dà huáng*)............................. 20g

Preparation notes: The ingredients are ground into powder and made into pills with honey. The normal dosage is 10g once or twice a day.

---

1. As the primary function here is to restrain, tonify, or soften, Paeoniae Radix alba *(bái sháo)* is preferred.

Actions: moistens the Intestines • drains heat • promotes the movement of qi • unblocks the bowels

Main pattern: heat-dryness blocking the physiological movement of fluids in the Spleen, known as Spleen bind

Key symptoms: constipation with hard stool that is difficult to expel • normal to frequent urination

Secondary symptoms: none noted

Tongue: dry • thin • yellow coating

Pulse: submerged • rapid or floating • choppy

Abdomen: palpable hard stool in bowels • soft abdominal wall

► CLINICAL NOTES

- For constipation and dry stools in patients with heat in the yang brightness where strong purgation is contraindicated. Urination is normal or even excessive, in contrast to severe yang brightness heat and dryness patterns where urination is reduced.

- Typical usage includes constipation in the elderly, post-operative or postpartum, characterized by signs of yang brightness excess in otherwise normal or even weak patients.

- Also used in patients suffering from hemorrhoids who require a laxative that does not aggravate the condition. For hemorrhoids add Persicae Semen (*táo rén*) and Angelicae sinensis Radix (*dāng guī*).

- Useful in patients with constipation who have a sedentary lifestyle, but who are neither excessively deficient nor have pronounced signs of damp-heat in the Intestines.

Contraindications: This formula drains heat excess and opens stagnation in the Intestines. It should not be used without modification in treating the very weak, or long term for habitual constipation. Contraindicated during pregnancy.

▶ FORMULAS WITH SIMILAR INDICATIONS

Moisten the Intestines Pill from *Master Shen's Book* (*rùn cháng wán*): For dry stools in patients with blood deficiency and stasis as reflected in dry skin and nails, palpitations, dizziness, forgetfulness, pale tongue, and a thin and rough pulse.

Five-Seed Pill (*wǔ rén wán*): For chronic constipation due to intense dryness of the Intestines, without any particular heat, that is marked by dry stools that are difficult to pass, dry tongue, and a thin and rough pulse.

─────────────────────── COMPOSITION ───────────────────────

Chief 君	Cannabis semen *(huǒ má rén)* ●	moistens the intestines, unblocks the bowels
Deputies 臣	Armeniacae Semen *(xìng rén)* ●	directs qi downward, moistens the intestines
	Paeoniae Radix alba *(bái sháo)* ● ●	nourishes the yin, harmonizes the interior
	Aurantii Fructus *(zhǐ shí)* ● ●	breaks up accumulation
Assistants 佐	Magnolia officinalis Cortex *(hòu pò)* ● ●	removes fullness and distention
	Rhei Radix et Rhizoma *(dà huáng)* ●	purgative function helps to unblock the bowels
Envoy 使	honey ●	harmonizes the effects of the other ingredients and moistens the Intestines

麥門冬湯（麦门冬汤）
Ophiopogonis Decoction
mài mén dōng tāng

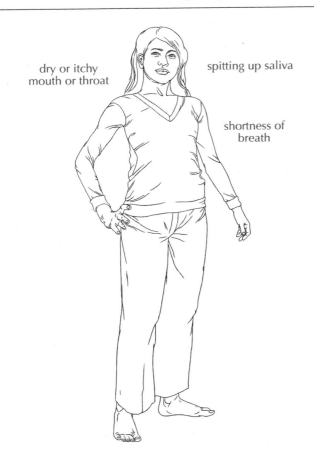

dry or itchy mouth or throat

spitting up saliva

shortness of breath

INGREDIENTS

Ophiopogonis Radix (*mài mén dōng*) 42-70g
Ginseng Radix (*rén shēn*) 9g
Nonglutinous rice (*jīng mǐ*) 6-15g
Jujubae Fructus (*dà zǎo*) .... 3-4 pieces
Glycyrrhizae Radix (*gān cǎo*) 6-9g
Pinelliae Rhizoma praeparatum (*zhì bàn xià*) 6-18g

Actions: benefits the Stomach • generates fluids • directs rebellious qi downward

Main patterns: Lung atrophy due to heat • throat obstruction

• Stomach and Lung yin deficiency accompanied by phlegm and rebellious qi

Key symptoms: spitting up saliva • coughing • dry or itchy mouth or throat • shortness of breath

Secondary symptoms: coughing up phlegm that is difficult to expectorate • thirst • fever • wheezing • hoarseness • nausea • facial flushing • heat in the palms and soles • dry skin

Tongue: dry body • scanty coating

Pulse: floating and deficient (acute conditions) • thin and weak (chronic conditions)

Abdomen: generally weak abdominal wall • hypertonicity of rectus abdominus muscle • discomfort or focal distention in epigastrium

▶ CLINICAL NOTES

• This formula treats chronic Stomach and Lung deficiency. These organs play an important role in directing qi and fluids downward but are easily affected by dryness and yin deficiency. If the yin of the Stomach and Lungs is damaged, the qi fails to be directed downward and rebels upward, and fluids do not transform. Key markers of this complex pattern are coughing up of frothy saliva in the presence of yin deficiency signs such as a dry mouth or throat, floating pulse, dry tongue, and facial flushing.

• This is an important formula for cough with phlegm that is difficult to expectorate. The cough may be acute or chronic, though absent any attendant exterior symptoms. While there will be sticky phlegm, the presence of any phlegm distinguishes this pattern from those of cough with more pronounced dryness. Another marker is focal distention or discomfort in the epigastrium, indicating that the qi cannot descend.

• This is also an important formula for throat obstruction characterized by dryness or itching of the throat accompanied by phlegm that is difficult to expectorate.

• This formula's ability to direct deficiency qi and fire downward makes it useful in treating a wide variety of problems rooted in Stomach or Lung yin deficiency. These include inverted menstruation, cough during pregnancy, morning sickness, wheezing, chronic bronchitis, pleurisy, atrophic gastritis, stomach and duodenal ulcers, esophagitis, and laryngitis.

Contraindications: dry cough with exterior symptoms • phlegm-dampness • Lung atrophy due to cold from deficiency

▶ FORMULAS WITH SIMILAR INDICATIONS

Lophatherum and Gypsum Decoction (*zhú yè shí gāo tāng*): For cough in the context of heat and yin and qi deficiency manifesting with fever or a flooding pulse and throat obstruction that is mild if it exists at all.

Pinellia and Magnolia Bark Decoction (*bàn xià hòu pò tāng*): For throat obstruction resulting from qi stagnation and excess phlegm characterized by itching in the throat but without dryness of the mouth or throat.

Lily Bulb Decoction to Preserve the Metal (*bǎi hé gù jīn tāng*): For cough with phlegm that is difficult to expectorate due to yin deficiency of the Lung and Kidneys. It addresses a deeper yin deficiency that can manifest with such signs as night sweats and steaming bones.

Clear Dryness and Rescue the Lungs Decoction (*qīng zào jiù fèi tāng*): Focuses on treating cough and other symptoms owing to Lung dryness and does not substantially address Stomach yin deficiency.

──────── COMPOSITION ────────

Chief 君	Ophiopogonis Radix (*mài mén dōng*)	clears heat from deficiency from the Stomach and generates fluids in the Stomach and Lungs
Deputy 臣	Ginseng Radix (*rén shēn*)	augments the qi, generates fluids, and revives the qi and yin
Assistants 佐	Nonglutinous rice (*jīng mǐ*)	
	Jujubae Fructus (*dà zǎo*)	assists the Stomach qi and generates fluids
	Glycyrrhizae Radix (*gān cǎo*)	
	Pinelliae Rhizoma praeparatum (*zhì bàn xià*)	facilitates the flow of Stomach qi and directs the qi downward

牡蠣散 （牡蛎散）
Oyster Shell Powder
mǔ lì sǎn

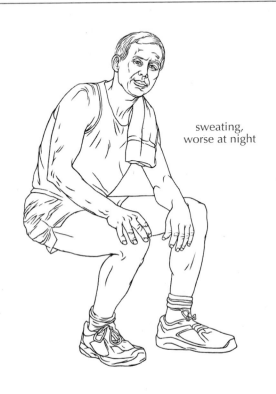

sweating, worse at night

Tongue: pale red

Pulse: thin • frail

Abdomen: no specific signs

▶ CLINICAL NOTES

• If this formula is to be used for night sweats, they must be associated with Heart qi deficiency. This type of sweating also occurs at night (which is not the case if solely due to Lung qi deficiency), yet there will be no signs of heat (distinguishing it from sweating due to damp-heat, yin deficiency, or blood stasis).

• Note that due to USDA restrictions, Tritici Fructus levis (*fú xiǎo mài*) cannot be imported into the U.S. as a bulk herb. In decoctions or regular powders, one useful substitute is Atractylodis macrocephalae Rhizoma (*bái zhú*) with a small amount of Schisandrae Fructus (*wǔ wèi zǐ*). Alternatively, a few grams of Tritici Fructus levis (*fú xiǎo mài*) in granule form can be added to the strained decoction, as granules can be imported.

Contraindications: sweating from yin or yang deficiency

▶ FORMULAS WITH SIMILAR INDICATIONS

Jade Windscreen Powder (*yù píng fēng sǎn*): For deficiency of protective qi characterized by allergies, recurrent colds or flu, and spontaneous sweating accompanied by aversion to drafts.

--- INGREDIENTS ---

Ostreae Concha (*mǔ lì*)... 15g
Astragali Radix (*huáng qí*) 9g
Ephedrae Radix (*má huáng gēn*)............................. 3g
Tritici Fructus levis (*fú xiǎo mài*)......................... 15g

Actions: inhibits sweating • stabilizes the exterior

Main patterns: spontaneous sweating due to unstable protective qi (associated with the Lungs) • night sweats due to constrained heat at the level of the nutritive qi (associated with the Heart)

Key symptoms: spontaneous sweating that worsens at night

Secondary symptoms: palpitations • easily startled • shortness of breath • irritability • general debility • lethargy

--- COMPOSITION ---

Chief 君	Ostreae Concha *(mǔ lì)*	●●	restrains the yin, anchors the floating yang, inhibits sweating, and relieves irritability
Deputy 臣	Astragali Radix *(huáng qí)*	●	strongly tonifies the Lung qi, strengthens the protective qi, and stabilizes the exterior
Assistants 佐	Ephedrae Radix *(má huáng gēn)*	●	assists the chief ingredient in augmenting the Heart qi, restraining sweat, and stabilizing the exterior
	Tritici Fructus levis *(fú xiǎo mài)*	●●	mildly nourishes the Heart qi and clears heat from constraint by venting it to the surface

木香檳榔丸（木香槟榔丸）
Aucklandia and Betel Nut Pill
mù xiāng bīng láng wán

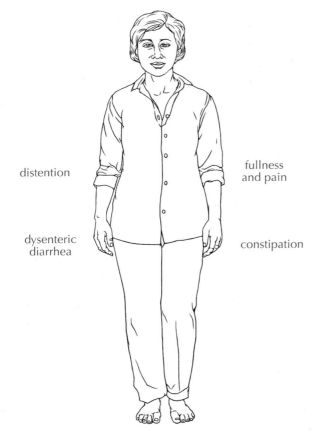

distention

fullness and pain

dysenteric diarrhea

constipation

INGREDIENTS

Aucklandiae Radix (*mù xiāng*) 30g
Arecae Semen (*bīng láng*) 30g
Rhei Radix et Rhizoma (*dà huáng*)..................................... 90g
Pharbitidis Semen (*qiān niú zǐ*)... 120g
Citri reticulatae viride Pericarpium (*qīng pí*)..................... 30g
Citri reticulatae Pericarpium (*chén pí*) 30g
dry-fried Cyperi Rhizoma (*chǎo xiāng fù*)........................ 120g
dry-fried Curcumae Rhizoma (*chǎo é zhú*) 30g
bran-fried Aurantii Fructus (*fū chǎo zhǐ ké*) 30g
Coptidis Rhizoma (*huáng lián*) 30g
Phellodendri Cortex (*huáng bǎi*).. 90g

Preparation notes: The ingredients are powdered and made into pills with water. The normal dosage is 6-9g taken 2-3 times a day with warm water or ginger tea.

Actions: promotes the movement of qi • guides out stagnation • purges accumulation • drains heat

Main pattern: accumulation of food obstructing the middle burner

Key symptoms: focal and generalized distention • fullness and pain in the epigastrium and abdomen

Secondary symptoms: constipation • dysenteric diarrhea with tenesmus • urinary difficulty • phlegm with cough and wheezing

Tongue: yellow, greasy coating

Pulse: submerged • excessive

Abdomen: no specific signs

► CLINICAL NOTES

• This formula disperses accumulation, obstruction, and damp-heat from the middle and lower burners, primarily the Stomach and Intestines. It is unsuitable for long-term use. Although it may seem incongruous that the formula can treat both constipation and diarrhea, it is important to understand that, in this situation, the two conditions stem from the same root: stagnation.

• While in a narrow sense the dispersing method refers to the treatment of food stagnation, in a broader sense it can be used as a method for treating various kinds of accumulations in the body. Given its qi and blood-breaking ingredients, contemporary practitioners have therefore extended the use of this formula to the treatment of ovarian cysts. For that purpose, Rhei Radix et Rhizoma (*dà huáng*), Coptidis Rhizoma (*huáng lián*), and Phellodendri Cortex (*huáng bǎi*) are omitted and herbs such as Angelicae sinensis Radix (*dāng guī*), Paeoniae Radix rubra (*chì sháo*), Moutan Cortex (*mǔ dān pí*), and Persicae Semen (*táo rén*) are added.

Contraindications: deficiency patterns

▶ FORMULAS WITH SIMILAR INDICATIONS

Unripe Bitter Orange Pill to Guide out Stagnation (*zhǐ shí*

dǎo zhì wán): For excess-type qi and food stagnation patterns that transform into heat stagnation patterns, but with less pronounced distention and pain and more signs of dampness.

COMPOSITION

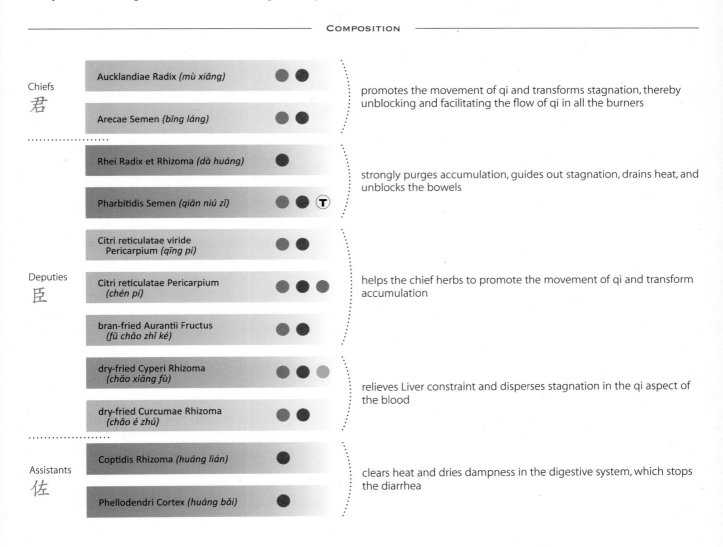

Role	Herb	Action
Chiefs 君	Aucklandiae Radix (*mù xiāng*) — Arecae Semen (*bīng láng*)	promotes the movement of qi and transforms stagnation, thereby unblocking and facilitating the flow of qi in all the burners
Deputies 臣	Rhei Radix et Rhizoma (*dà huáng*) — Pharbitidis Semen (*qiān niú zǐ*) (T)	strongly purges accumulation, guides out stagnation, drains heat, and unblocks the bowels
	Citri reticulatae viride Pericarpium (*qīng pí*) — Citri reticulatae Pericarpium (*chén pí*) — bran-fried Aurantii Fructus (*fū chǎo zhǐ ké*)	helps the chief herbs to promote the movement of qi and transform accumulation
	dry-fried Cyperi Rhizoma (*chǎo xiāng fù*) — dry-fried Curcumae Rhizoma (*chǎo é zhú*)	relieves Liver constraint and disperses stagnation in the qi aspect of the blood
Assistants 佐	Coptidis Rhizoma (*huáng lián*) — Phellodendri Cortex (*huáng bǎi*)	clears heat and dries dampness in the digestive system, which stops the diarrhea

平胃散
Calm the Stomach Powder
píng wèi sǎn

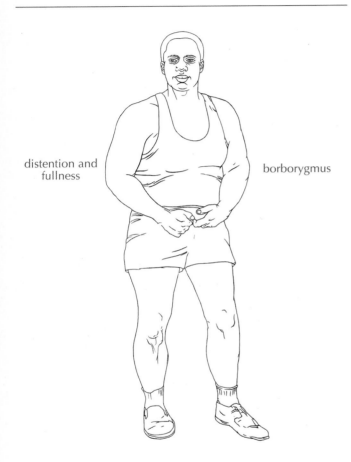

distention and fullness

borborygmus

INGREDIENTS

dry-fried Atractylodis Rhizoma (*chǎo cāng zhú*) 15-21g

ginger-fried Magnoliae officinalis Cortex (*jiāng chǎo hòu pò*) 9g

Citri reticulatae Pericarpium (*chén pí*) 9g

Glycyrrhizae Radix praeparata (*zhì gān cǎo*) 3-6g

Zingiberis Rhizoma recens (*shēng jiāng*) 3-6g

Jujubae Fructus (*dà zǎo*) .... 2 pieces

Actions: dries dampness • improves the Spleen's ability to transform and transport • promotes the movement of qi • harmonizes the Stomach

---

Main pattern: dampness stagnating in the Spleen and Stomach

Key symptoms: distention and fullness in the epigastrium and abdomen • borborygmus after eating

Secondary symptoms: loss of taste and appetite • heavy sensation in the limbs • loose stools or diarrhea • increased desire to sleep • nausea and vomiting • belching • acid reflux

Tongue: thick, white, greasy coating

Pulse: moderate • slippery

Abdomen: fullness and distention around the umbilicus • epigastric fullness

▶ CLINICAL NOTES

- This is the main formula for excess dampness hampering the transporting and transforming functions of the middle burner. The pattern's key markers are a greasy tongue coating and fullness and distention around the umbilicus extending toward the epigastrium.

- Because the middle burner is the fulcrum of the qi dynamic, this formula can treat a very wide range of manifestations. For instance, it is a key formula for facilitating labor if the cause of the delay is dampness-induced qi stagnation.

- This formula can be flexibly modified. For example, for abdominal distention with nausea and vomiting, omit Jujubae Fructus (*dà zǎo*) and add Aucklandiae Radix (*mù xiāng*) and Amomi Fructus (*shā rén*); for Spleen deficiency with hard focal distention, add Atractylodis macrocephalae Rhizoma (*bái zhú*) and Aurantii Fructus immaturus (*zhǐ shí*); for abdominal distention and diarrhea, nausea, vomiting, and a thick, greasy, white tongue coating, omit Jujubae Fructus (*dà zǎo*) and add Pogostemonis/Agastaches Herba (*huò xiāng*) and Pinelliae Rhizoma praeparatum (*zhì bàn xià*); for concomitant food stagnation with sour regurgitation, omit Jujubae Fructus (*dà zǎo*) and add Crataegi Fructus (*shān zhā*), Massa medicata fermentata (*shén qū*), Hordei Fructus germinatus (*mài yá*), and Amomi Fructus (*shā rén*).

Contraindications: yin or blood deficiency • use cautiously during pregnancy

► FORMULAS WITH SIMILAR INDICATIONS

Patchouli/Agastache Powder to Rectify the Qi (*huò xiāng zhèng qì sǎn*): For wind-cold-dampness in the exterior complicated by dampness in the middle burner which presents as headaches, digestive upset or chills and fevers.

Six-Gentlemen Decoction with Aucklandia and Amomum (*xiāng shā liù jūn zǐ tāng*): For qi deficiency of the Spleen and Stomach with qi stagnation and phlegm-dampness. Deficiency is reflected in such signs as a soft and weak pulse, shortness of breath, or spontaneous sweating.

Pinellia Decoction to Drain the Epigastrium (*bàn xià xiè xīn tāng*): For cold-heat complex or damp-heat in the Stomach in the context of Spleen yang deficiency. This pattern can also manifest with diarrhea and borborygmus, but these symptoms stem from deficiency cold rather than damp excess; that is, the diarrhea is watery rather than explosive and does not relieve the sensation of stagnation. Furthermore, abdominal palpation points to stagnation in the epigastrium rather than the abdomen.

──────── COMPOSITION ────────

Chief 君	dry-fried Atractylodis Rhizoma (*chǎo cāng zhú*)	dispels dampness and strengthens the transportive function of the Spleen
Deputy 臣	ginger-fried Magnoliae officinalis Cortex (*jiāng chǎo hòu pò*)	moves the qi, disperses fullness, directs the qi downward, and transforms dampness
Assistant 佐	Citri reticulatae Pericarpium (*chén pí*)	regulates the qi and harmonizes the Stomach
	Glycyrrhizae Radix praeparata (*zhì gān cǎo*)	
Envoys 使	Zingiberis Rhizoma recens (*shēng jiāng*)	tonifies the Spleen; harmonizes the actions of the other herbs and enhances their Spleen-strengthening properties
	Jujubae Fructus (*dà zǎo*)	

普濟消毒飲（普济消毒饮）
Universal Benefit Drink to Eliminate Toxin
pǔ jì xiāo dú yǐn

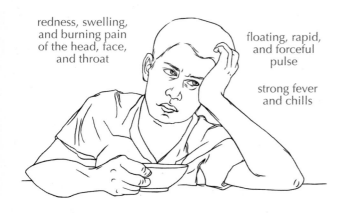

redness, swelling, and burning pain of the head, face, and throat

floating, rapid, and forceful pulse

strong fever and chills

INGREDIENTS

Scutellariae Radix (*huáng qín*) 15g
Coptidis Rhizoma (*huáng lián*) 15g
Ginseng Radix (*rén shēn*) 3g
Citri reticulatae Exocarpium rubrum (*jú hóng*) 6g
Glycyrrhizae Radix (*gān cǎo*) 6g
Scrophulariae Radix (*xuán shēn*) 6g
Bupleuri Radix (*chái hú*) 6g
Platycodi Radix (*jié gěng*) 6g
Forsythiae Fructus (*lián qiào*) 3g
Isatidis /Baphicacanthis Radix (*bǎn lán gēn*)....................... 3g
Lasiosphaera/Calvatia (*mǎ bó*)... 3g
Arctii Fructus (*niú bàng zǐ*) 3g
Menthae haplocalycis Herba (*bò hé*) 3g
dry-fried Bombyx batryticatus (*chǎo jiāng cán*) 2g
Cimicifugae Rhizoma (*shēng má*).. 2g

Actions: clears heat • eliminates fire toxin • disperses wind-heat

Main pattern: acute, massive febrile disorder of the head due to a seasonal epidemic toxin associated with wind-heat and phlegm-dampness

Key symptoms: strong fever and chills • redness, swelling, and burning pain of the head, face, and throat

Secondary symptoms: inability to open the eyes • dysfunction of the throat • dryness and thirst

Tongue: red body • powdery-white or yellow coating

Pulse: floating • rapid • forceful

Abdomen: no specific signs

▶ CLINICAL NOTES

• For acute feverish disorders presenting with accumulation of heat toxin in the head such as mumps, swollen and painful lymph glands, tonsillitis, or infections of the mouth.

Contraindications: Use cautiously in treating patients with yin deficiency.

▶ FORMULAS WITH SIMILAR INDICATIONS

Sweet Dew Special Pill to Eliminate Toxin (*gān lù xiāo dú dān*): For initial-stage damp-heat toxin epidemic disorders where dysfunction of the throat is accompanied by afternoon fevers, thirst but not necessarily a strong desire to drink, and a greasy, white, or slightly yellow tongue coating.

Immortals' Formula for Sustaining Life (*xiān fāng huó mìng yǐn*): For sores and swellings owing to accumulation of toxic heat caused by stasis of blood and stagnation of qi in the absence of systemic fever.

Bupleurum Decoction to Clear the Liver (*chái hú qīng gān tang*): Primarily for ear problems or recurrent throat infections due to excess heat in the Liver and Gallbladder channels, but can also be applied to toxic swellings along the course of the Liver and Gallbladder channels, tinnitus, dizziness, headache, irritability, or rib pain.

COMPOSITION

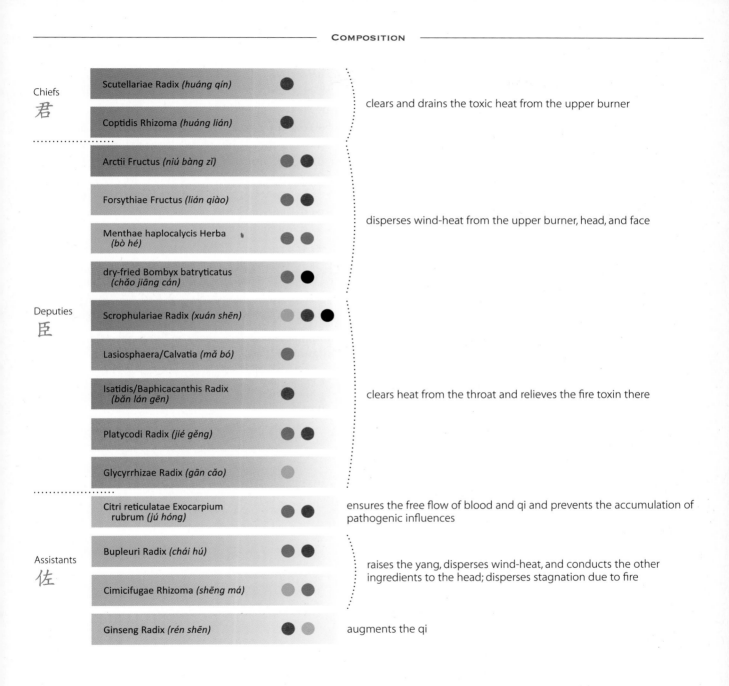

Chiefs 君

Scutellariae Radix *(huáng qín)*
Coptidis Rhizoma *(huáng lián)*

clears and drains the toxic heat from the upper burner

Deputies 臣

Arctii Fructus *(niú bàng zǐ)*
Forsythiae Fructus *(lián qiào)*
Menthae haplocalycis Herba *(bò hé)*
dry-fried Bombyx batryticatus *(chǎo jiāng cán)*

disperses wind-heat from the upper burner, head, and face

Scrophulariae Radix *(xuán shēn)*
Lasiosphaera/Calvatia *(mǎ bó)*
Isatidis/Baphicacanthis Radix *(bǎn lán gēn)*
Platycodi Radix *(jié gěng)*
Glycyrrhizae Radix *(gān cǎo)*

clears heat from the throat and relieves the fire toxin there

Assistants 佐

Citri reticulatae Exocarpium rubrum *(jú hóng)*

ensures the free flow of blood and qi and prevents the accumulation of pathogenic influences

Bupleuri Radix *(chái hú)*
Cimicifugae Rhizoma *(shēng má)*

raises the yang, disperses wind-heat, and conducts the other ingredients to the head; disperses stagnation due to fire

Ginseng Radix *(rén shēn)*

augments the qi

牽正散（牽正散）
Lead to Symmetry Powder
qiān zhèng sǎn

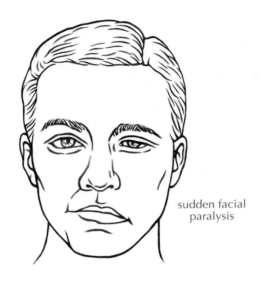

sudden facial paralysis

INGREDIENTS

Typhonii Rhizoma (*bái fù zǐ*)

Bombyx batryticatus (*bái jiāng cán*)

Scorpio (*quán xiē*), minus the tail

Preparation notes: The tail is removed from the Scorpio (*quán xiē*) and equal parts of the three herbs are ground into a powder. Three grams of the powder are washed down with warm rice wine each time. Note that all of these ingredients must be sterilized before use.

Actions: dispels wind • transforms phlegm • stops spasms

Main pattern: sequelae of channel stroke with symptoms confined to the head and face

Key symptoms: sudden facial paralysis • deviation of the eyes and mouth • facial muscle twitch

Tongue: no special signs

Pulse: should not be frail, minute, or hidden

Abdomen: should not be lax

▶ CLINICAL NOTES

• This formula is specific for facial paralysis due to wind-phlegm obstructing the channels and collaterals without any internal symptoms.

→ For very chronic and stubborn cases, one should add herbs to dispel phlegm and drive out lifeless blood from the channels such as Gastrodiae Rhizoma (*tiān má*), Pheretima (*dì lóng*), Scolopendra (*wú gōng*), Carthami Flos (*hóng huā*), and Persicae Semen (*táo rén*), along with tonifying herbs such as Astragali Radix (*huáng qí*) and Angelicae sinensis Radix (*dāng guī*).

→ For acute cases, herbs that expel wind-dampness, such as Notopterygii Rhizoma seu Radix (*qiāng huó*) and Angelicae dahuricae Radix (*bái zhǐ*), are often added. Alternatively, Saposhnikoviae Radix (*fáng fēng*) can be used if these herbs are considered overly drying.

Contraindications: deficiency conditions • wind-heat or phlegm-heat

──────────────────── COMPOSITION ────────────────────

Chief
君   Typhonii Rhizoma *(bái fù zǐ)*   ● ● Ⓣ   dispels wind and transforms phlegm

Deputy
臣   Bombyx batryticatus   ● ●   extinguishes internal wind, dispels external wind, and transforms phlegm;
            (bái jiāng cán)   eliminates wind-phlegm and unblocks the collaterals

Assistant
佐   Scorpio *(quán xiē)*   ● ● Ⓣ   extinguishes wind and stops spasms, unblocks the collaterals, arrests
                                                              wind, and alleviates facial paralysis

羌活勝濕湯（羌活胜湿汤）
Notopterygium Decoction to Overcome Dampness
qiāng huó shèng shī tāng

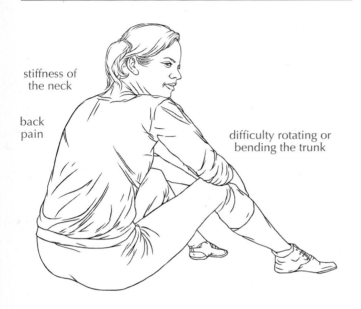

stiffness of the neck

back pain

difficulty rotating or bending the trunk

INGREDIENTS

Notopterygii Rhizoma seu Radix (*qiāng huó*) 3-6g
Angelicae pubescentis Radix (*dú huó*) 3-6g
Ligustici Rhizoma (*gǎo běn*) 1.5-3g
Saposhnikoviae Radix (*fáng fēng*) 1.5-3g
Chuanxiong Rhizoma (*chuān xiōng*) 1.5-3g
Viticis Fructus (*màn jīng zǐ*) 1-3g
Glycyrrhizae Radix praeparata (*zhì gān cǎo*) 1.5-3g

Actions: expels wind and dampness

Main pattern: wind-dampness lodging in the exterior (channels and muscle layer)

Key symptoms: stiffness of the neck • back pain • difficulty rotating or bending the trunk

Secondary symptoms: heavy and painful head • generalized sensation of heaviness • generalized pain • mild fever • chills

Tongue: white, greasy coating

Pulse: floating and lax • floating and soft

Abdomen: no specific signs

▶ CLINICAL NOTES

- This is a formula for wind-dampness lodging in the channels and muscle layer of the body's exterior. It is especially suitable for problems in the greater yang channels such as headaches, neck stiffness, and temporomandibular joint syndrome.

- The source text suggests that bodily heaviness and a sinking feeling in the lower back can be attributed to cold-dampness in the channel and should be treated by adding 1.5g of Stephaniae tetrandrae Radix (*hàn fáng jǐ*). For mild cases, add 1.5g of Aconiti Radix lateralis praeparata (*zhì fù zǐ*); for more severe cases, add 1.5g of Aconiti Radix praeparata (*zhì chuān wū*).

Contraindications: yin deficiency • excess heat

▶ FORMULAS WITH SIMILAR INDICATIONS

Nine-Herb Decoction with Notopterygium (*jiǔ wèi qiāng huó tāng*): For wind-cold-dampness invading the body's exterior with heat constraint in the interior. This manifests with chills and fevers, headache, absence of sweating, bitter taste, and slight thirst.

Pubescent Angelica and Taxillus Decoction (*dú huó jì shēng tāng*): For painful obstruction with Kidney and Liver deficiency manifesting with difficulty moving the joints, particularly in the lower body.

——— COMPOSITION ———

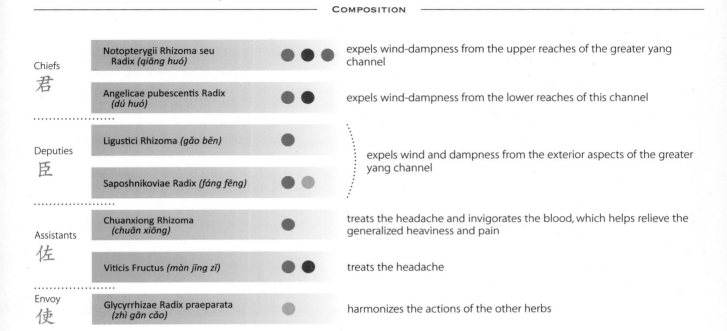

Chiefs 君	Notopterygii Rhizoma seu Radix *(qiāng huó)*	● ● ●	expels wind-dampness from the upper reaches of the greater yang channel
	Angelicae pubescentis Radix *(dú huó)*	● ●	expels wind-dampness from the lower reaches of this channel
Deputies 臣	Ligustici Rhizoma *(gǎo běn)*	●	expels wind and dampness from the exterior aspects of the greater yang channel
	Saposhnikoviae Radix *(fáng fēng)*	● ●	
Assistants 佐	Chuanxiong Rhizoma *(chuān xiōng)*	●	treats the headache and invigorates the blood, which helps relieve the generalized heaviness and pain
	Viticis Fructus *(màn jīng zǐ)*	● ●	treats the headache
Envoy 使	Glycyrrhizae Radix praeparata *(zhì gān cǎo)*	●	harmonizes the actions of the other herbs

青黛散
Indigo Powder
qīng dài săn

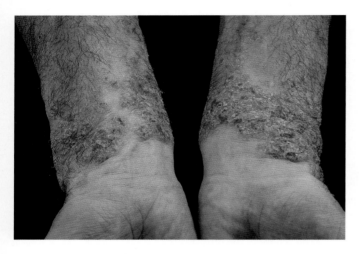

INGREDIENTS

Indigo naturalis (*qīng dài*) 60g

Gypsum fibrosum (*shí gāo*) 120g

Talcum (*huá shí*) 120g

Phellodendri Cortex (*huáng băi*) 60g

Preparation notes: Grind the herbs to a fine powder and process through an 80*mu* (80 openings per inch) sieve.

Actions: gathers in dampness • relieves itching • clears heat • resolves toxicity

Main pattern: damp-heat skin disorders

Key symptoms: weeping • erosion • heat • swelling • itching • pain

▶ CLINICAL NOTES

• Treats all manner of damp-heat skin disorders. These sores are red, itching, weeping, and sometimes painful. Examples include eczema, herpes zoster and simplex, and contact dermatitis (including plant-based contact dermatitis such as poison ivy).

• Sprinkle the powder onto damp sores and reapply four or five times a day. For less damp lesions, mix with a liquid adjuvant and spread on a gauze pad which is then applied to the affected area. Change the dressing once per day.

• Liquid adjuvants can include tea water, egg white, or a tea made from Taraxaci Herba (*pú gōng yīng*), Portulacae Herba (*mă chǐ xiàn*), or Isatidis Folium (*dà qīng yè*). Alternatively, the fresh juice of these herbs can also be used. To make a more viscous plaster, combine with an appropriate ointment such as Lithospermum/Arnebia and Tangkuei Ointment (*zǐ dāng gāo*) or with sesame oil or petroleum jelly (or a facsimile thereof).

Contraindications: none noted

▶ FORMULAS WITH SIMILAR INDICATIONS

Golden-Yellow Powder (*jīn huáng săn*): Especially for reducing swelling and dispersing knots as well as clearing heat and dampness. It is best suited for toxic swellings such as boils and furuncles and swellings from trauma and infection.

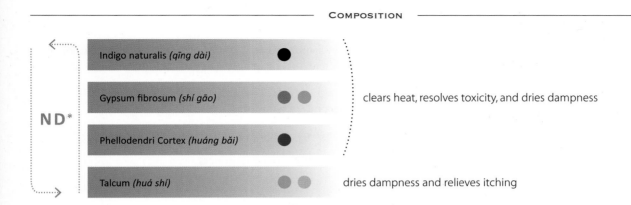

———— COMPOSITION ————

N D*

Indigo naturalis *(qīng dài)*

Gypsum fibrosum *(shí gāo)* — clears heat, resolves toxicity, and dries dampness

Phellodendri Cortex *(huáng bǎi)*

Talcum *(huá shí)* — dries dampness and relieves itching

*herb roles are not differentiated

青蒿鱉甲湯（青蒿鳖甲汤）
Sweet Wormwood and Soft-Shelled Turtle Shell Decoction [Version 1]
qīng hāo biē jiǎ tang

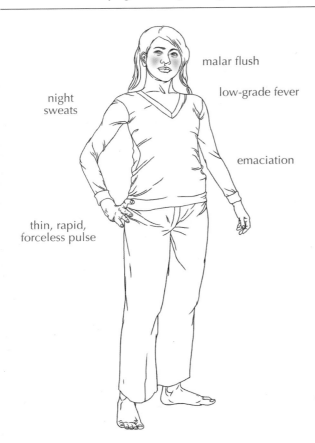

malar flush

low-grade fever

night sweats

emaciation

thin, rapid, forceless pulse

pathogen disease when the heat has depleted the yin and fluids

Key symptoms: low-grade fever • night sweats • emaciation with no loss of appetite • nighttime fever with morning coolness

Secondary symptoms: malar flush

Tongue: red body • scanty coating

Pulse: thin • rapid • forceless

▶ CLINICAL NOTES

- This formula is specific for heat stagnating within the deep collaterals. The typical manifestation is night fevers and morning coolness with no sweating as the fever recedes, reflecting the diurnal movement of the body's yang qi, which at times aggravates and at times reduces the manifestations of constraint.

- Indicated for low-grade fevers in tuberculosis, fevers of unknown origin, and the recovery phase of infectious diseases. The formula can also address Liver yin deficiency giving rise to menopausal flushing, emotion-related disorders, post-operative fevers, or chronic pyelonephritis.

Contraindications: early stages of a warm-heat pathogen disorder when the pathogenic influence is still in the qi level, and also in cases with spasms or convulsions

▶ FORMULAS WITH SIMILAR INDICATIONS

Great Tonify the Yin Pill (*dà bǔ yīn wán*): For a pattern of pure yin deficiency with exuberant fire that exhibits signs such as steaming bones, afternoon tidal fevers, night sweats, and often a strong, flooding pulse in the proximal positions. This pattern exhibits no symptoms of heat lurking in the yin aspect, such as nighttime heat with morning coolness.

*Cool the Bones Powder (*qīng gǔ sǎn*): For yin-deficiency fevers that appear to arise from within the bones and are accompanied by sweating, emaciation, and other signs of deficiency heat.

INGREDIENTS

Trionycis Carapax (*biē jiǎ*) 15g

Artemisiae annuae Herba (*qīng hāo*) 6g

Rehmanniae Radix (*shēng dì huáng*) 12g

Anemarrhenae Rhizoma (*zhī mǔ*) 6g

Moutan Cortex (*mǔ dān pí*) 9g

Actions: nourishes the yin • vents heat

Main pattern: heat lurking in the yin aspects of the body; this pattern usually occurs during the later stages of a warm-heat

*Large Gentian and Soft-Shelled Turtle Shell Powder (*qín jiāo biē jiǎ sǎn*): Treats yin deficiency, external wind, and lurking internal heat that exist in a patient with deficiency of the exterior. Often the patient is chronically ill and there are also symptoms of wind attacking a weakened exterior, such as joint or lower back pain.

COMPOSITION

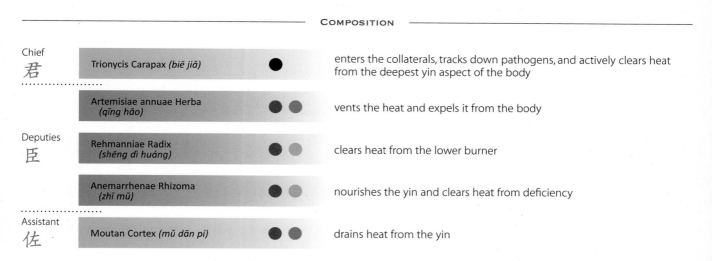

Chief 君	Trionycis Carapax *(biē jiǎ)*	●	enters the collaterals, tracks down pathogens, and actively clears heat from the deepest yin aspect of the body
	Artemisiae annuae Herba *(qīng hāo)*	● ●	vents the heat and expels it from the body
Deputies 臣	Rehmanniae Radix *(shēng dì huáng)*	● ●	clears heat from the lower burner
	Anemarrhenae Rhizoma *(zhī mǔ)*	● ●	nourishes the yin and clears heat from deficiency
Assistant 佐	Moutan Cortex *(mǔ dān pí)*	● ●	drains heat from the yin

清氣化痰丸（清气化痰丸）
Clear the Qi and Transform Phlegm Pill
qīng qì huà tán wán

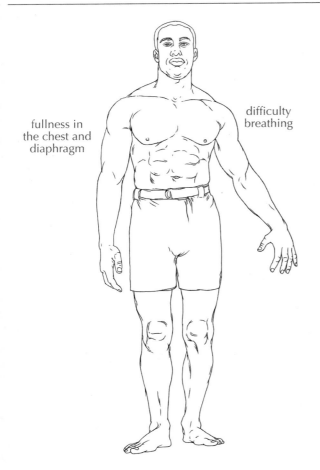

fullness in the chest and diaphragm

difficulty breathing

INGREDIENTS

Arisaema cum Bile (*dǎn nán xīng*)..................................... 9g

Pinelliae Rhizoma praeparatum (*zhì bàn xià*)...................... 9g

Trichosanthis Semen (*guā lóu rén*).................................... 6g

Scutellariae Radix (*huáng qín*) 6g

Citri reticulatae Pericarpium (*chén pí*).............................. 6g

Armeniacae Semen (*xìng rén*) 6g

Aurantii Fructus immaturus (*zhǐ shí*) 6g

Poria (*fú líng*) 6g

Actions: clears heat • transforms phlegm • directs rebellious qi downward • stops coughing

Main pattern: internal clumping of phlegm-heat

Key symptoms: productive cough with yellow, viscous sputum that is difficult to expectorate • fullness in the chest and diaphragm • difficulty breathing

Secondary symptoms: focal distention • nausea • vomiting • irritability • insomnia

Tongue: yellow, greasy coating

Pulse: rapid • slippery

Abdomen: discomfort in epigastrium

> ► **CLINICAL NOTES**

- This formula is mainly used to treat productive cough with yellow sputum. This pattern often occurs during wind-warmth disorders when wind has been dispelled from the exterior but phlegm remains and combines with excess internal heat.

- The formula can also be used to treat warm-dryness disorders where wind has been dispelled but dryness remains, manifesting as a dry, painful throat, cough with yellow sputum, and stabbing pains in the flanks.

- Other possible indications are manifestations of rebellious qi, such as nausea and vomiting, from damp-heat obstructing the middle burner. For this purpose, consider adding Bambusae Caulis in taeniam (*zhú rú*) and Perillae Caulis (*zǐ sū gěng*). Also, the formula can treat phlegm-heat obstructing the Triple Burner, causing insomnia and palpitations, by substituting Poriae Sclerotium pararadicis (*fú shén*) for Poria (*fú líng*) and adding Acori tatarinowii Rhizoma (*shí chāng pǔ*), Polygalae Radix (*yuǎn zhì*), and a small amount of Coptidis Rhizoma (*huáng lián*).

- Wind-cold exterior patterns that progress into phlegm-heat in the Lungs are also treated with this formula.

- This formula is drying and is used in situations where a heat pathogen has, in many cases, already compromised the yin and fluids of the Lungs. If this is a concern, including herbs such as Mori Cortex (*sāng bái pí*), Anemarrhenae Rhizoma (*zhī mǔ*), and Phragmitis Rhizoma (*lú gēn*) to protect the yin and fluids is advised.

Contraindications: cough where the exterior has not yet been resolved

▶ FORMULAS WITH SIMILAR INDICATIONS

Ephedra, Apricot Kernel, Gypsum, and Licorice Decoction (*má xìng shí gān tāng*): For heat in the chest and Lungs and cold fettering the exterior as reflected in wheezing, irritability, and slight sweating. While this pattern may present with some phlegm, it is not a phlegm-heat pattern and presents with only a slight amount of phlegm and a thin tongue coating.

Arrest Wheezing Decoction (*dìng chuǎn tāng*): For phlegm-heat in the Lungs and wind-cold fettering the exterior that causes the Lung qi to rebel upward. In this pattern the ascent of qi manifests with wheezing—rather than coughing—as the main symptom.

COMPOSITION

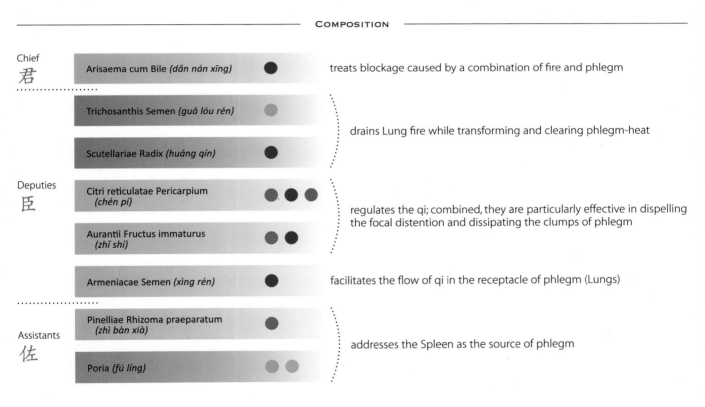

Chief 君	Arisaema cum Bile (*dǎn nán xīng*)	treats blockage caused by a combination of fire and phlegm
	Trichosanthis Semen (*guā lóu rén*)	drains Lung fire while transforming and clearing phlegm-heat
	Scutellariae Radix (*huáng qín*)	
Deputies 臣	Citri reticulatae Pericarpium (*chén pí*)	regulates the qi; combined, they are particularly effective in dispelling the focal distention and dissipating the clumps of phlegm
	Aurantii Fructus immaturus (*zhǐ shí*)	
	Armeniacae Semen (*xìng rén*)	facilitates the flow of qi in the receptacle of phlegm (Lungs)
Assistants 佐	Pinelliae Rhizoma praeparatum (*zhì bàn xià*)	addresses the Spleen as the source of phlegm
	Poria (*fú líng*)	

清暑益氣湯 （清暑益气汤）
Clear Summerheat and Augment the Qi Decoction
qīng shǔ yì qì tāng

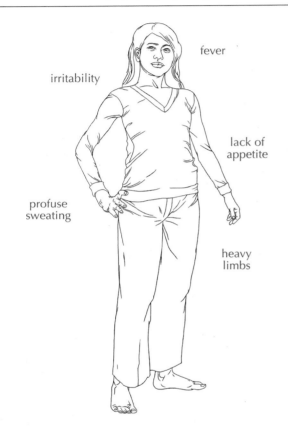

fever

irritability

lack of appetite

profuse sweating

heavy limbs

Actions: clears summerheat • augments the qi • nourishes the yin • generates fluids

Main pattern: summerheat injuring the qi and fluids

Key symptoms: fever • profuse sweating • thirst • irritability • heavy limbs • lack of appetite

Secondary symptoms: dark urine • loose stools • shortness of breath • apathy

Tongue: thin body • white or yellow and greasy coating

Pulse: deficient • rapid

Abdomen: no specific signs

► CLINICAL NOTES

• Indicated for summertime colds and fevers presenting with heat, dampness, and qi deficiency. Qi deficiency is a very important indication for this formula. One should thus look for a deficient pulse and sweating that is more profuse than would be expected by the low fever usually present in qi deficient summerheat patterns.

• May also be used in the aftermath of summerheat fevers to clear remaining pathogens while engendering fluids and augmenting qi.

Contraindications: summerheat patterns without deficiency • while most summerheat patterns carry some dampness, this formula is inappropriate for patterns where dampness is prominent

► FORMULAS WITH SIMILAR INDICATIONS

*White Tiger plus Ginseng Decoction (*bái hǔ jiā rén shēn tāng*): For dry-heat patterns with qi deficiency.

Lophatherum and Gypsum Decoction (*zhú yè shí gāo tāng*: For lingering dry-heat in the Stomach that has not been completely cleared, leading to rebelliousness. This is reflected in such signs as vomiting, difficulty falling asleep, or burning in the epigastrium.

INGREDIENTS

Panacis quinquefolii Radix (*xī yáng shēn*) 4.5-6g

Citrulli Exocarpium (*xī guā*) 24-30g

Nelumbinis Caulis (*lián gěng*) 12-15g

Dendrobii Herba (*shí hú*) 12-15g

Ophiopogonis Radix (*mài mén dōng*) 6-9g

Lophateri Herba (*dàn zhú yè*) 4.5-6g

Anemarrhenae Rhizoma (*zhī mǔ*) 4.5-6g

Coptidis Rhizoma (*huáng lián*) 2-3g

Glycyrrhizae Radix (*gān cǎo*) 2-3g

Nonglutinous rice (*jīng mǐ*) 12-15g

──────── **COMPOSITION** ────────

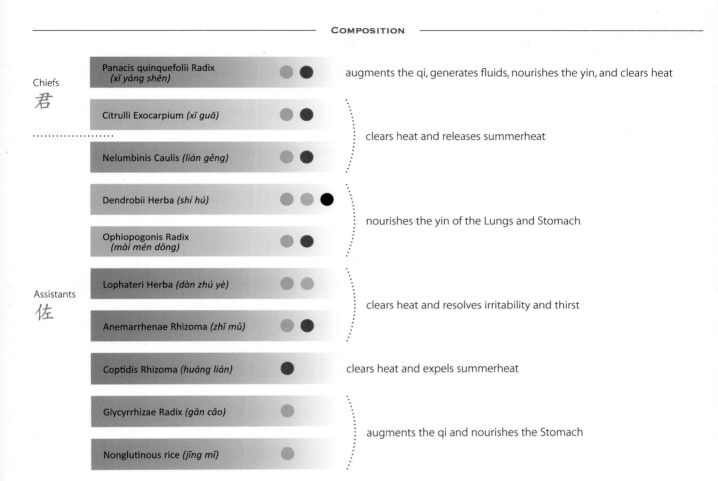

Chiefs
君

Panacis quinquefolii Radix
(*xī yáng shēn*) ● ● — augments the qi, generates fluids, nourishes the yin, and clears heat

Citrulli Exocarpium (*xī guā*) ● ●

clears heat and releases summerheat

Nelumbinis Caulis (*lián gěng*) ● ●

Dendrobii Herba (*shí hú*) ● ● ●

nourishes the yin of the Lungs and Stomach

Ophiopogonis Radix
(*mài mén dōng*) ● ●

Assistants
佐

Lophateri Herba (*dàn zhú yè*) ● ●

clears heat and resolves irritability and thirst

Anemarrhenae Rhizoma (*zhī mǔ*) ● ●

Coptidis Rhizoma (*huáng lián*) ● — clears heat and expels summerheat

Glycyrrhizae Radix (*gān cǎo*) ●

augments the qi and nourishes the Stomach

Nonglutinous rice (*jīng mǐ*) ●

清胃散
Clear the Stomach Powder
qīng wèi sǎn

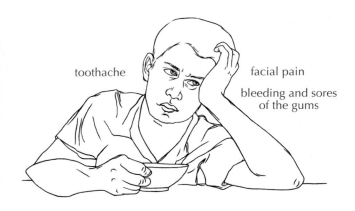

toothache   facial pain

bleeding and sores
of the gums

▸ INGREDIENTS

Coptidis Rhizoma (*huáng lián*) 6g
Cimicifugae Rhizoma (*shēng má*) 9g
Moutan Cortex (*mǔ dān pí*) 9g
Rehmanniae Radix (*shēng dì huáng*) 6-9g
Angelicae sinensis radicis Corpus (*dāng guī shēn*) 9g

Actions: drains Stomach fire • cools the blood • nourishes the yin

Main patterns: heat accumulation in the Stomach

Key symptoms: toothache (especially when the pain extends into the head) • bleeding and sores of the gums • facial pain

Secondary symptoms: swollen, painful tongue, lips, or jaw • fever • bad breath

Tongue: red body • scanty coating

Pulse: large • rapid

Abdomen: no specific signs

▸ CLINICAL NOTES

• This is a key formula for treating toothache, swollen gums, and bleeding of the gums due to blazing fire from fire constraint in the Stomach. Typically, disorders are of acute onset and the painful areas respond favorably to cold and worsen with heat. The combination of Coptidis Rhizoma (*huáng lián*) and Cimicifugae Rhizoma (*shēng má*) is effective in resolving the constraint and venting the blazing fire via the exterior.

• The formula can also be used to treat trigeminal neuralgia due to wind-heat in the Stomach channel.

Contraindications: toothache due to wind-cold • tooth and gum problems due to Kidney deficiency

▸ FORMULAS WITH SIMILAR INDICATIONS

Drain the Yellow Powder (*xiè huáng sǎn*): For a pattern of heat lurking in the Stomach with less intense heat signs. This formula employs mostly mild, acrid-dispersing herbs to clear heat and is far less likely to injure the patient's yin.

*Jade Woman Decoction (*yù nū jiān*): For Stomach fire arising from Kidney yin deficiency. It directs deficiency fire downward rather than venting it via the exterior. This formula's yin-nourishing properties are frequently applied to wasting and thirsting disorder.

───────────────────────── COMPOSITION ─────────────────────────

Chief
君

Coptidis Rhizoma *(huáng lián)* ● — attacks the Stomach fire and drains the accumulation of heat

Dep/Env
臣/使

Cimicifugae Rhizoma *(shēng má)* ● ● — raises and disperses the heat and resolves toxicity

Moutan Cortex *(mǔ dān pí)* ● ●

Assistants
佐

Rehmanniae Radix
(shēng dì huáng) ● ●

⎫
⎬ cools the blood and nourishes the yin
⎭

Angelicae sinensis radicis
Corpus *(dāng guī shēn)* ● ● — reduces swelling and alleviates pain by harmonizing the blood

清營湯（清营汤）
Clear the Nutritive Level Decoction
qīng yíng tāng

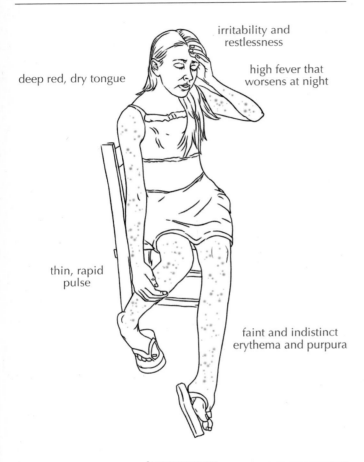

irritability and restlessness

deep red, dry tongue

high fever that worsens at night

thin, rapid pulse

faint and indistinct erythema and purpura

Actions: clears the nutritive level • relieves fire toxin • drains heat • nourishes the yin

Main pattern: heat in the nutritive level

Key symptoms: high fever that worsens at night • irritability and restlessness • faint and indistinct erythema and purpura

Secondary symptoms: little thirst • confusion or loss of consciousness

Tongue: deep red • dry

Pulse: thin • rapid

Abdomen: no specific signs

► **CLINICAL NOTES**

- This is the key formula for treating heat at the nutritive level. It cools the blood, augments the yin and fluids, resolves heat toxin, prevents blood stasis, and turns pathogenic heat back toward the qi aspect. From there it can be eliminated by venting to the exterior or draining it through the bowels or urine. These strategies can be used in all cases of heat at the nutritive level irrespective of the cause. With appropriate modifications the formula can thus be used in treating such diverse problems as skin disorders due to fire toxin, menstrual irregularities, or fevers due to lurking pathogens.

- In the course of warm pathogen disorders, the key symptoms indicating that heat is entering the nutritive aspect are a worsening of the fever at night, a dry, scarlet tongue body, and a thin, rapid pulse. Symptoms indicating heat in the qi aspect, such as a yellow tongue coating or thirst, disappear as the pattern changes to one affecting the nutritive aspect. It is considered an encouraging sign if these symptoms reappear as a consequence of administering the formula.

Contraindications: white and slippery tongue coating, indicating dampness

---

INGREDIENTS

Bubali Cornu (*shuǐ niú jiǎo*) 30g
Scrophulariae Radix (*xuán shēn*)..................................... 9g
Rehmanniae Radix (*shēng dì huáng*)............................ 15-21g
Ophiopogonis Radix (*mài mén dōng*) 9g
Lonicerae Flos (*jīn yín huā*) 9g
Forsythiae Fructus (*lián qiào*) 6-9g
Coptidis Rhizoma (*huáng lián*) 5g
Lophatheri Herba (*dàn zhú yè*).................................... 3-5g
Salviae miltiorrhizae Radix (*dān shēn*)......................... 6-9g

COMPOSITION

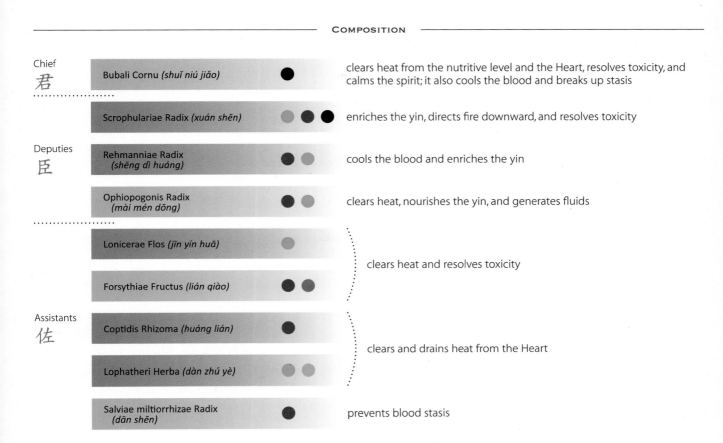

Chief
君

Bubali Cornu (shuǐ niú jiǎo) — clears heat from the nutritive level and the Heart, resolves toxicity, and calms the spirit; it also cools the blood and breaks up stasis

Scrophulariae Radix (xuán shēn) — enriches the yin, directs fire downward, and resolves toxicity

Deputies
臣

Rehmanniae Radix (shēng dì huáng) — cools the blood and enriches the yin

Ophiopogonis Radix (mài mén dōng) — clears heat, nourishes the yin, and generates fluids

Lonicerae Flos (jīn yín huā)

Forsythiae Fructus (lián qiào)

— clears heat and resolves toxicity

Assistants
佐

Coptidis Rhizoma (huáng lián)

Lophatheri Herba (dàn zhú yè)

— clears and drains heat from the Heart

Salviae miltiorrhizae Radix (dān shēn) — prevents blood stasis

清燥救肺湯 (清燥救肺汤)
Clear Dryness and Rescue the Lungs Decoction
qīng zào jiù fèi tāng

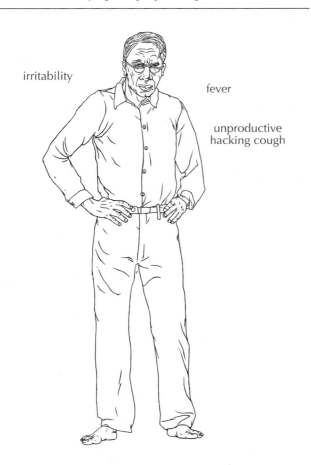

irritability

fever

unproductive hacking cough

Actions: clears dryness • moistens the Lungs

Main pattern: warm-dryness attacking the Lungs with damage to both the qi and yin

Key symptoms: fever • unproductive hacking cough • wheezing • irritability

Secondary symptoms: headache • dry and parched throat • dry nasal passages • sensation of fullness in the chest • hypochondriac pain • thirst

Tongue: dry body • scanty coating

Pulse: deficient • large • rapid

Abdomen: no specific signs

▶ CLINICAL NOTES

- This formula is prescribed for disorders caused by exposure to dry environmental conditions (including seasonal and indoor dryness). The dryness leads to Lung qi constraint and severely damages the fluids, which in turn leads to rebellious qi. Key marker is the presence of both thirst and cough.

- By extension, this formula is used for treatment of skin conditions such as sunburn with dryness and heat damaging the collaterals of the skin.

- This same presentation can occur at the tail end of Lung-heat disorders where the drying nature of a heat pathogen coupled with aggressive treatment have damaged the Lung yin and fluids. This formula can be used for patients in these situations when they have a cough with little or no sputum, thirst, and signs of considerable heat.

Contraindications: Spleen and Stomach deficiency

▶ FORMULAS WITH SIMILAR INDICATIONS

Mulberry Leaf and Apricot Kernel Decoction (*sāng xìng tāng*): For warm-dryness at the protective rather than qi level as reflected in fever and chills as well as a dry cough and a floating pulse.

──── INGREDIENTS ────

Mori Folium (*sāng yè*)	9g
Gypsum fibrosum (*shí gāo*)	8g
Ophiopogonis Radix (*mài mén dōng*)	4g
Asini Corii Colla (*ē jiāo*) ..... [dissolve in strained decoction]	3g
dry-fried Sesami Semen nigrum (*chǎo hēi zhī má*)	3g
Armeniacae Semen (*xìng rén*)	2g
honey-prepared Eriobotryae Folium (*mì zhì pí pá yè*)	3g
Ginseng Radix (*rén shēn*)	2g
Glycyrrhizae Radix (*gān cǎo*)	3g

Glehnia and Ophiopogonis Decoction (*shā shēn mài mén dōng tāng*): For dry disorders with damage to the fluids but without any exterior symptoms or qi level heat as reflected in a dry cough without sputum, fever, thirst, and a deep, thin pulse.

COMPOSITION

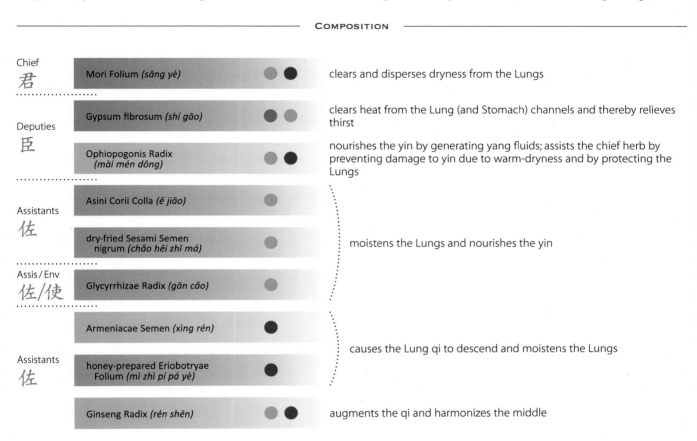

Chief 君	Mori Folium (*sāng yè*)	clears and disperses dryness from the Lungs
Deputies 臣	Gypsum fibrosum (*shí gāo*)	clears heat from the Lung (and Stomach) channels and thereby relieves thirst
	Ophiopogonis Radix (*mài mén dōng*)	nourishes the yin by generating yang fluids; assists the chief herb by preventing damage to yin due to warm-dryness and by protecting the Lungs
Assistants 佐	Asini Corii Colla (*ē jiāo*)	moistens the Lungs and nourishes the yin
	dry-fried Sesami Semen nigrum (*chǎo hēi zhī má*)	
Assis/Env 佐/使	Glycyrrhizae Radix (*gān cǎo*)	
Assistants 佐	Armeniacae Semen (*xìng rén*)	causes the Lung qi to descend and moistens the Lungs
	honey-prepared Eriobotryae Folium (*mì zhì pí pá yè*)	
	Ginseng Radix (*rén shēn*)	augments the qi and harmonizes the middle

人參敗毒散（人参败毒散）
Ginseng Powder to Overcome Pathogenic Influences
rén shēn bài dú săn

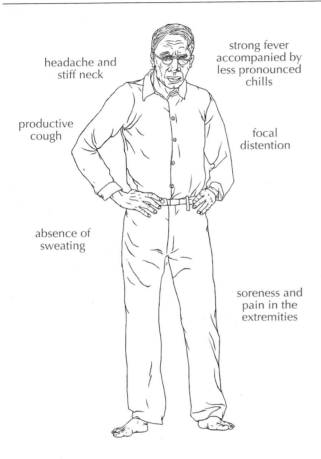

- headache and stiff neck
- strong fever accompanied by less pronounced chills
- productive cough
- focal distention
- absence of sweating
- soreness and pain in the extremities

INGREDIENTS

Notopterygii Rhizoma seu Radix (*qiāng huó*)......................9g
Angelicae pubescentis Radix (*dú huó*) 9g
Chuanxiong Rhizoma (*chuān xiōng*) 9g
Bupleuri Radix (*chái hú*)..9g
Platycodi Radix (*jié gěng*)...9g
Aurantii Fructus (*zhǐ ké*)...9g
Peucedani Radix (*qián hú*)..9g
Ginseng Radix (*rén shēn*)..9g
Poria (*fú líng*)...9g

Glycyrrhizae Radix (*gān căo*)...3-6g
Zingiberis Rhizoma recens (*shēng jiāng*)......................... 2-3g
Menthae haplocalycis Herba (*bò hé*)................................ 2-3g

Actions: releases wind-cold-dampness from the exterior • dispels wind and dampness • augments the qi

Main patterns: externally-contracted wind-cold-dampness in patients with a qi deficient constitution • pattern may additionally be complicated by phlegm obstruction and qi stagnation

Key symptoms: strong fever accompanied by relatively less pronounced chills • absence of sweating • soreness and pain in the extremities

Secondary symptoms: headache and stiff neck • productive cough • focal distention • fullness of the chest • nasal congestion

Tongue: pale body • greasy, white coating

Pulse: floating and soggy • weak or deficient with stronger pressure

Abdomen: no specific signs

▶ CLINICAL NOTES

- Originally designed as a pediatric formula, its use has been expanded to include a wider range of wind-cold-damp disorders. It is now used to treat this pattern in patients with underlying qi deficiency and phlegm-dampness obstructing the qi dynamic, regardless of age. It is also used in treating postpartum women and those recovering from debilitating illness.

- Used for early-stage wind-cold-damp dysenteric disorders with exterior symptoms.

- Used for very early-stage measles (before the rash has begun to surface) characterized by moderate fever and chills, no significant thirst, loose stools, a white tongue coating, and a thin, weak pulse.

- Used for deep-seated sores and boils in patients with qi deficiency.

Contraindications: externally-contracted heat or damp-heat • externally-contracted disorders in yin deficient patients

▶ FORMULAS WITH SIMILAR INDICATIONS

*Ginseng and Perilla Leaf Drink (shēn sū yǐn): For patterns with more pronounced qi deficiency and obstruction of the qi dynamic by phlegm and thin mucus characterized by roughly equal fever and chills, headache, nasal congestion, productive cough, stifling sensation in the chest, and a frail pulse.

COMPOSITION

Role	Herb		Actions
Chiefs 君	Notopterygii Rhizoma seu Radix (qiāng huó)	●●●	dispels wind-cold from the exterior, dispels dampness, alleviates pain
	Angelicae pubescentis Radix (dú huó)	●●	
Deputies 臣	Chuanxiong Rhizoma (chuān xiōng)	●	helps chief herbs to release the exterior, move the blood, dispel wind and relieve pain
	Bupleuri Radix (chái hú)	●●	releases the exterior, reduces fever, and expels pathogenic influences
	Menthae haplocalycis Herba (bò hé)	●●	
Assistants 佐	Platycodi Radix (jié gěng)	●●	regulates the flow of qi in the chest, improves circulation of Lung qi, expels phlegm
	Aurantii Fructus (zhǐ ké)	●●	
	Peucedani Radix (qián hú)	●●	
	Poria (fú líng)	●●	transforms phlegm and strengthens the Spleen
	Zingiberis Rhizoma recens (shēng jiāng)	●	
	Ginseng Radix (rén shēn)	●●	strengthens normal qi to expel pathogenic influences, generates fluids, strengthens the body's resistance to invasion
Envoy 使	Glycyrrhizae Radix (gān cǎo)	●	harmonizes the actions of the other herbs

潤腸丸（润肠丸）
Moisten the Intestines Pill
from *Master Shen's Book*
rùn cháng wán

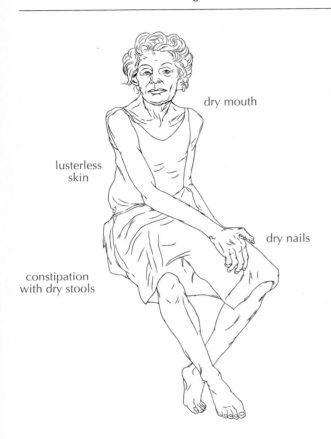

dry mouth

lusterless skin

dry nails

constipation with dry stools

Secondary symptoms: dizziness • forgetfulness • palpitations • shortness of breath

Tongue: dry • thin • little coating

Pulse: thin • rough

Abdomen: dry skin • palpable hard stool in bowels • weak abdominal muscles

► CLINICAL NOTES

- Mainly used for chronic constipation associated with debility and dryness due to deficiency of blood and fluids.
- This formula has a mild action and may take some time to work.

Contraindications: should not be prescribed in cases that require purging

► FORMULAS WITH SIMILAR INDICATIONS

Hemp Seed Pill (*má zǐ rén wán*): For dry-stool constipation with frequent urination from heat-dryness blocking the movement of fluids.

--- INGREDIENTS ---

Cannabis Semen (*huǒ má rén*)... 15g

Persicae Semen (*táo rén*)... 9g

Angelicae sinensis Radix (*dāng guī*) 9g

Rehmanniae Radix (*shēng dì huáng*)................................. 30g

Aurantii Fructus (*zhǐ ké*)... 9g

Actions: moistens the Intestines • unblocks the bowels

Main patterns: constipation due to desiccated intestines

Key symptoms: constipation with dry stools • lusterless skin • dry nails • dry mouth

COMPOSITION

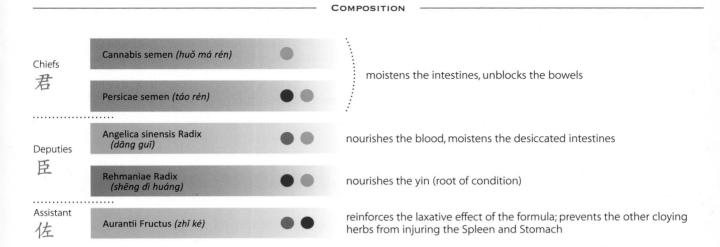

Chiefs
君

Cannabis semen *(huǒ má rén)*

Persicae semen *(táo rén)*

moistens the intestines, unblocks the bowels

Deputies
臣

Angelica sinensis Radix
(dāng guī)

nourishes the blood, moistens the desiccated intestines

Rehmaniae Radix
(shēng dì huáng)

nourishes the yin (root of condition)

Assistant
佐

Aurantii Fructus *(zhǐ ké)*

reinforces the laxative effect of the formula; prevents the other cloying herbs from injuring the Spleen and Stomach

三仁湯（三仁汤）
Three-Seed Decoction
sān rén tāng

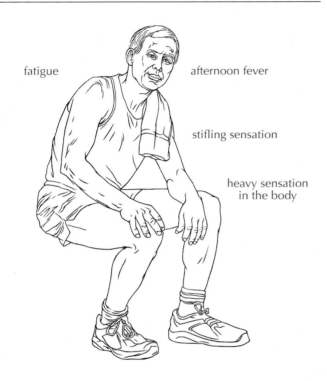

fatigue

afternoon fever

stifling sensation

heavy sensation in the body

INGREDIENTS

Armeniacae Semen (*xìng rén*) 15g
Amomi Fructus rotundus (*bái dòu kòu*) 6g
Magnoliae officinalis Cortex (*hòu pò*) 6g
Pinelliae Rhizoma praeparatum (*zhì bàn xià*) 15g
Coicis Semen (*yì yǐ rén*) 18g
Tetrapanacis Medulla (*tōng cǎo*) 6g
Lophateri Herba (*dàn zhú yè*) 6g
Talcum (*huá shí*) 18g

Actions: disseminates the qi • facilitates the qi dynamic • clears damp-warmth

Main pattern: early-stage damp-warmth or summerheat-warmth in which dampness predominates and the pathogenic influences are lodged in the protective and qi levels

Key symptoms: afternoon fever • fatigue • heavy sensation in the body • stifling sensation in chest or upper abdomen

Secondary symptoms: chills or cool extremities • headache • pale yellow complexion • generalized pain • loss of appetite • absence of thirst

Tongue: white coating

Pulse: wiry • thin • soggy

Abdomen: fullness in the diaphragmatic area

▶ CLINICAL NOTES

- This formula treats damp-heat obstructing the Triple Burner with dampness significantly more pronounced than heat. Such disorders tend to linger and are often difficult to dislodge. The manifestation can resemble a lesser yang disorder with heat from constraint and cold extremities; a yin deficiency disorder with heat that becomes more pronounced in the evenings; and also a yang brightness disorder with afternoon fevers. In each case, the differentiation is based on the signs of dampness that manifest as a heavy sensation in the body or a stifling sensation in the chest or upper abdomen in combination with a soggy pulse and a white tongue coating.

- Because it focuses on unblocking the qi dynamic of the upper and middle burners, this formula's range of indications is extremely wide, encompassing acute and chronic inflammatory conditions throughout both the body's exterior and the internal organs. For instance, for early stage damp-warmth disorders characterized by pronounced Lung organ system symptoms such as headache, chills and fever, and coughing, one can add herbs that release the exterior such as Pogostemonis/Agastaches Herba (*huò xiāng*) and Sojae Semen praeparatum (*dàn dòu chǐ*); for alternating heat and cold, add Tsaoko Fructus (*cǎo guǒ*) and Artemisiae annuae Herba (*qīng hao*); for foul turbidity with a very greasy tongue coating, fatigue, and heavyheadedness, add Acori tatarinowii Rhizoma (*shí chāng pǔ*) and Eupatorii Herba (*pèi lán*).

• This formula is not indicated for damp-warmth disorders with significantly more heat than dampness, as reflected in a clearly yellow tongue coating.

Contraindications: cold damage disorders at the lesser yang stage • yin deficiency • internal clumping in the Intestines

▶ FORMULAS WITH SIMILAR INDICATIONS

Nine-Herb Decoction with Notopterygium (*jiǔ wèi qiāng huó* *tāng*): For damp-cold at the qi level obstructing the body's exterior with heat in the interior. The presentation includes headaches, chills and fevers, body and joint pain, a wiry and slippery pulse, and a white or normal tongue coating.

Sweet Dew Special Pill to Eliminate Toxin (*gān lù xiāo dú dān*): For the early stage of a qi aspect damp-warmth epidemic disorder flooding all three burners and presenting with equally pronounced heat and dampness.

────────── COMPOSITION ──────────

Chiefs 君	Armeniacae Semen *(xìng rén)*	●	dredges the Lung qi, opens what is clogged, and facilitates the downward movement of qi and fluids
	Amomi Fructus rotundus *(bái dòu kòu)*	● ●	transforms turbid dampness and revives the Spleen; treats the upper burner by spreading the qi in the chest
	Coicis Semen *(yì yǐ rén)*	● ●	leaches out dampness through the urine; treats the middle burner by strengthening the Spleen
Deputies 臣	Tetrapanacis Medulla *(tōng cǎo)*	● ●	leaches out dampness through the urine and clears heat
	Lophateri Herba *(dàn zhú yè)*	● ●	
	Talcum *(huá shí)*	● ●	
Assistants 佐	Magnoliae officinalis Cortex *(hòu pò)*	● ●	treats epigastric and abdominal distention due to dampness or phlegm
	Pinelliae Rhizoma praeparatum *(zhì bàn xià)*	●	

三子養親湯（三子养亲汤）
Three-Seed Decoction to Nourish One's Parents
sān zǐ yǎng qīn tāng

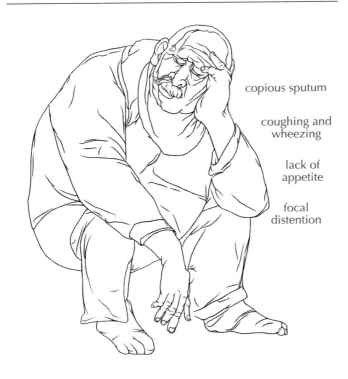

copious sputum

coughing and wheezing

lack of appetite

focal distention

INGREDIENTS

Sinapis Semen (*bái jiè zǐ*) 6-9g
Perillae Fructus (*zǐ sū zǐ*) 6-9g
Raphani Semen (*lái fú zǐ*) 6-9g

Preparation notes: The ingredients should be placed in a cheese-cloth bag and decocted for approximately 10 minutes. Can be taken throughout the day as a tea.

Actions: directs the qi downward • transforms phlegm • reduces harbored food

Main pattern: phlegm clogging the Lungs along with qi stagnation in the middle burner and diaphragm

Key symptoms: coughing and wheezing • copious sputum • focal distention in the chest • lack of appetite

Secondary symptoms: indigestion • belching with taste of previously eaten food • bloating • lack of appetite

Tongue: white, greasy coating

Pulse: slippery

Abdomen: no specific signs

▶ CLINICAL NOTES

- This formula treats phlegm clogging the Lungs in combination with qi stagnation caused by harbored food. It is most often seen in those with long-standing deficiency of middle burner qi and blood and is commonly found among the elderly and others with sedentary lifestyles and poor dietary habits.

- To treat deficiency patterns the formula is often modified to include such herbs as Atractylodis macrocephalae Rhizoma (*bái zhú*) and Glycyrrhizae Radix (*gān cǎo*) to tonify the middle burner and Atractylodis Rhizoma (*cāng zhú*) to increase the formula's ability to dry dampness. This strategy is usually followed by switching to a formula such as Six-Gentlemen Decoction (*liù jūn zǐ tāng*) that both tonifies the middle burner and transforms phlegm-dampness.

Contraindications: deficiency cold

▶ FORMULAS WITH SIMILAR INDICATIONS

Preserve Harmony Pill (*bǎo hé wán*): For harbored food causing stagnation in the middle burner that manifests with vomiting, diarrhea, or nausea.

──────────── COMPOSITION ────────────

| Sinapis Semen *(bái jiè zǐ)* | ● | penetrates the yin and restores movement to the yang |

| Perillae Fructus *(zǐ sū zǐ)* | ● | directs the Lung qi downward and thereby stops the coughing and wheezing; excels at directing rebellious qi downward, thus dispersing phlegm and calming wheezing, while moistening and facilitating Intestinal movement |

| Raphani Semen *(lái fú zǐ)* | ● ● | enters the Lung channel to direct the qi downward and transform phlegm; mobilizes the Spleen channel to promote the flow of Spleen qi and reduce harbored food |

桑菊飲 （桑菊饮）
Mulberry Leaf and Chrysanthemum Drink
sāng jú yǐn

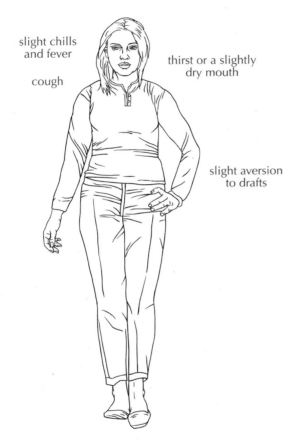

slight chills and fever

cough

thirst or a slightly dry mouth

slight aversion to drafts

Actions: disperses wind and clears heat • stop~~~ • disseminates Lung qi

Main patterns: early stage of a warm patho~~~ • wind-heat invading the Lungs

Key symptoms: slight aversion to drafts~~~ fever • cough

Secondary symptoms: may have thirs~~~ mouth

Tongue: red tip • thin, white coating

Pulse: floating • rapid (especially in right distal position)

Abdomen: no specific signs

► CLINICAL NOTES

- Specific for cough at the early stage of a wind-heat disorder. Must be modified for more severe disorders, when pathogens are already entering the qi or nutritive aspects (as indicated by higher fever, phlegm, or blood-streaked sputum) or when the fluids have already been damaged (as indicated by pronounced thirst).

- Can also be used for eye disorders due to wind-heat and a hacking cough due to external invasion of dryness.

- This formula consists of light and mild-acting herbs that treat the exterior. It should be decocted only for a short time, usually 15 minutes.

Contraindications: cough due to wind-cold

► FORMULAS WITH SIMILAR INDICATIONS

Honeysuckle and Forsythia Powder (*yín qiào sǎn*): For sore throat, higher fever, and stronger systemic signs of wind-heat disorders.

Mulberry Leaf and Apricot Kernel Decoction (*sāng xìng tāng*): For externally-contracted warm-dryness with dry nose or throat, thirst, and irritability and restlessness.

INGREDIENTS

Mori Folium (*sāng yè*)	7.5g
Chrysanthemi Flos (*jú huā*)	3g
Forsythiae Fructus (*lián qiào*) clear heat	5g
Menthae haplocalycis Herba (*bò hé*) [add near end]	2.5g
Platycodi Radix (*jié gěng*) stop cough	6g
Armeniacae Semen (*xìng rén*) stop cough	6g
Phragmitis Rhizoma (*lú gēn*) clear heat	6g
Glycyrrhizae Radix (*gān cǎo*)	2.5g

Preparation notes: Do not cook for more than 20 minutes.

COMPOSITION

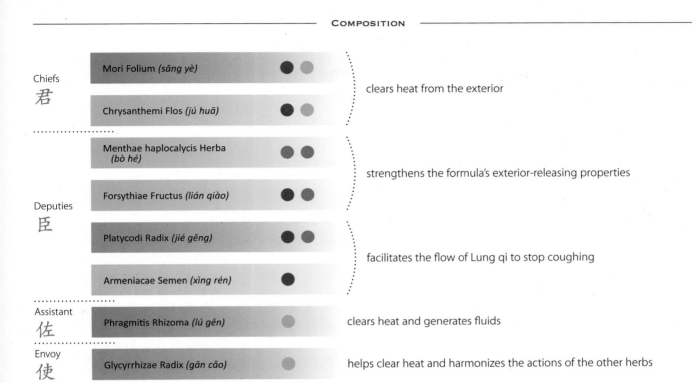

Chiefs
君

Mori Folium (*sāng yè*) ⬤⬤

Chrysanthemi Flos (*jú huā*) ⬤⬤

clears heat from the exterior

Deputies
臣

Menthae haplocalycis Herba (*bò hé*) ⬤⬤

Forsythiae Fructus (*lián qiào*) ⬤⬤

strengthens the formula's exterior-releasing properties

Platycodi Radix (*jié gěng*) ⬤⬤

Armeniacae Semen (*xìng rén*) ⬤

facilitates the flow of Lung qi to stop coughing

Assistant
佐

Phragmitis Rhizoma (*lú gěn*) ⬤

clears heat and generates fluids

Envoy
使

Glycyrrhizae Radix (*gān cǎo*) ⬤

helps clear heat and harmonizes the actions of the other herbs

桑杏湯 （桑杏汤）
Mulberry Leaf and Apricot Kernel Decoction
sāng xìng tāng

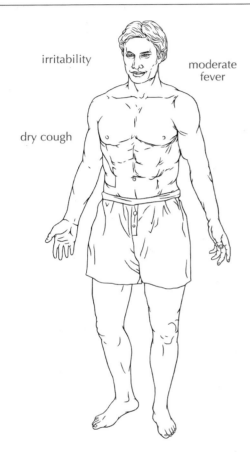

irritability

moderate fever

dry cough

INGREDIENTS

Mori Folium (*sāng yè*) 3g
Gardeniae Fructus (*zhī zǐ*)................................. 3g
Sojae Semen praeparatum (*dàn dòu chǐ*) 3g
Armeniacae Semen (*xìng rén*) 4.5g
Fritillariae thunbergii Bulbus (*zhè bèi mǔ*)............ 3g
Glehniae Radix (*běi shā shēn*)............................ 6g
Pyri Exocarpium (*lí pí*)...................................... 3g

Actions: clears and disperses warm-dryness

Main pattern: externally-contracted warm-dryness injuring the Lung qi at the protective and superficial qi levels

Key symptoms: moderate fever • dry cough (hacking or with scanty, thick, and sticky sputum) • irritability

Secondary symptoms: headache • thirst • cough with blood-streaked sputum

Tongue: red body • thin, dry, white coating

Pulse: floating • rapid • rough (especially at the right proximal position)

Abdomen: no specific signs

▶ CLINICAL NOTES

- For dryness entering the protective level causing constraint in the Lung collaterals and damaging the fluids. A key marker is a dry cough accompanied by exterior signs and symptoms such as fever and chills or headache, irritability, and a floating, rapid or rough pulse (especially at the right proximal position).

- With the addition of herbs to clear heat and engender fluids such as Trichosanthis Radix (*tiān huā fěn*) and Phragmitis Rhizoma (*lú gēn*), this formula can be used to treat the latter stages of heat-toxin rash disorders such as measles and chicken pox. For this purpose, the formula is used after the heat toxin has been completely expressed and the rash has subsided. The goal of treatment is to clear heat remnants and engender fluids to replace those that have been damaged during the course of the illness.

Contraindications: cases with injury to the yin

▶ FORMULAS WITH SIMILAR INDICATIONS

Apricot Kernel and Perilla Leaf Powder (*xìng sū sǎn*): For externally-contracted cool-dryness with dryness of the throat or nose and a dry cough but with more pronounced chills, no irritability, and a wiry pulse.

Mulberry Leaf and Chrysanthemum Drink (*sāng jú yǐn*): For externally-contracted wind-heat at the protective level damaging the Lung collaterals. This pattern presents with coughing at the onset of the disorder and with heat that is more prominent than dryness.

Clear Dryness and Rescue the Lungs Decoction (*qīng zào jiù fèi tāng*): For externally-contracted heat-dryness at the qi level with more pronounced heat that has already severely damaged the body fluids and manifests with rebellious qi. This pattern presents with cough and wheezing as well as thirst; exterior symptoms are mild or altogether absent.

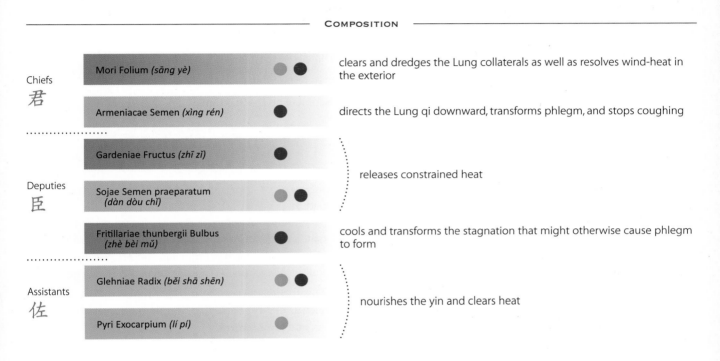

COMPOSITION

Chiefs 君	Mori Folium (*sāng yè*)	clears and dredges the Lung collaterals as well as resolves wind-heat in the exterior
	Armeniacae Semen (*xìng rén*)	directs the Lung qi downward, transforms phlegm, and stops coughing
Deputies 臣	Gardeniae Fructus (*zhī zǐ*)	releases constrained heat
	Sojae Semen praeparatum (*dàn dòu chǐ*)	
	Fritillariae thunbergii Bulbus (*zhè bèi mǔ*)	cools and transforms the stagnation that might otherwise cause phlegm to form
Assistants 佐	Glehniae Radix (*běi shā shēn*)	nourishes the yin and clears heat
	Pyri Exocarpium (*lí pí*)	

沙參麥門冬湯（沙参麦门冬汤）
Glehnia and Ophiopogonis Decoction
shā shēn mài mén dōng tāng

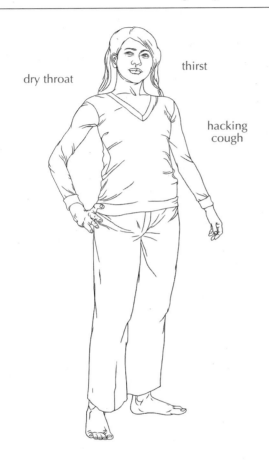

dry throat

thirst

hacking cough

Main pattern: injury to the Lungs, Stomach, and fluids from dryness

Key symptoms: dry throat • thirst • fever • hacking cough with scanty sputum • red tongue with scanty coating

Secondary symptoms: none noted

Tongue: red body • scanty coating

Pulse: rapid • thin

Abdomen: no specific signs

► CLINICAL NOTES

- The key clinical marker here is that the patient has all the signs of upper and middle burner dryness as this pattern is internal dryness that develops in the aftermath of an attack of external dryness. These patients usually have a tendency toward yin deficiency. When pronounced coughing is the main complaint, add Fritillariae cirrhosae Bulbus (*chuān bèi mǔ*) and Armeniacae Semen (*xìng rén*).

- This formula is used in modern times to treat disorders such as dry-type atrophic rhinitis, pulmonary tuberculosis, and mouth sores.

Contraindications: heat excess damaging the body fluids

► FORMULAS WITH SIMILAR INDICATIONS

Clear Dryness and Rescue the Lungs Decoction (*qīng zào jiù fèi tāng*): For conditions when excess heat is still present. This pattern is marked by headache, fullness in the chest and hypochondria, hacking cough, and other signs of dryness.

INGREDIENTS

Adenophorae Radix (*nán shā shēn*) 9g

Ophiopogonis Radix (*mài mén dōng*) 9g

Polygonati odorati Rhizoma (*yù zhú*) 6g

Mori Folium (*sāng yè*) 4.5g

Trichosanthis Radix (*tiān huā fěn*) 4.5g

Lablab Semen album (*biǎn dòu*) 4.5g

Glycyrrhizae Radix (*gān cǎo*) 3g

Actions: clears and nourishes the Lungs and Stomach • generates fluids • moistens dryness

─── COMPOSITION ───

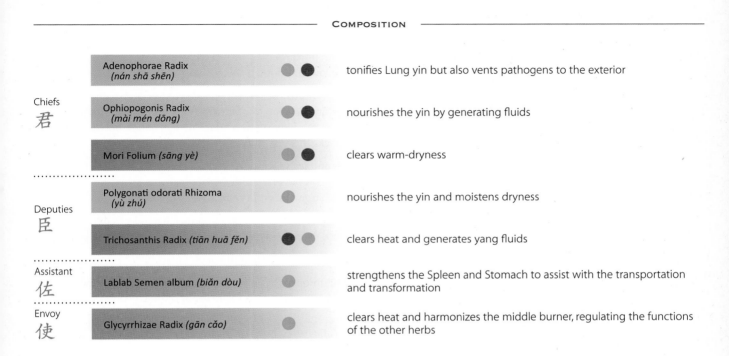

Chiefs
君

Adenophorae Radix
(nán shā shēn)
tonifies Lung yin but also vents pathogens to the exterior

Ophiopogonis Radix
(mài mén dōng)
nourishes the yin by generating fluids

Mori Folium (sāng yè)
clears warm-dryness

Deputies
臣

Polygonati odorati Rhizoma
(yù zhú)
nourishes the yin and moistens dryness

Trichosanthis Radix (tiān huā fěn)
clears heat and generates yang fluids

Assistant
佐

Lablab Semen album (biǎn dòu)
strengthens the Spleen and Stomach to assist with the transportation and transformation

Envoy
使

Glycyrrhizae Radix (gān cǎo)
clears heat and harmonizes the middle burner, regulating the functions of the other herbs

少腹逐瘀湯（少腹逐瘀汤）
Drive Out Stasis from the Lower Abdomen Decoction
shào fù zhú yū tāng

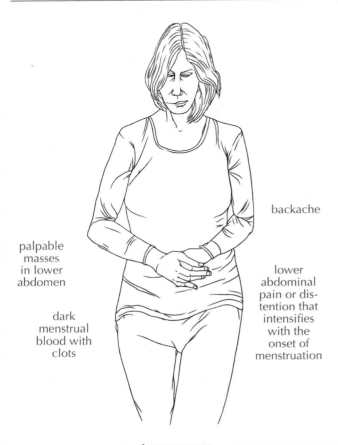

palpable masses in lower abdomen

backache

dark menstrual blood with clots

lower abdominal pain or distention that intensifies with the onset of menstruation

Actions: invigorates the blood • dispels blood stasis • warms the menses • alleviates pain

Main pattern: cold-induced blood stasis accumulation in the lower abdomen

Key symptoms: palpable masses in lower abdomen • lower abdominal pain or distention that intensifies with the onset of menstruation • dark menstrual blood with clots • backache

Secondary symptoms: aversion to cold • low or depressed mood • cold extremities • irregular menstruation • vaginal discharge • infertility • habitual miscarriage

Tongue: dark body • stasis spots • distended sublingual veins • white coating

Pulse: deep and tight or rough • forceful

Abdomen: pain on palpation in the lower abdomen • palpable masses in the lower abdomen

▶ CLINICAL NOTES

- This formula is designed to treat blood stasis in the lower abdomen due to cold. The focus is on dispelling the stasis and invigorating the blood, not on tonifying the yang. This cold-stasis excess pattern occurs primarily in women. Typical indications include palpable masses, pain in the lower abdomen that is relieved by warmth, and irregular menstruation with dark clots and pain at the onset of bleeding.

- When deficiency patterns involving blood and essence deficiency as well as cold lead to a similar presentation, more powerfully tonifying formulas such as Tangkuei and Peony Powder (*dāng guī sháo yào săn*), Flow-Warming Decoction (*wēn jīng tāng*), or even a modification of Rhubarb and Ground Beetle Pill (*dà huáng zhè chóng wán*) are indicated.

Contraindications: deficiency patterns • irregular periods or blood stasis due to heat

▶ FORMULAS WITH SIMILAR INDICATIONS

Peach Pit Decoction to Order the Qi (*táo hé chéng qì tāng*):

── INGREDIENTS ──

dry-fried Foeniculi Fructus (*chăo xiăo huí xiāng*) 1.5g
dry-fried Zingiberis Rhizoma (*chăo gān jiāng*)..................... 3g
Corydalis Rhizoma (*yán hú suŏ*) 3g
Angelicae sinensis Radix (*dāng guī*) 9g
Chuanxiong Rhizoma (*chuān xiōng*) 3g
Myrrha (*mò yào*).. 6g
Cinnamomi Cortex (*ròu guì*) 3g
Paeoniae Radix rubra (*chì sháo*)..................................... 6g
Typhae Pollen (*pú huáng*).. 9g
dry-fried Trogopterori Faeces (*chăo wŭ líng zhī*) 6g

For blood stasis in the lower abdomen due to heat. The lower abdomen will typically be tender to the touch and there may be heat signs like facial flushing, headache, or dizziness.
Tangkuei and Peony Powder (*dāng guī sháo yào sǎn*): For blood stasis in the lower abdomen with blood deficiency, water buildup, and Spleen-Liver disharmony. The most common manifestation is lower abdominal pain in the presence of qi and blood deficiency symptoms.

COMPOSITION

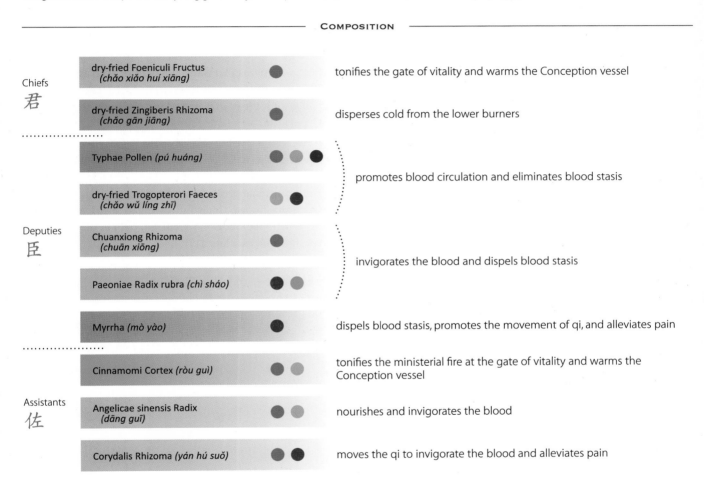

Chiefs 君	dry-fried Foeniculi Fructus (*chǎo xiǎo huí xiāng*)	tonifies the gate of vitality and warms the Conception vessel
	dry-fried Zingiberis Rhizoma (*chǎo gān jiāng*)	disperses cold from the lower burners
Deputies 臣	Typhae Pollen (*pú huáng*)	promotes blood circulation and eliminates blood stasis
	dry-fried Trogopterori Faeces (*chǎo wǔ líng zhī*)	
	Chuanxiong Rhizoma (*chuān xiōng*)	invigorates the blood and dispels blood stasis
	Paeoniae Radix rubra (*chì sháo*)	
	Myrrha (*mò yào*)	dispels blood stasis, promotes the movement of qi, and alleviates pain
Assistants 佐	Cinnamomi Cortex (*ròu guì*)	tonifies the ministerial fire at the gate of vitality and warms the Conception vessel
	Angelicae sinensis Radix (*dāng guī*)	nourishes and invigorates the blood
	Corydalis Rhizoma (*yán hú suǒ*)	moves the qi to invigorate the blood and alleviates pain

芍藥甘草湯（芍药甘草汤）
Peony and Licorice Decoction
sháo yào gān cǎo tāng

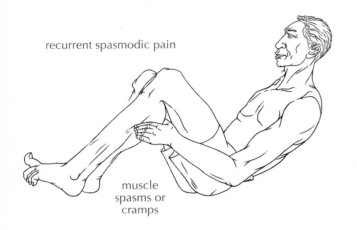

recurrent spasmodic pain

muscle
spasms or
cramps

───── INGREDIENTS ─────

[1]Paeoniae Radix (*sháo yào*) 12g
Glycyrrhizae Radix praeparata (*zhì gān cǎo*) 12g

Actions: nourishes the blood • augments the yi • moderates painful spasms • alleviates pain

Main patterns: blood deficiency • injury to the fluids

Key symptoms: muscle spasms or cramps • recurrent spasmodic pain

Secondary symptoms: irritability

Tongue: scanty coating

Pulse: wiry in middle position

Abdomen: hypertonicity of rectus abdominis muscle or relaxed abdomen with palpable tightness in the depth

► CLINICAL NOTES

• The classic indication of this formula is cramping of the leg muscles. This may be acute or chronic and accompanied by

pain and difficulty in walking or in flexing and extending the leg. Today the formula is used for a wide range of problems presenting with muscle spasms or pain in the abdomen involving the gastrointestinal, urinary, or reproductive systems. The characteristic presentation of such pain is that it is cramp-like and recurrent. The formula can be combined with herbs that drain heat such as Coptidis Rhizoma (*huáng lián*) if the pain is from heat; with herbs that warm the interior such as Zingiberis Rhizoma (*gān jiāng*) and Aconiti Radix lateralis praeparata (*zhì fù zǐ*) if the pain is from cold; and with herbs such as Cyperi Rhizoma (*xiāng fù*) and Bupleuri Radix (*chái hú*) if the pain is associated with Liver qi constraint.

• Because of its ability to relieve muscle spasms and tension, the formula's indications have been extended to include conditions that present with spasms with little or no pain (such as asthma or infertility owing to obstructive spasms of the fallopian tubes) or recurrent pain in the absence of spasm (such as sciatica).

Contraindications: Long-term use is contraindicated due to the known side effects of Glycyrrhizae Radix (*gān cǎo*), which can lead to water retention and a subsequent rise in blood pressure.

───

1. As the primary function here is to restrain, tonify, or soften, Paeoniae Radix alba (*bái sháo*) is preferred.

COMPOSITION

Chief 君	Paeoniae Radix alba *(bái sháo)*	●●	nourishes the blood and preserves the yin; enters the Spleen, softens the Liver, and alleviates pain
Deputy 臣	Glycyrrhizae Radix praeparata *(zhì gān cǎo)*	●	augments the qi of the the Spleen and moderates urgency

參附湯（参附汤）
Ginseng and Aconite Accessory Root Decoction
shēn fù tang

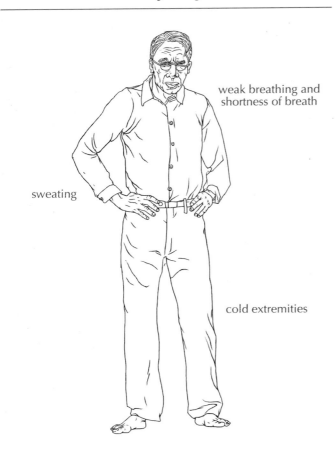

weak breathing and shortness of breath

sweating

cold extremities

INGREDIENTS

Ginseng Radix (*rén shēn*)... 9-12g
Aconiti Radix lateralis praeparata (*zhì fù zǐ*) 9-15g

Actions: restores the yang • strongly tonifies the source qi • rescues the qi from collapse due to devastated yang

Main patterns: yang abandonment • severe deficiency of the source qi with sudden collapse of the yang qi

Key symptoms: cold extremities • sweating • weak breathing and shortness of breath

Secondary symptoms: dizziness • extremely pale complexion

Tongue: pale

Pulse: faint

Abdomen: lacking in tone • cold and sweaty

▶ CLINICAL NOTES

• This is the main formula for yang abandonment, characterized by incessant and severe sweating, cold body, and weak breathing. It is a very strong tonic designed for the treatment of acute and perilous conditions and should not be administered long term. At present, patients for whom this formula is indicated should be sent to the emergency room. We've included it in this handbook in case that cannot be done.

Contraindications: other types of abandonment disorders (qi, blood, yin)

▶ FORMULAS WITH SIMILAR INDICATIONS

Frigid Extremities Decoction (*sì nì tāng*): This formula is similar in action but focuses less on tonifying the source qi and more on warming the middle burner. Its scope of indications is wider and not limited to acute abandonment disorders.

COMPOSITION

Chief 君	Ginseng Radix *(rén shēn)*	● ●	warms and stimulates the fire at the gate of vitality so that it reaches the extremities
Deputy 臣	Aconiti Radix lateralis praeparata *(zhì fù zǐ)*	● Ⓣ	warms the middle burner and eliminates cold, strengthens the Spleen's functions of transforming and transporting

参苓白术散（參苓白朮散）
Ginseng, Poria, and White Atractylodes Powder
shēn líng bái zhú sǎn

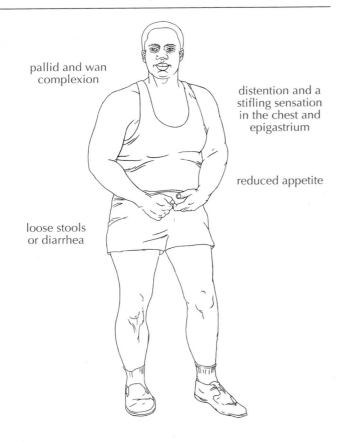

pallid and wan complexion

distention and a stifling sensation in the chest and epigastrium

reduced appetite

loose stools or diarrhea

INGREDIENTS

Ginseng Radix (*rén shēn*) 15g
Atractylodis macrocephalae Rhizoma (*bái zhú*) 15g
Poria (*fú líng*) 15g
Glycyrrhizae Radix praeparata (*zhì gān cǎo*) 9g
Dioscoreae Rhizoma (*shān yào*) 15g
Lablab Semen album (*biǎn dòu*) 12g
Nelumbinis Semen (*lián zǐ*) 9g
Coicis Semen (*yì yǐ rén*) 9g
Amomi Fructus (*shā rén*) 6g

Platycodi Radix (*jié gěng*) 6g

Actions: augments the qi • strengthens the Spleen • leaches out dampness • stops diarrhea

Main pattern: Spleen qi deficiency leading to internally-generated dampness

Key symptoms: loose stools or diarrhea • reduced appetite • distention and a stifling sensation in the chest and epigastrium • pallid and wan complexion

Secondary symptoms: coughing up copious amounts of white sputum • vomiting • dryness of the throat • bland taste in the mouth • weakness of the extremities • weight loss • edema

Tongue: pale body • white coating

Pulse: thin and moderate • deficient and moderate

Abdomen: soft abdomen • splashing sounds in epigastrium

► CLINICAL NOTES

• Specific for qi deficiency accompanied by significant amounts of dampness and phlegm that the body seeks to expel via the Lungs or Large Intestine. The presentation for this formula should include symptoms such as chronic diarrhea or soft, copious amounts of white sputum, discharge, edema, or obesity.

• The formula's ability to contain essence even as it facilitates the resolution of dampness makes it ideal as a base formula for Spleen yin deficiency and for treating disorders such as diabetes or proteinuria characterized by leakage of essence and qi deficiency/dampness.

Contraindications: heat from yin deficiency

► FORMULAS WITH SIMILAR INDICATIONS

Four-Gentlemen Decoction (*sì jūn zǐ tāng*): Focuses on tonifying the Spleen and Stomach in patients with pallor, fatigue, lack of appetite, and the avoidance of physical activity but less pronounced presence of phlegm-dampness.

Six-Gentlemen Decoction (*liù jūn zǐ tāng*): Focuses on tonifying the Spleen and Stomach in patients with pallor, fatigue, lack of appetite, and the avoidance of physical activity who also have signs that indicate the presence of phlegm-dampness such as nausea and fullness after eating, soft stools, or coughing.

COMPOSITION

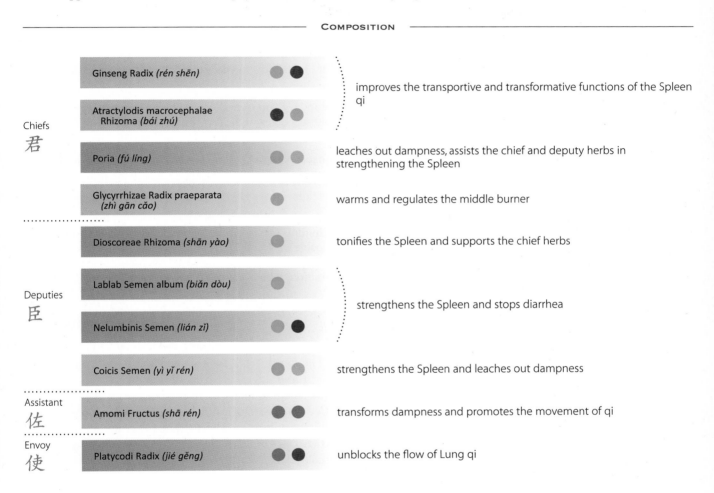

Chiefs
君

Ginseng Radix (*rén shēn*) — improves the transportive and transformative functions of the Spleen qi

Atractylodis macrocephalae Rhizoma (*bái zhú*)

Poria (*fú líng*) — leaches out dampness, assists the chief and deputy herbs in strengthening the Spleen

Glycyrrhizae Radix praeparata (*zhì gān cǎo*) — warms and regulates the middle burner

Deputies
臣

Dioscoreae Rhizoma (*shān yào*) — tonifies the Spleen and supports the chief herbs

Lablab Semen album (*biǎn dòu*)

Nelumbinis Semen (*lián zǐ*) — strengthens the Spleen and stops diarrhea

Coicis Semen (*yì yǐ rén*) — strengthens the Spleen and leaches out dampness

Assistant
佐

Amomi Fructus (*shā rén*) — transforms dampness and promotes the movement of qi

Envoy
使

Platycodi Radix (*jié gěng*) — unblocks the flow of Lung qi

腎氣丸（肾气丸）
Kidney Qi Pill
shèn qì wán

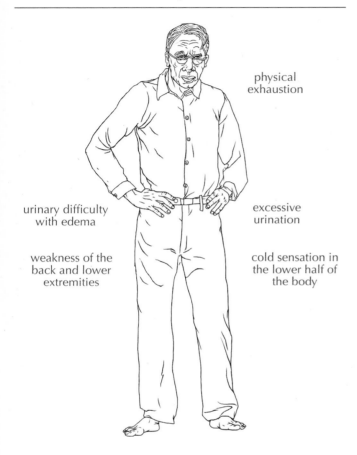

physical exhaustion

urinary difficulty with edema

excessive urination

weakness of the back and lower extremities

cold sensation in the lower half of the body

INGREDIENTS

Rehmanniae Radix (*shēng dì huáng*) 24g

Corni Fructus (*shān zhū yú*) 12g

Dioscoreae Rhizoma (*shān yào*) 12g

¹Aconiti Radix lateralis praeparata (*zhì fù zǐ*) 3g

Cinnamomi Ramulus (*guì zhī*) 3g

Alismatis Rhizoma (*zé xiè*) 9g

Poria (*fú líng*) 9g

1. This ingredient may be difficult to obtain because of legal issues. Psoraleae Fructus *(bǔ gǔ zhī)*, Cynomorii Herba *(suǒ yáng)*, or Epimedii Herba *(yín yáng huò)* may be substituted.

Moutan Cortex (*mǔ dān pí*) 9g

Actions: warms and tonifies the Kidney yang

Main pattern: Kidney yang deficiency with insufficient fire at the gate of vitality

Key symptoms: physical exhaustion • weakness of the back and lower extremities • cold sensation in the lower half of the body • urinary difficulty with edema • excessive urination

Secondary symptoms: loss of libido • impotence • thirst • pitting edema of the feet and ankles • soft stools • deafness • tinnitus

Tongue: pale, wet body • thin coating • possible cracks

Pulse: empty • frail • submerged and faint at the proximal position

Abdomen: weak abdomen • hypertonicity of rectus abdominis muscle in the lower abdomen accompanied by a palpable weakness in the area between the muscles • pencil-line tightness of linea alba below the umbilicus • palpable pulsations between umbilicus and pubic bone

► CLINICAL NOTES

• This is the main formula for Kidney yang deficiency. The key marker for this formula is the combination of three interrelated manifestations: (i) an excess of pathological fluids, often combined with dryness due to lack of physiological fluids, such as edema or puffiness with dry, brittle, and itchy skin; (ii) symptoms indicating deficiency of fire at the gate of vitality such as aversion to cold, exhaustion, or impotence; (iii) symptoms pointing to the Kidneys as the root of the disorder such as urinary dysfunction (with increased or decreased urination), low back pain, weak knees, hypertonicity and/or weakness of the lower abdomen, hearing loss, and tinnitus.

• Patients may also have a floating deficient yang with symptoms such as a flushed face, wheezing, severe sweating, insomnia, or hypertension. Heat associated with unanchored deficient yang may also manifest in the lower abdomen or the Kidney system. This is exemplified by the low-grade inflammatory signs and symptoms associated with conditions such as chronic prostatitis, chronic pyelonephritis, or pelvic inflammatory disease. Unlike conditions due to yin-deficiency fire, these will present with weak and cold lower extremities and a deficient, rootless pulse.

- While the original formula specifies Rehmanniae Radix (*shēng dì huáng*) and Cinnamomi Ramulus (*guì zhī*), many physicians prefer to substitute Rehmanniae Radix praeparata (*shú dì huáng*) and Cinnamomi Cortex (*ròu guì*). The difference is that the original formula focuses more on fluid disorders and stagnation of the body fluids, including blood stasis, thus its use of Cinnamomi Ramulus (*guì zhī*); the later variation focuses on tonification of essence and on warming of the vitality-gate yang.

Contraindications: yin deficiency with deficiency heat

▶ FORMULAS WITH SIMILAR INDICATIONS

True Warrior Decoction (*zhēn wǔ tāng*): Focuses on lesser yin-warp disorders with flooding of the entire body by pathogenic fluids. This pattern is characterized by manifestations of severe yin excess including abdominal pain that is aggravated by cold, deep aching and heaviness in the extremities, and a pale or dark, swollen tongue.

Restore the Right [Kidney] Pill (*yòu guī wán*): Focuses on Kidney tonification without either draining pathogenic water or leading floating yang back to its source in the lower burner. This formula is indicated for chronic disorders characterized by weakness and exhaustion in addition to cold.

--- COMPOSITION ---

Chiefs 君	Aconiti Radix lateralis praeparata (*zhì fù zǐ*)	● Ⓣ	tonifies the source fire, dispels cold, and eliminates dampness
	Cinnamomi Ramulus (*guì zhī*)	● ●	benefits the joints, warms the channels, and unblocks the vessels
Deputies 臣	Rehmanniae Radix (*shēng dì huáng*)	● ●	enriches the yin and generates fluids
	Corni Fructus (*shān zhū yú*)	●	tonifies the Liver and benefits the Spleen in order to tonify and reinforce the essence and blood
	Dioscoreae Rhizoma (*shān yào*)	●	
Assistants 佐	Alismatis Rhizoma (*zé xiè*)	● ●	unblocks and regulates the water passageways
	Poria (*fú líng*)	● ●	strengthens the Spleen and drains dampness
	Moutan Cortex (*mǔ dān pí*)	● ●	clears heat and quells Liver fire

身痛逐瘀湯（身痛逐瘀汤）
Drive Out Stasis from a Painful Body Decoction
shēn tōng zhú yū tāng

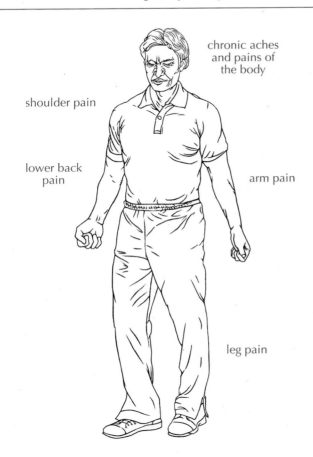

chronic aches and pains of the body

shoulder pain

lower back pain

arm pain

leg pain

INGREDIENTS

Gentianae macrophyllae Radix (*qín jiāo*) 3g
Chuanxiong Rhizoma (*chuān xiōng*) 6g
Persicae Semen (*táo rén*) 9g
Carthami Flos (*hóng huā*) 9g
Glycyrrhizae Radix (*gān cǎo*) 6g
Notopterygii Rhizoma seu Radix (*qiāng huó*) 3g
Myrrha (*mò yào*) 6g
Angelicae sinensis Radix (*dāng guī*) 9g
dry-fried Trogopterori Faeces (*chǎo wǔ líng zhī*) 6g

Cyperi Rhizoma (*xiāng fù*) 3g
Cyathulae Radix (*chuān niú xī*) 9g
Pheretima (*dì lóng*) 6g

Actions: invigorates the blood • promotes the movement of qi • dispels blood stasis • unblocks the collaterals • unblocks painful obstruction • alleviates pain

Main pattern: painful obstruction due to the stasis of qi and blood in the channels and collaterals

Key symptoms: shoulder pain • arm pain • lower back pain • leg pain • chronic aches and pains of the body

Secondary symptoms: systemic signs and symptoms of qi stagnation and blood stasis

Tongue: dark body • stasis spots • distended sublingual veins • white coating

Pulse: rough • forceful

Abdomen: As the stasis is in the channels, no abdominal signs need be present. However, it is common for the patient to have pain on pressure in the lower abdomen or visible nevi on the chest or abdominal wall.

▶ CLINICAL NOTES

• This formula treats painful obstruction due to blood stasis. This type of painful obstruction is chronic and will not respond well to formulas for wind-cold-damp painful obstruction. The pain is usually fixed and may wake the patient at night. There may be some heat due to constraint. Although the pain may be aggravated by cold, sensitivity to changes in the weather is not a prominent feature of this condition.

• When it is necessary to strongly dispel wind, cold, or dampness, this formula can be combined with one that specifically targets that type of painful obstruction pattern, or herbs such as Clematidis Radix (*wēi líng xiān*), Saposhnikoviae Radix (*fáng fēng*), or Acanthopanacis Cortex (*wǔ jiā pí*) can be added.

Contraindications: stagnation in the channels and collaterals arising from deficiency

▶ FORMULAS WITH SIMILAR INDICATIONS

Remove Painful Obstruction Decoction (*juān bì tāng*): For painful obstruction due to wind, cold, and dampness in patients with blood and qi deficiency.

Pubescent Angelica and Taxillus Decoction (*dú huó jì shēng tāng*): For painful obstruction due to wind, cold, and dampness in patients with Kidney and Liver deficiency.

COMPOSITION

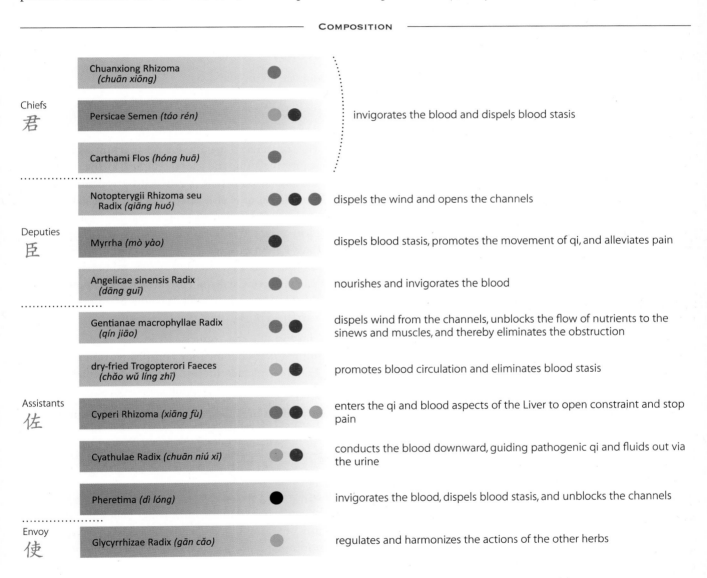

Chiefs
君

Chuanxiong Rhizoma (*chuān xiōng*)

Persicae Semen (*táo rén*)

Carthami Flos (*hóng huā*)

invigorates the blood and dispels blood stasis

Deputies
臣

Notopterygii Rhizoma seu Radix (*qiāng huó*)

dispels the wind and opens the channels

Myrrha (*mò yào*)

dispels blood stasis, promotes the movement of qi, and alleviates pain

Angelicae sinensis Radix (*dāng guī*)

nourishes and invigorates the blood

Gentianae macrophyllae Radix (*qín jiāo*)

dispels wind from the channels, unblocks the flow of nutrients to the sinews and muscles, and thereby eliminates the obstruction

dry-fried Trogopterori Faeces (*chǎo wǔ líng zhī*)

promotes blood circulation and eliminates blood stasis

Assistants
佐

Cyperi Rhizoma (*xiāng fù*)

enters the qi and blood aspects of the Liver to open constraint and stop pain

Cyathulae Radix (*chuān niú xī*)

conducts the blood downward, guiding pathogenic qi and fluids out via the urine

Pheretima (*dì lóng*)

invigorates the blood, dispels blood stasis, and unblocks the channels

Envoy
使

Glycyrrhizae Radix (*gān cǎo*)

regulates and harmonizes the actions of the other herbs

生化湯（生化汤）
Generating and Transforming Decoction
shēng huà tāng

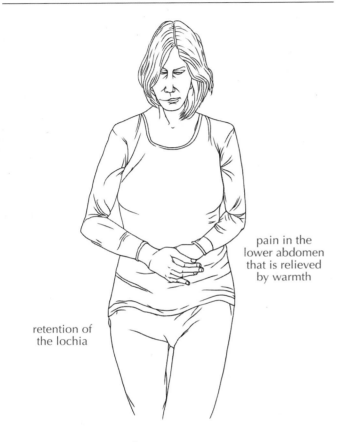

pain in the lower abdomen that is relieved by warmth

retention of the lochia

INGREDIENTS

Angelicae sinensis Radix (*dāng guī*).............................15-24g
Chuanxiong Rhizoma (*chuān xiōng*)...............................6-9g
Persicae Semen (*táo rén*)...4.5-6g
Zingiberis Rhizoma praeparata (*páo jiāng*).....................1-2g
Glycyrrhizae Radix praeparata (*zhì gān cǎo*)..................1-2g

Actions: invigorates the blood • transforms and dispels blood stasis • warms the menses • alleviates pain

Main pattern: postpartum blood stagnation in the uterus due to cold taking advantage of blood deficiency

Key symptoms: retention of the lochia • pain in the lower abdomen that is relieved by warmth

Secondary symptoms: uterine bleeding that is dark in color and may have dark clots

Tongue: dark body • stasis spots • dark, distended sublingual veins

Pulse: thin, submerged, rough • deep, tight, wiry • slow and thin or wiry

Abdomen: no specific signs

▶ CLINICAL NOTES

• This formula is specific for postpartum women with scanty bleeding and clots, retained lochia, and lower abdominal pain that is relieved by warmth. Because the normal qi is also often deficient after giving birth, the formula is often combined with Ginseng Radix (*rén shēn*) or Jade Windscreen Powder (*yù píng fēng sǎn*) with the addition of other blood-invigorating herbs such as Leonuri Herba (*yì mǔ cǎo*), Salviae miltiorrhizae Radix (*dān shēn*), or Carthami Flos (*hóng huā*) as appropriate. It should not be prescribed as a matter of course but only if warranted by the presentation.

• This formula can also treat deficiency-cold blood stasis in the lower abdomen for non-postpartum conditions. Examples include uterine fibroids, dysmenorrhea, and disorders that occur after abortion or miscarriage.

Contraindications: blood stasis due to heat • postpartum hemorrhage • pregnancy

▶ FORMULAS WITH SIMILAR INDICATIONS

Flow-Warming Decoction (*wēn jīng tāng*): Can also be used for postpartum patterns involving deficiency cold but focuses on warming and opening the qi dynamic rather than transforming blood stasis. Typically, there will be signs of dryness and yin deficiency heat even though the abdominal pain and stasis are clearly due to cold.

Sudden Smile Powder (*shī xiào sǎn*): For postpartum patterns characterized by significant amounts of pain and no deficiency.

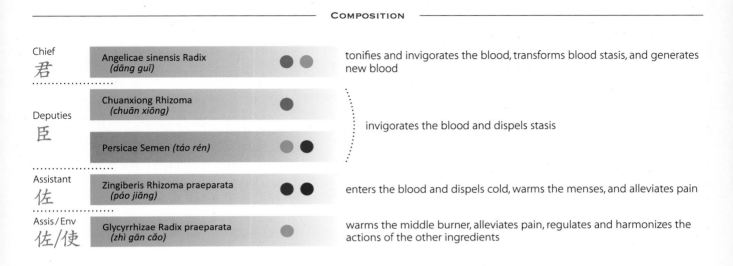

COMPOSITION

Chief 君 — Angelicae sinensis Radix (dāng guī) — tonifies and invigorates the blood, transforms blood stasis, and generates new blood

Deputies 臣 — Chuanxiong Rhizoma (chuān xiōng) / Persicae Semen (táo rén) — invigorates the blood and dispels stasis

Assistant 佐 — Zingiberis Rhizoma praeparata (páo jiāng) — enters the blood and dispels cold, warms the menses, and alleviates pain

Assis/Env 佐/使 — Glycyrrhizae Radix praeparata (zhì gān cǎo) — warms the middle burner, alleviates pain, regulates and harmonizes the actions of the other ingredients

生脈散 （生脉散）
Generate the Pulse Powder
shēng mài sǎn

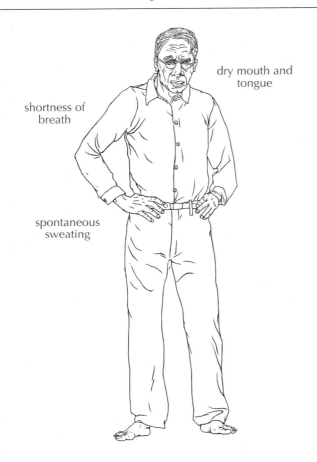

dry mouth and tongue

shortness of breath

spontaneous sweating

Secondary symptoms: chronic cough with sparse sputum that is difficult to expectorate • laconic speech

Tongue: pale red body • dry, thin coating

Pulse: deficient and rapid • deficient and thin

Abdomen: weak and soft abdomen

► CLINICAL NOTES

- Originally for damage to qi and body fluids, specifically of the Lungs, following various types of warm pathogen disorders (e.g., summerheat stroke) or chronic illness.

- In contemporary practice, this has become one of the most important formulas for treating various types of heart disease, including the aftermath of myocardial infarction. It is particularly indicated for patterns presenting with palpitations, a stifling sensation in the chest, shortness of breath, sweating, a dry mouth and thirst, poor sleep, a pale red and dry tongue, and a slow-irregular or consistently-irregular pulse. Usually blood-moving herbs such as Salviae miltiorrhizae Radix (*dān shēn*) are added in these situations.

- Modern-day practitioners often use this formula to treat chronic cough that presents with signs of yin and qi deficiency, such as scanty phlegm that is difficult to expectorate, dry mouth, and shortness of breath. Often herbs to moisten the Lung and relieve cough, such as Armeniacae Semen (*xìng rén*) and Mori Cortex (*sāng bái pí*), are included for this purpose.

- Due to its astringent nature, the formula must not be used in cases where external pathogens are still present in the exterior. It can, however, be used to tonify Lung qi and yin in order to prevent external invasion in deficient individuals.

Contraindications: exterior excess patterns • patterns lacking damage to the fluids

► FORMULAS WITH SIMILAR INDICATIONS

Ginseng and Aconite Accessory Root Decoction (*shēn fù tāng*): For sudden exhaustion of the yang qi with severe sweating and shock but no signs of dryness.

INGREDIENTS

Ginseng Radix (*rén shēn*).. 9g
Ophiopogonis Radix (*mài mén dōng*) 15g
Schisandrae Fructus (*wǔ wèi zǐ*)... 6g

Actions: augments the qi • generates fluids • preserves the yin • relieves cough • mitigates excessive sweating

Main pattern: simultaneous deficiency of qi and yin, primarily of the Lungs

Key symptoms: spontaneous sweating • shortness of breath • dry mouth and tongue

Frigid Extremities Decoction (*sì nì tāng*): For extremely weak yang qi with internal ascent of yin cold manifesting as a pulse that is thin and weak with pronounced signs of internal cold, such as cold extremities.

Prepared Licorice Decoction (*zhì gān cǎo tāng*): Often used for deficiency of qi and blood following an illness, this formula puts more emphasis on tonification of the blood than does Generate the Pulse Powder (*shēng mài sǎn*).

COMPOSITION

Chief 君	Ginseng Radix (*rén shēn*)	● ●	strongly tonifies the source qi, generates fluids, and calms the spirit
Deputy 臣	Ophiopogonis Radix (*mài mén dōng*)	● ●	nourishes the yin, moistens the Lungs, benefits the Stomach and generates fluids, and clears heat from the Heart
Assistant 佐	Schisandrae Fructus (*wǔ wèi zǐ*)	● ●	restrains the leakage of Lung qi and generates fluids in the Kidneys

十全大補湯（十全大补汤）
All-Inclusive Great Tonifying Decoction
shí quán dà bǔ tāng

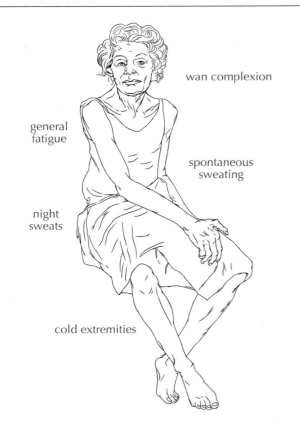

wan complexion

general fatigue

spontaneous sweating

night sweats

cold extremities

Actions: warms and augments the qi • tonifies the blood

Main pattern: combined deficiency of qi and blood that is often seen in consumptive or long-term disorders

Key symptoms: wan complexion • general fatigue • spontaneous sweating • night sweats • cold extremities

Secondary symptoms: reduced appetite • dizziness • palpitations • lassitude • dyspnea • sores that do not heal • irregular periods • continuous spotting from uterine bleeding

Tongue: pale • scanty coating

Pulse: deep • thin • frail

Abdomen: weak abdomen • tension in rectus abdominis muscle • periodic palpable pulsations in upper abdomen

► CLINICAL NOTES

- Tonifies qi and blood as well as Kidney yang and thus has the ability to increase vitality and promote the growth of new tissue. It is primarily used in the aftermath of serious illness, major surgery, or the treatment of severe, chronic disorders.

- Modern uses include the supportive treatment of chemotherapy and radiotherapy and major surgery. In these cases, patients should begin taking the formula 1-2 weeks before surgery or before treatment commences. Some practitioners limit this use to before, between, and following these conventional medical treatments to avoid unwanted interactions.

Contraindications: yin deficiency • any excess pattern

► FORMULAS WITH SIMILAR INDICATIONS

Eight-Treasure Decoction (*bā zhēn tāng*): For milder qi and blood deficiency patterns, with no prominent signs of cold.

*Ginseng Decoction to Nourish Luxuriance (*rén shēn yǎng róng tāng*): This formula treats similar disorders but focuses on the Heart spirit, and is for patterns that manifest with Heart symptoms such as fright palpitations as well as nonhealing sores.

INGREDIENTS

Ginseng Radix (*rén shēn*)... 6g
Atractylodis macrocephalae Rhizoma (*bái zhú*) 9g
Poria (*fú líng*)... 9g
Glycyrrhizae Radix praeparata (*zhì gān cǎo*) 3g
Rehmanniae Radix praeparata (*shú dì huáng*) 9-12g
Paeoniae Radix alba (*bái sháo*)...................................... 9g
Angelicae sinensis Radix (*dāng guī*) 9g
Chuanxiong Rhizoma (*chuān xiōng*) 6g
Cinnamomi Cortex (*ròu guì*) 3-6g
Astragali Radix (*huáng qí*) 12-15g
Zingiberis Rhizoma recens (*shēng jiāng*).................... 3 pieces
Jujubae Fructus (*dà zǎo*)....................................... 2 pieces

———— COMPOSITION ————

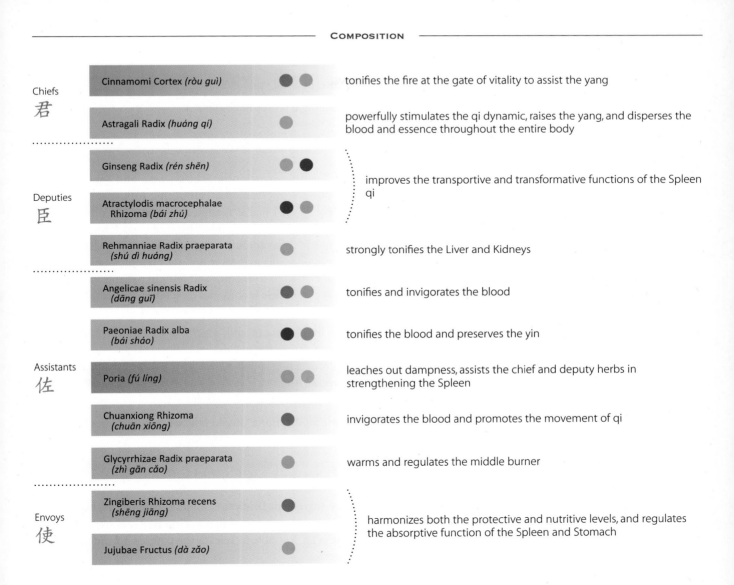

Chiefs 君

Cinnamomi Cortex (ròu guì) — tonifies the fire at the gate of vitality to assist the yang

Astragali Radix (huáng qí) — powerfully stimulates the qi dynamic, raises the yang, and disperses the blood and essence throughout the entire body

Deputies 臣

Ginseng Radix (rén shēn)

Atractylodis macrocephalae Rhizoma (bái zhú) — improves the transportive and transformative functions of the Spleen qi

Rehmanniae Radix praeparata (shú dì huáng) — strongly tonifies the Liver and Kidneys

Angelicae sinensis Radix (dāng guī) — tonifies and invigorates the blood

Paeoniae Radix alba (bái sháo) — tonifies the blood and preserves the yin

Assistants 佐

Poria (fú líng) — leaches out dampness, assists the chief and deputy herbs in strengthening the Spleen

Chuanxiong Rhizoma (chuān xiōng) — invigorates the blood and promotes the movement of qi

Glycyrrhizae Radix praeparata (zhì gān cǎo) — warms and regulates the middle burner

Envoys 使

Zingiberis Rhizoma recens (shēng jiāng)

Jujubae Fructus (dà zǎo) — harmonizes both the protective and nutritive levels, and regulates the absorptive function of the Spleen and Stomach

十味敗毒散（十味败毒散）
Ten-Ingredient Powder to Overcome Toxicity
shí wèi bài dú sǎn

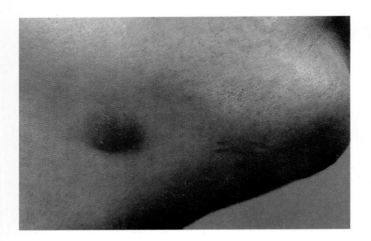

---- INGREDIENTS ----

Bupleuri Radix (*chái hú*)..6g
Angelicae pubescentis Radix (*dú huó*) 3-6g
[1]Cerasi Cortex (*yīng pí*)..6-9g
Saposhnikoviae Radix (*fáng fēng*)..............................3-6g
Platycodi Radix (*jié gěng*)...6g
Chuanxiong Rhizoma (*chuān xiōng*) 3-6g
Poria (*fú líng*)..6-9g
Schizonepetae Herba (*jīng jiè*)...................................2-3g
Glycyrrhizae Radix (*gān cǎo*)......................................2-3g
Zingiberis Rhizoma (*gān jiāng*)..................................2-3g

Actions: dispels wind and transforms dampness • clears heat • resolves toxicity

Main pattern: heat toxin flushing through the exterior aspects of the body

Key symptoms: initial stages of painful and hot toxic sores

Secondary symptoms: fever and chills • hot, itchy rash

---

1. Because this herb is difficult to obtain in the West, Lonicerae Flos *(jīn yín huā)* and Gleditsiae Spina *(zào jiǎo cì)* may be substituted to increase the formula's ability to clear heat, resolve toxicity, and thrust out pus.

Tongue: This is an external pattern that has not yet affected the tongue, although a thin, white or yellow coating may appear

Pulse: floating • rapid

Abdomen: no specific signs

▶ CLINICAL NOTES

- This is a variation of Schizonepeta and Saposhnikovia Powder to Overcome Pathogenic Influences (*jīng fáng bài dú sǎn*) that is intended to treat acute onset of pus-filled sores accompanied by chills and fever. It is often used for acute outbreaks of boils, carbuncles, or sties, even if chills and fever are not present. Conversely, it is also used to treat chills and fever in patients who have no apparent skin lesions, but have internal infections such as ear infections (inner and outer) or sinusitis.

- This formula's ability to dispel dampness, heat, and wind from the exterior of the body is also helpful in the treatment of acute outbreaks of hot hives and red, itching, eczematous skin rashes, even though no pus formation is involved in these disorders.

Contraindications: should not be used once sores have burst and released pus • not for long-term use

▶ FORMULAS WITH SIMILAR INDICATIONS

Five-Ingredient Drink to Eliminate Toxin (*wǔ wèi xiāo dú yǐn*): Has a much stronger ability to clear heat and resolve toxicity but is far less able to release the pathogen from the body's exterior.

Immortals' Formula for Sustaining Life (*xiān fāng huó mìng yǐn*): Treats red, hot swellings in their initial stage where there may be associated symptoms of fever and chills. However, frequently the pattern is related to an internal disharmony. By contrast, Ten-Ingredient Powder to Overcome Toxicity (*shí wèi bài dú sǎn*) primarily treats external patterns and lays a much stronger emphasis on releasing pathogens from the exterior.

COMPOSITION

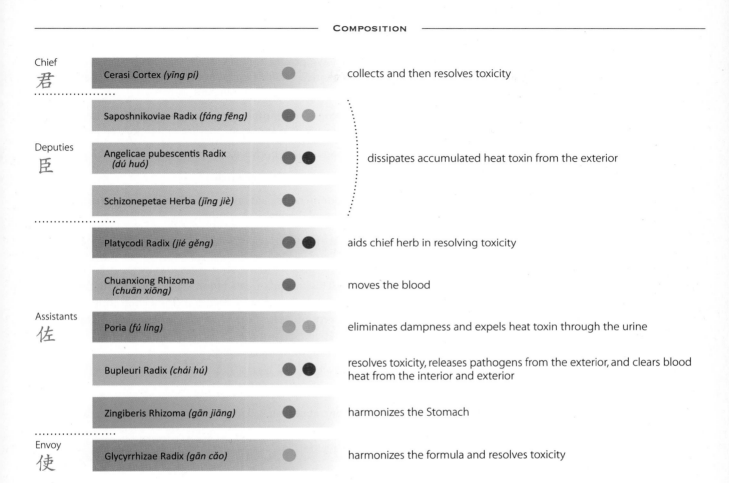

Chief
君

Cerasi Cortex (yīng pí) — collects and then resolves toxicity

Deputies
臣

Saposhnikoviae Radix (fáng fēng)

Angelicae pubescentis Radix (dú huó)

Schizonepetae Herba (jīng jiè) — dissipates accumulated heat toxin from the exterior

Assistants
佐

Platycodi Radix (jié gěng) — aids chief herb in resolving toxicity

Chuanxiong Rhizoma (chuān xiōng) — moves the blood

Poria (fú líng) — eliminates dampness and expels heat toxin through the urine

Bupleuri Radix (chái hú) — resolves toxicity, releases pathogens from the exterior, and clears blood heat from the interior and exterior

Zingiberis Rhizoma (gān jiāng) — harmonizes the Stomach

Envoy
使

Glycyrrhizae Radix (gān cǎo) — harmonizes the formula and resolves toxicity

失笑散
Sudden Smile Powder
shī xiào sǎn

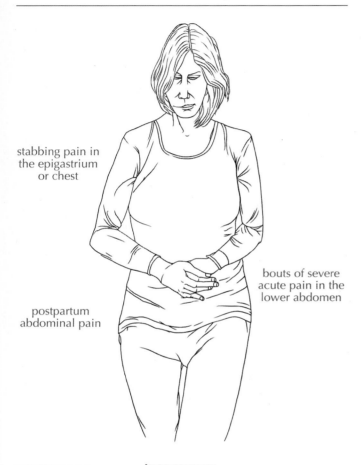

stabbing pain in the epigastrium or chest

bouts of severe acute pain in the lower abdomen

postpartum abdominal pain

Main pattern: retention of static blood which obstructs the vessels that serve the lower abdomen

Key symptoms: bouts of severe acute pain in the lower abdomen • stabbing pain in the epigastrium or chest • postpartum abdominal pain

Secondary symptoms: irregular menstruation • long menstrual cycle • dysmenorrhea • retention of lochia

Tongue: dark body • stasis spots

Pulse: thin, wiry, or rough

Abdomen: no pain on pressure in either epigastrium or lower abdomen

► CLINICAL NOTES

• This formula treats blood stasis obstructing the vessels, especially when it occurs in the Penetrating and Conception vessels below and the terminal yin vessels in the abdomen and chest. This allows the formula to treat the symptoms noted above.

• A key clinical marker for this formula is pain that is severe, acute in onset, colicky, and fixed in location.

Contraindications: pregnancy • Stomach deficiency

► FORMULAS WITH SIMILAR INDICATIONS

Generating and Transforming Decoction (*shēng huà tāng*): For postpartum patterns due to deficiency cold with less severe pain.

Salvia Drink (*dān shēn yǐn*): For blood stasis and qi stagnation that give rise to pain in the epigastrium that radiates into the chest.

INGREDIENTS

Trogopterori Faeces (*wǔ líng zhī*)...................................... 8-12g
Typhae Pollen (*pú huáng*)... 8-12g

Preparation notes: When decocted at the above dosage, the substances should be placed in a cheesecloth bag. Alternatively, and commonly after both ingredients are ground into powder, 6g of the result are chased with either Chinese yellow wine or vinegar.

Actions: invigorates the blood • dispels blood stasis • disperses accumulations • alleviates pain

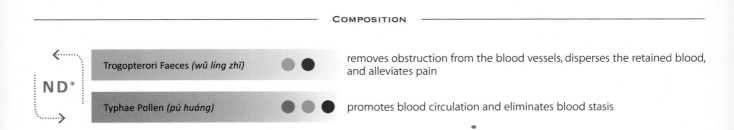

COMPOSITION

N D*

Trogopterori Faeces *(wŭ líng zhī)* — removes obstruction from the blood vessels, disperses the retained blood, and alleviates pain

Typhae Pollen *(pú huáng)* — promotes blood circulation and eliminates blood stasis

*herb roles are not differentiated

四君子湯(四君子汤)
Four-Gentlemen Decoction
sì jūn zǐ tāng

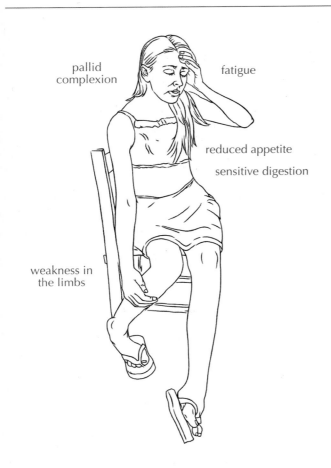

pallid complexion

fatigue

reduced appetite

sensitive digestion

weakness in the limbs

INGREDIENTS

Ginseng Radix (*rén shēn*)..9g
Atractylodis macrocephalae Rhizoma (*bái zhú*)..................9g
Poria (*fú líng*)...9g
Glycyrrhizae Radix praeparata (*zhì gān cǎo*)....................6-9g

Actions: tonifies the qi • strengthens the Spleen

Main pattern: Spleen qi deficiency

Key symptoms: pallid complexion • fatigue • reduced appetite • sensitive digestion • weakness in the limbs

Secondary symptoms: low and soft voice • abdominal fullness • nausea • loose stools • borborygmus

Tongue: pale and swollen body • tooth marks • scanty coating

Pulse: deficient • frail • deep

Abdomen: weak abdomen • splashing sounds • discomfort in epigastrium • pencil-line tightness of linea alba between umbilicus and xiphoid process

▶ CLINICAL NOTES

• This is the primary formula for middle burner qi deficiency accompanied by dampness. Its balanced combination is ideal for treating the root, while specific symptoms or manifestations may be addressed by way of appropriate additions. Japanese Kampo physicians regularly add Zingiberis Rhizoma recens (*shēng jiāng*) and Jujubae Fructus (*dà zǎo*) to harmonize the nutritive and protective aspects.

• Patients for whom this formula is indicated often present with sensitive digestive systems or other sensitivities. Because the middle burner harmonizes the function of all the organ systems and this formula is considered to be especially balanced in terms of its composition, it can help to moderate such sensitivities.

Contraindications: full heat • yin deficiency patterns

▶ FORMULAS WITH SIMILAR INDICATIONS

Ginseng, Poria, and White Atractylodes Powder (*shēn líng bái zhú sǎn*): For middle burner yang deficiency patterns with more pronounced dampness and phlegm marked by very loose stools or diarrhea and a stifling sensation in the chest and epigastrium. Also addresses water swelling due to Spleen qi deficiency.

Regulate the Middle Pill (*lǐ zhōng wán*): For middle burner qi and yang deficiency with signs of cold-induced stagnation or transformation failure. Important signs of this pattern include diarrhea with watery stools, nausea and vomiting, abdominal pain, and a pale tongue with a white coating.

─────────────── COMPOSITION ───────────────

Chief
君
Ginseng Radix *(rén shēn)*

improves the transportive and transformative functions of the Spleen qi

Deputy
臣
Atractylodis macrocephalae Rhizoma *(bái zhú)*

Assistant
佐
Poria *(fú líng)*

leaches out dampness, assists the chief and deputy herbs in strengthening the Spleen

Envoy
使
Glycyrrhizae Radix praeparata *(zhì gān cǎo)*

warms and regulates the middle burner

四逆散
Frigid Extremities Powder
sì nì sǎn

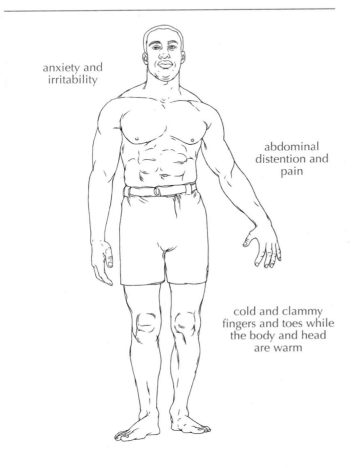

anxiety and irritability

abdominal distention and pain

cold and clammy fingers and toes while the body and head are warm

— INGREDIENTS —

Bupleuri Radix (*chái hú*)..........................9-12g
Aurantii Fructus immaturus (*zhǐ shí*)..........9-12g
Paeoniae Radix alba (*bái sháo*)................12-24g
Glycyrrhizae Radix praeparata (*zhì gān cǎo*)....6-9g

Preparation notes: When taken as a powder, equal amounts of each ingredient are used.

Actions: vents pathogenic qi • releases constraint • spreads Liver qi • regulates the Spleen

Main pattern: yang- or hot-type inversion (陽厥 *yáng jué*) due to internal constraint of yang qi that manifests as yang failing to reach the extremities

Key symptoms: cold and clammy fingers and toes while the body and head are warm • anxiety and irritability • abdominal distention and pain

Secondary symptoms: fullness in the chest and epigastrium • palpitations • insomnia • fatigue • frequent sighing or taking deep breaths • depressive moods • cough • diarrhea alternating with constipation • nausea • urinary difficulty

Tongue: red with a yellow coating

Pulse: wiry

Abdomen: focal distention in epigastrium • noticeable tension in rectus abdominis muscle • fullness and distention in hypochondrium

▶ CLINICAL NOTES

- Dredges the Liver and regulates the qi in the abdomen. Palpable tension in the rectus abdominus muscle or a wiry pulse is widely considered to be a necessary sign for prescribing this formula, particularly in Japan.

- Particularly useful for patterns that combine signs of internal tension with both heat/dryness and cold/dampness such as smelly, pain-free diarrhea; constipation with hard, pellet-like stools alternating with diarrhea; one-sided sinusitis or rhinitis with yellow mucus due to heat in the Gallbladder; inflammatory disorders in the abdomen accompanied by pain and obstruction such as pancreatitis, gastritis, colitis, obstructed ovarian ducts, or calculi in both the biliary or urinary systems.

- Used for erectile dysfunction in men characterized by failure of ministerial fire to extend to the penis.

- Frequently used in the treatment of emotional distress marked by tension that is directed inward such as melancholia or depression with bouts of anger and irritability.

- Where pain is an important aspect of the presentation, Bupleurum Powder to Dredge the Liver (*chái hú shū gān sǎn*) is the preferred variation of this formula because of its stronger qi and blood regulating functions.

Contraindications: qi constraint associated with yin deficiency • long-term use

▶ FᴏRᴍᴜʟAꜱ ᴡɪᴛʜ SɪᴍɪʟAR IɴᴅɪᴄAᴛɪᴏɴꜱ ⇢

Minor Bupleurum Decoction (*xiǎo chái hú tāng*): For cold constraining the lesser yang warp with alternating chills and fever, bitter taste, and a dry throat. Constipation, diarrhea, bloating, and cold extremities are not regarded as key symptoms of this formula.

Cᴏᴍᴘᴏꜱɪᴛɪᴏɴ

Chief 君	Bupleuri Radix *(chái hú)*	harmonizes and resolves the lesser yang, disperses pathogens and vents the exterior
Deputy 臣	Aurantii Fructus immaturus *(zhǐ shí)*	directs qi downward and unbinds focal distention; with Bupleuri Radix, improves the transporting function of the Spleen and readjusts the pivot of the qi dynamic
Assistant 佐	Paeoniae Radix *(bái sháo)*	augments the yin and nourishes the blood; with Bupleuri Radix, dredges the Liver qi and regulates the Spleen
Envoy 使	Glycyrrhizae Radix praeparata *(zhì gān cǎo)*	harmonizes the effects of the other ingredients

四逆湯（四逆汤）
Frigid Extremities Decoction
sì nì tāng

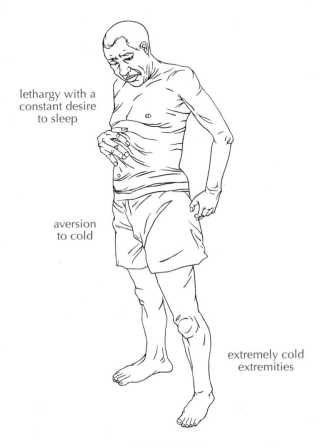

lethargy with a constant desire to sleep

aversion to cold

extremely cold extremities

INGREDIENTS

[1]Aconiti Radix lateralis (*fù zǐ*)...5-15g

Zingiberis Rhizoma (*gān jiāng*)..5-9g

Glycyrrhizae Radix praeparata (*zhì gān cǎo*).......................6g

Actions: rescues devastated yang • warms the middle burner • stops diarrhea

Main patterns: lesser yin warp disorders • interior deficiency cold

1. This ingredient may be difficult to obtain because of legal issues. No substitute is useful in this context.

Key symptoms: extremely cold extremities • aversion to cold • lethargy with a constant desire to sleep

Secondary symptoms: lying down in fetal position • vomiting • diarrhea with undigested food particles • painful and cold abdomen • increased urination • absence of thirst

Tongue: pale • little or thin, white coating

Pulse: thin • submerged • faint

Abdomen: weak muscle tone • skin folds can be easily lifted up • splashing sounds

▶ CLINICAL NOTES

• This is the main formula for treating lesser yin warp patterns characterized by cold and cyanotic extremities, lethargy with a desire to sleep or lie down, and a faint and thin pulse. Because the cold in the extremities results from a lack of yang qi, it may extend all the way to the elbows or knees. The lower extremities in particular will be cold. Deficiency of yang in the interior manifests as diarrhea, vomiting, or increased urination. There may be many additional signs of yang deficiency such as spontaneous sweating, dyspnea, a weak and laconic voice, a heavy body, or increased salivation.

• The typical pulse for which this formula is indicated is deep, faint, and thin, reflecting that there is insufficient yang to warm and move the blood. The pulse may become so faint as to be imperceptible. It may also be very superficial and weak, or suddenly become large and superficial but feel deficient on pressure. This indicates that yang is floating to the exterior as the cold in the interior is increasing.

• False heat or floating yang may manifest as flushing, headaches, irritability, or the floating pulse described above. It can be distinguished from true heat by signs that indicate the presence of severe cold in the interior such as watery diarrhea, cold extremities, and lack of thirst.

Contraindications: true heat and false cold characterized by cold extremities, thirst with a desire to drink cool beverages, dark urine, and a red tongue with a yellow coating

▶ FORMULAS WITH SIMILAR INDICATIONS

True Warrior Decoction (*zhēn wǔ tāng*): For lesser yin patterns characterized by significant accumulation of water in the interior.

Regulate the Middle Pill (*lǐ zhōng wán*): For middle burner deficiency-cold diarrhea that comes and goes in relation to factors such as food intake, climate, or physical and mental exhaustion without the more pronounced lesser yin warp signs.

Ginseng and Aconite Accessory Root Decoction (*shēn fù tāng*): For abandoned yang patterns with such symptoms as wheezing, sweating, and a very faint pulse.

───── COMPOSITION ─────

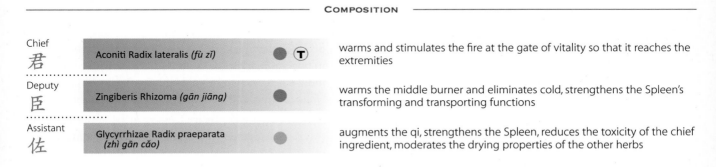

Chief 君	Aconiti Radix lateralis *(fù zǐ)*	● Ⓣ	warms and stimulates the fire at the gate of vitality so that it reaches the extremities
Deputy 臣	Zingiberis Rhizoma *(gān jiāng)*	●	warms the middle burner and eliminates cold, strengthens the Spleen's transforming and transporting functions
Assistant 佐	Glycyrrhizae Radix praeparata *(zhì gān cǎo)*	●	augments the qi, strengthens the Spleen, reduces the toxicity of the chief ingredient, moderates the drying properties of the other herbs

四神丸
Four-Miracle Pill
sì shén wán

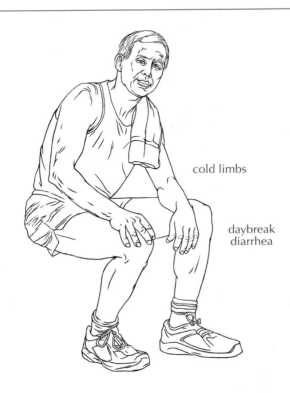

cold limbs

daybreak diarrhea

INGREDIENTS

Psoraleae Fructus (*bǔ gǔ zhī*) 12g

Evodiae Fructus (*wú zhū yú*) 3g

Myristicae Semen (*ròu dòu kòu*) 6g

Schisandrae Fructus (*wǔ wèi zǐ*).. 6g

Zingiberis Rhizoma recens (*shēng jiāng*)................................ 3g

Jujubae Fructus (*dà zǎo*).. 6 pieces

Actions: warms and tonifies the Spleen and Kidneys • binds the Intestines • stops diarrhea

Main patterns: diarrhea owing to insufficient fire at the gate of vitality • yang deficiency cold of the Spleen and Kidney

Key symptoms: daybreak diarrhea

Secondary symptoms: lack of interest in food • undigested food in stools • low back soreness • cold limbs • fatigue

• lethargy • abdominal pain that is eased by warmth

Tongue: pale body • thin and white coating

Pulse: submerged • slow • forceless

Abdomen: no specific signs

▶ CLINICAL NOTES

• This formula is specific for diarrhea due to Kidney and Spleen yang deficiency. Although it is said to typically occur at daybreak, this is not always the case. Equally important markers are watery diarrhea with undigested food, a tendency to be cold and tired, pale tongue with a white coating, and a submerged, forceless pulse.

• Can also be used to treat excessive urination or sweating (Myristicae Semen (*ròu dòu kòu*) is usually omitted) or other outcomes of deficiency cold of the Spleen and Kidney such as asthma, sweating, headache, low back pain, fever, cramps, and abdominal pain. It is not uncommon for symptoms related to this pattern to be most prominent in the early morning.

• Patients should be advised to avoid raw or cooling foods while taking this formula.

Contraindications: accumulation or stagnation in the Stomach or Intestines

▶ FORMULAS WITH SIMILAR INDICATIONS

*True Man's Decoction to Nourish the Organs (*zhēn rén yǎng zàng tāng*): Focuses on stopping unremitting diarrhea due to abandonment with persistent abdominal pain, a wan complexion, and lethargy.

Ginseng, Poria, and White Atractylodes Powder (*shēn líng bái zhú sǎn*): For diarrhea due to Spleen earth encumbered by phlegm-dampness with soft stools that may contain mucus. Symptoms typically worsen in relation to dietary irregularities or exhaustion, but cold is not a prominent sign.

Chief 君	Psoraleae Fructus *(bǔ gǔ zhī)*	● ● ●	tonifies the gate of vitality, benefits the Spleen, secures the primal yang, and stops the diarrhea
Deputy 臣	Myristicae Semen *(ròu dòu kòu)*	● ●	warms the Spleen and Kidneys and binds up the Intestines
Assistants 佐	Evodiae Fructus *(wú zhū yú)*	● ●	disperses cold in the middle burner
	Schisandrae Fructus *(wǔ wèi zǐ)*	● ●	strengthens the deputy's ability to bind up the Intestines
Envoys 使	Zingiberis Rhizoma recens *(shēng jiāng)*	●	disperses cold and activates the metabolism of water
	Jujubae Fructus *(dà zǎo)*	●	nourishes the Spleen and Stomach

四物湯（四物汤）
Four-Substance Decoction
sì wù tāng

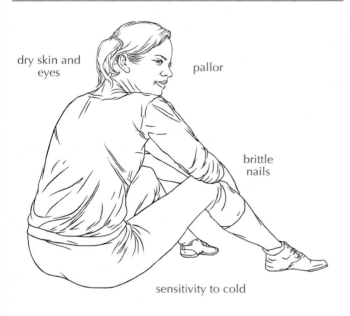

dry skin and eyes

pallor

brittle nails

sensitivity to cold

INGREDIENTS

Rehmanniae Radix praeparata (*shú dì huáng*) 12g
Paeoniae Radix alba (*bái sháo*).. 9-12g
Angelicae sinensis Radix (*dāng guī*) 9g
Chuanxiong Rhizoma (*chuān xiōng*) 6-9g

Actions: tonifies the blood • regulates the Liver

Main pattern: generalized blood deficiency and stagnation

Key symptoms: pallor • sensitivity to cold • brittle nails • dry skin and eyes

Secondary symptoms: dizziness • blurred vision • heavy head • generalized muscle tension • insomnia • palpitations • numbness • irregular menstruation with scanty flow or amenorrhea • menorrhagia • hard abdominal masses with recurrent pain • restless fetus disorder

Tongue: pale

Pulse: thin and wiry • thin and choppy

Abdomen: periumbilical and lower abdominal pain on deep pressure • periumbilical pulsations

► CLINICAL NOTES

• This is the primary formula for Liver blood deficiency. It thus addresses a wide variety of gynecological disorders. A small number of core modifications are sufficient to treat most conditions:

→ For heavy bleeding, reduce the dosage of Chuanxiong Rhizoma (*chuān xiōng*) and add Artemisiae argyi Folium (*ài yè*) and Asini Corii Colla (*ē jiāo*); or add qi tonics such as Ginseng Radix (*rén shēn*) or Astragali Radix (*huáng qí*).

→ For painful menstruation, add Linderae Radix (*wū yào*), Cyperi Rhizoma (*xiāng fù*), and Citri reticulatae viride Pericarpium (*qīng pí*) if qi stagnation is evident; or Corydalis Rhizoma (*yán hú suǒ*), Persicae Semen (*táo rén*), and Carthami Flos (*hóng huā*) if blood stasis is pronounced.

→ For pronounced heat prior to menstruation, add herbs that clear and drain heat such as Moutan Cortex (*mǔ dān pí*), Lycii Cortex (*dì gǔ pí*), or Phellodendri Cortex (*huáng bǎi*).

Contraindications: acute or severe blood loss • dampness with abdominal fullness, poor appetite, and loose stools

► FORMULAS WITH SIMILAR INDICATIONS

Restore the Spleen Decoction (*guī pí tāng*): For blood deficiency patterns with more pronounced deficiencies of Heart blood and Spleen qi.

———————————————————————— COMPOSITION ————————————————————————

Chief
君   Rehmanniae Radix praeparata   ●   strongly tonifies the Liver and Kidneys
           (shú dì huáng)
....

Deputies
臣   Paeoniae Radix alba (bái sháo)   ● ●   tonifies the blood and preserves the yin

           Angelicae sinensis Radix   ● ●   tonifies and invigorates the blood
           (dāng guī)
....
Assistant
佐   Chuanxiong Rhizoma   ●   invigorates the blood and promotes the movement of qi
           (chuān xiōng)

酸棗仁湯（酸枣仁汤）
Sour Jujube Decoction
suān zǎo rén tāng

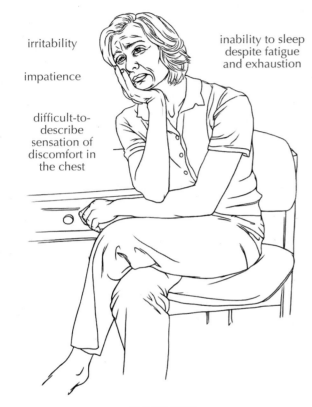

irritability

impatience

difficult-to-describe sensation of discomfort in the chest

inability to sleep despite fatigue and exhaustion

INGREDIENTS

Ziziphi spinosae Semen (*suān zǎo rén*)	12-18g
Poria (*fú líng*)	6g
Anemarrhenae Rhizoma (*zhī mǔ*)	6g
Chuanxiong Rhizoma (*chuān xiōng*)	6g
Glycyrrhizae Radix (*gān cǎo*)	3g

Actions: nourishes the blood • calms the spirit • clears heat • eliminates irritability

Main patterns: deficiency overwork (虛勞 *xū láo*) • deficiency irritability

Key symptoms: inability to sleep despite fatigue and exhaustion • irritability • impatience • difficult to describe sensation of discomfort in the chest

Secondary symptoms: palpitations • anxiety • hot flushes • night sweats • dizziness • vertigo • dry throat and mouth

Tongue: dry body • red tip • scanty coating

Pulse: thin • rapid • forceless

Abdomen: weak abdominal wall • palpable periumbilical pulsations

► CLINICAL NOTES

- This is an important formula for insomnia. Typically, patients will find it difficult to sleep even when they are exhausted. They may wake with night sweats; they are mentally frustrated but not excessively restless physically. The root cause is Liver constraint arising from deficiency and fire from constraint harassing the Heart. For this reason, the formula can also be used to treat menopausal hot flushes, anxiety, mild pain, and even hypersomnia.

- The original indication of this formula is a condition known as deficiency irritability arising from the presence of formless heat in the chest. The patient will often experience this as an ill-defined discomfort in the region of the chest, while the practitioner will not find signs of phlegm-fire, dampness, blood stasis, or any other fullness that could account for this discomfort.

- Additions should be made based on the precise causes of constraint: for deficiency of fluids, add Rehmanniae Radix (*shēng dì huáng*), Scrophulariae Radix (*xuán shēn*), and Ophiopogonis Radix (*mài mén dōng*); for blood stasis, add Paeoniae Radix rubra (*chì sháo*), Angelicae sinensis Radix (*dāng guī*), and Moutan Cortex (*mǔ dān pí*); for dampness and phlegm, add Pinelliae Rhizoma praeparatum (*zhì bàn xià*), Polygalae Radix (*yuǎn zhì*), and Acori tatarinowii Rhizoma (*shí chāng pǔ*); and for fire, add Gypsum fibrosum (*shí gāo*), Gardeniae Fructus (*zhī zǐ*), and Sojae Semen praeparatum (*dàn dòu chǐ*).

- For best effects, many modern physicians increase the dosage of the main herb significantly. If fire from constraint is predominant, it is best to use untreated Ziziphi spinosae Semen (*suān zǎo rén*). If deficiency is predominant, use the dry-fried herb.

Contraindications: loose stools

▶ FORMULAS WITH SIMILAR INDICATIONS

*Gardenia and Prepared Soybean Decoction (*zhī zǐ chǐ tāng*): For deficiency irritability from fire without form in the epigastrium and diaphragm areas harassing the Heart. This is characterized by great difficulty falling asleep.

*Coptis and Ass-Hide Gelatin Decoction (*huáng lián ē jiāo tāng*): For Heart fire in the context of blood deficiency. This pattern presents with severe dryness and severe restlessness and agitation.

Licorice, Wheat, and Jujube Decoction (*gān mài dà zǎo tāng*): For deficiency of nutritive qi unable to control the yang. This pattern is characterized by loss of control over the emotions.

COMPOSITION

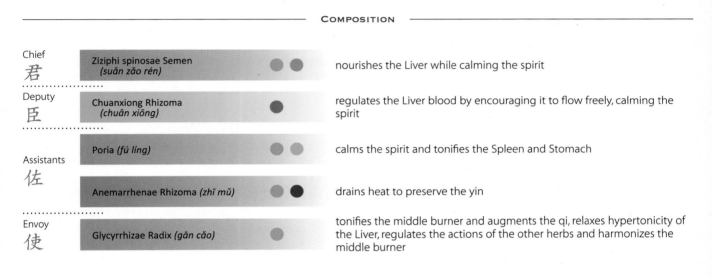

Chief 君	Ziziphi spinosae Semen (*suān zǎo rén*)	nourishes the Liver while calming the spirit
Deputy 臣	Chuanxiong Rhizoma (*chuān xiōng*)	regulates the Liver blood by encouraging it to flow freely, calming the spirit
Assistants 佐	Poria (*fú líng*)	calms the spirit and tonifies the Spleen and Stomach
	Anemarrhenae Rhizoma (*zhī mǔ*)	drains heat to preserve the yin
Envoy 使	Glycyrrhizae Radix (*gān cǎo*)	tonifies the middle burner and augments the qi, relaxes hypertonicity of the Liver, regulates the actions of the other herbs and harmonizes the middle burner

桃核承氣湯（桃核承气汤）
Peach Pit Decoction to Order the Qi
táo hé chéng qì tāng

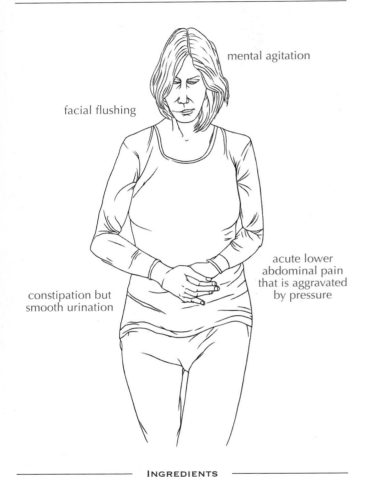

mental agitation

facial flushing

acute lower abdominal pain that is aggravated by pressure

constipation but smooth urination

INGREDIENTS

Persicae Semen (*táo rén*).. 12g
Rhei Radix et Rhizoma (*dà huáng*).................................. 12g
Cinnamomi Ramulus (*guì zhī*)... 6g
Natrii Sulfas (*máng xiāo*) .... [add to strained decoction] 6g
Glycyrrhizae Radix praeparata (*zhì gān cǎo*) 6g

Actions: drains heat • breaks up blood stasis

Main pattern: blood buildup (蓄血 *xù xuè*) in the lower burner caused by the accumulation of blood stasis and heat

Key symptoms: acute lower abdominal pain that is aggravated by pressure • constipation but smooth urination • facial flushing • mental agitation

Secondary symptoms: headache • dizziness • tinnitus • nighttime fevers • irritability • restlessness • insomnia • thirst • delirious speech • dysmenorrhea • amenorrhea • dark or black stools

Tongue: dry body • white coating • visible and enlarged sublingual veins

Pulse: submerged and full • choppy

Abdomen: generally strong abdomen • hardness and distention in the lower abdomen with resistance to pressure • hypertonicity of rectus abdominis muscle

▶ CLINICAL NOTES

• This is the main formula for acute blood stasis with excess heat in the lower abdomen. Key markers are acute lower abdominal pain, an abdomen that is firm but elastic without palpable masses, and pain upon the application of pressure in the lower abdomen. This is typically accompanied by heat excess surging upward as reflected in such symptoms as facial flushing, dizziness, headaches, tinnitus, palpitations, delirious speech, restlessness, or a burning sensation in the skin. The extremities may be cold or even numb, but the patient will have an aversion to warmth.

• This formula is indicated for patients with a strong constitution but has a very wide range of application in clinical practice, from the treatment of acute trauma to gynecological disorders, cardiovascular problems, neurological disorders, mental-emotional problems, or bleeding with dark purple blood.

• This formula is generally indicated for acute problems. If there are exterior symptoms, the pathogen should be released from the exterior before using this formula. It is considered a good sign if the patient's stools become dark or loose after taking this formula.

Contraindications: pregnancy • deficiency patterns • chronic diarrhea

► FORMULAS WITH SIMILAR INDICATIONS

Cinnamon Twig and Poria Pill (*guì zhī fú líng wán*): For blood stasis in the lower abdomen without constipation or excess heat.

Tangkuei and Peony Powder (*dāng guī sháo yào sǎn*): For blood stasis in the lower abdomen with blood deficiency, water buildup, and Spleen-Liver disharmony.

─────────────────────── COMPOSITION ───────────────────────

Chiefs 君	Persicae Semen (*táo rén*)		breaks up and eliminates blood stasis
	Rhei Radix et Rhizoma (*dà huáng*)		attacks and purges accumulations and cleanses pathogenic heat
Deputy 臣	Cinnamomi Ramulus (*guì zhī*)		warms the sinews, unblocks the vessels, and dispels retained blood from the lower burner
Assistant 佐	Natrii Sulfas (*máng xiāo*)		softens areas of hardness and dispels accumulation
Assis/Env 佐/使	Glycyrrhizae Radix praeparata (*zhì gān cǎo*)		protects the Stomach and calms the middle burner by moderating the harsh properties of the other ingredients in the formula

天麻鈎藤飲 （天麻钩藤饮）
Gastrodia and Uncaria Drink
tiān má gōu téng yǐn

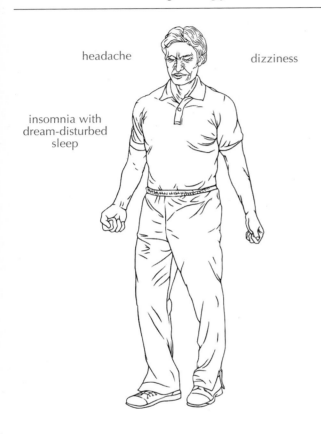

headache

dizziness

insomnia with
dream-disturbed
sleep

INGREDIENTS

Gastrodiae Rhizoma (*tiān má*)...9g
Uncariae Ramulus cum Uncis (*gōu téng*) 12-15g
Haliotidis Concha (*shí jué míng*).................. [cook first] 18-24g
Gardeniae Fructus (*zhī zǐ*)..9g
Scutellariae Radix (*huáng qín*) 9g
Leonuri Herba (*yì mǔ cǎo*)... 9-12g
Cyathulae Radix (*chuān niú xī*)..12g
Eucommiae Cortex (*dù zhòng*)... 9-12g
Taxilli Herba (*sāng jì shēng*)... 9-24g
Polygoni multiflori Caulis (*yè jiāo téng*) 9-30g
Poriae Sclerotium pararadicis (*fú shén*)......................... 9-15g

Actions: calms the Liver • extinguishes wind • clears heat • invigorates the blood • tonifies the Liver and Kidneys

Main pattern: ascendant Liver yang leading to internal stirring of Liver wind with signs of blood stasis and water accumulation

Key symptoms: headache • dizziness • insomnia with dream-disturbed sleep

Secondary symptoms: vertigo • tinnitus • blurred vision • sensation of heat rushing to the head • numbness • twitching and spasms in the extremities • hemiplegia

Tongue: red body • thin, yellow coating

Pulse: wiry • rapid

Abdomen: palpable muscle tension extending from the left ribcage toward the umbilicus

▶ CLINICAL NOTES

• This formula focuses on treating the branches in patterns characterized by hyperactivity of Liver yang against a background of yin deficiency. It was specifically designed to treat hypertension, utilizing pharmacological knowledge about the effect of individual constituents. It is used today for similar disorders such as menopausal hot flushes, migraine headaches, or Meniere's disease. Once the initial symptoms have subsided, herbs such as Paeoniae Radix alba (*bái sháo*), Angelicae sinensis Radix (*dāng guī*), and Rehmanniae Radix (*shēng dì huáng*) can be added to address the root.

• For arteriosclerosis, the source text recommends the addition of Rosae rugosae Flos (*méi guī huā*) and Sargassum (*hǎi zǎo*) because both contain rutin.

Contraindications: Liver fire • damp-heat

▶ FORMULAS WITH SIMILAR INDICATIONS

Antelope Horn and Uncaria Decoction (*líng jiǎo gōu téng tāng*): For Liver wind caused by heat in the nutritive and blood aspects.

Sedate the Liver and Extinguish Wind Decoction (*zhèn gān xī fēng tāng*): For internal Liver wind with qi and heat surging upward in the Penetrating vessel. This formula focuses on directing yang and blood downward rather than on venting heat and extinguishing wind. It subdues the spirit with a preponderance of heavy substances, in contrast to Gastrodia and Uncaria Drink (*tiān má gōu téng yǐn*), which utilizes more spirit-quieting herbs.

COMPOSITION

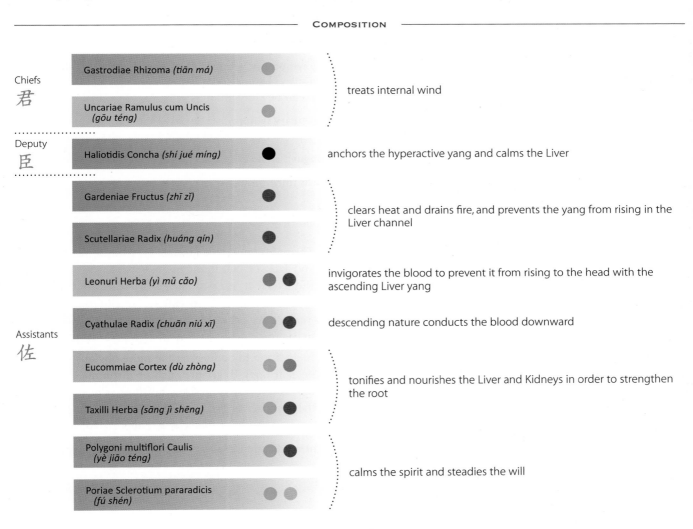

Chiefs 君

Gastrodiae Rhizoma (*tiān má*)

Uncariae Ramulus cum Uncis (*gōu téng*)

⟩ treats internal wind

Deputy 臣

Haliotidis Concha (*shí jué míng*) — anchors the hyperactive yang and calms the Liver

Assistants 佐

Gardeniae Fructus (*zhī zǐ*)

Scutellariae Radix (*huáng qín*)

⟩ clears heat and drains fire, and prevents the yang from rising in the Liver channel

Leonuri Herba (*yì mǔ cǎo*) — invigorates the blood to prevent it from rising to the head with the ascending Liver yang

Cyathulae Radix (*chuān niú xī*) — descending nature conducts the blood downward

Eucommiae Cortex (*dù zhòng*)

Taxilli Herba (*sāng jì shēng*)

⟩ tonifies and nourishes the Liver and Kidneys in order to strengthen the root

Polygoni multiflori Caulis (*yè jiāo téng*)

Poriae Sclerotium pararadicis (*fú shén*)

⟩ calms the spirit and steadies the will

天王補心丹（天王补心丹）
Emperor of Heaven's Special Pill to Tonify the Heart
tiān wáng bǔ xīn dān

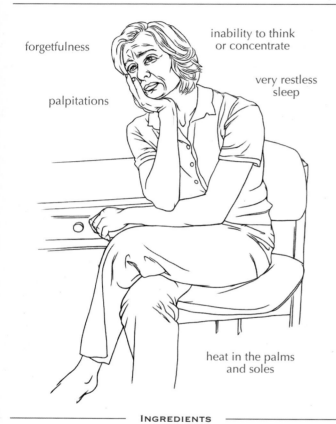

forgetfulness

inability to think or concentrate

palpitations

very restless sleep

heat in the palms and soles

INGREDIENTS

Rehmanniae Radix (*shēng dì huáng*)	12-24g
Ginseng Radix (*rén shēn*)	6-12g
Asparagi Radix (*tiān mén dōng*)	6g
Ophiopogonis Radix (*mài mén dōng*)	6g
Scrophulariae Radix (*xuán shēn*)	6-15g
Salviae miltiorrhizae Radix (*dān shēn*)	6-15g
Poria (*fú líng*)	6-15g
Polygalae Radix (*yuǎn zhì*)	6-15g
Angelicae sinensis Radix (*dāng guī*)	6g
Schisandrae Fructus (*wǔ wèi zǐ*)	6-15g
Platycladi Semen (*bǎi zǐ rén*)	6g
Ziziphi spinosae Semen (*suān zǎo rén*)	6g

Platycodi Radix (*jié gěng*)......................................3-15g

Preparation notes: Commonly taken in pill form.

Actions: enriches the yin • nourishes the blood • clears heat • calms the spirit

Main patterns: yin and blood deficiency leading to a restless state of mind • Heart and Kidneys failing to communicate

Key symptoms: irritability • palpitations • heat in the palms and soles • fatigue • very restless sleep • inability to think or concentrate • forgetfulness

Secondary symptoms: • anxiety • sores of the mouth and tongue • low-grade fever • night sweats • dry stools

Tongue: red body • scanty coating

Pulse: thin • rapid

▶ CLINICAL NOTES

- This is an important formula for treating yin deficiency and lack of communication between the Heart and Kidneys that leads to flaring of Heart fire. Symptoms such as difficulty to concentrate, forgetfulness, a thin and weak pulse, dry stools, and a dry tongue are important indicators.

- In addition to addressing the more obvious symptoms of deficiency Heart fire such as insomnia, irritability, difficulty in concentrating, hot flushes or night sweats, the formula can also be used to treat chronic or recurrent urticaria, chronic conjunctivitis, mouth sores, or infertility.

Contraindications: Spleen and Stomach deficiency patterns

▶ FORMULAS WITH SIMILAR INDICATIONS

Restore the Spleen Decoction (*guī pí tāng*): For dual deficiency of the qi and blood of the Heart and Spleen characterized by reduced appetite, loose stools, a pale tongue, and a thin, frail pulse.

Prepared Licorice Decoction (*zhì gān cǎo tāng*): For deficiency of yin-blood and qi that gives rise to upper burner symptoms such as anxiety, insomnia, palpitations, and dry mouth.

COMPOSITION

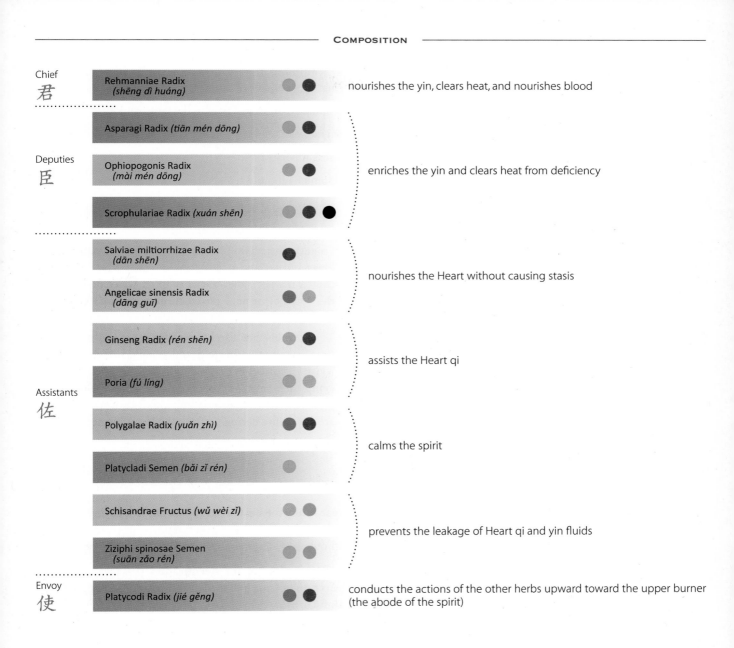

Chief
君
Rehmanniae Radix (*shēng dì huáng*) — nourishes the yin, clears heat, and nourishes blood

Deputies
臣
Asparagi Radix (*tiān mén dōng*)
Ophiopogonis Radix (*mài mén dōng*)
Scrophulariae Radix (*xuán shēn*) — enriches the yin and clears heat from deficiency

Assistants
佐
Salviae miltiorrhizae Radix (*dān shēn*)
Angelicae sinensis Radix (*dāng guī*) — nourishes the Heart without causing stasis

Ginseng Radix (*rén shēn*)
Poria (*fú líng*) — assists the Heart qi

Polygalae Radix (*yuǎn zhì*)
Platycladi Semen (*bǎi zǐ rén*) — calms the spirit

Schisandrae Fructus (*wǔ wèi zǐ*)
Ziziphi spinosae Semen (*suān zǎo rén*) — prevents the leakage of Heart qi and yin fluids

Envoy
使
Platycodi Radix (*jié gěng*) — conducts the actions of the other herbs upward toward the upper burner (the abode of the spirit)

通關丸（通关丸）
Open the Gate Pill
tōng guān wán

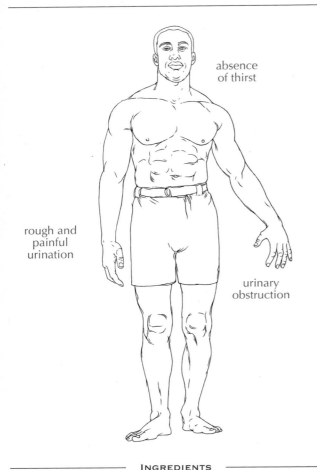

absence of thirst

rough and painful urination

urinary obstruction

---

lower burner and obstructing the qi transformation of the Bladder

Key symptoms: urinary obstruction • rough and painful urination • absence of thirst

Secondary symptoms: pain in the lower abdomen

Tongue: yellow, greasy coating

Pulse: slippery • rapid

Abdomen: rebound tenderness in the lower abdomen

▶ Clinical Notes

• Urinary obstruction here is due to heat collecting in the lower burner and obstructing qi transformation. A key clinical marker is the absence of thirst, which distinguishes this form of urinary obstruction from those caused by excess heat in the upper or middle burners.

• This formula can also be used for sores and pain in the lower extremities due to heat flowing downward into the Kidney channel or to guide yin fire downward to treat symptoms such as headache, wheezing, palpitations, paraesthesia, and chronic bulging disorders when these are due to fire flaring up from the lower burner.

Contraindications: deficiency cold patterns

▶ Formulas with Similar Indications

Great Tonify the Yin Pill (*dà bǔ yīn wán*): For flaring of yin fire due to Kidney and essence deficiency. This pattern presents without obstruction of the qi transformation in the Bladder.

Eight-Herb Powder for Rectification (*bā zhèng sǎn*): For Heart heat flowing into the lower burner causing damp-heat painful urinary dribbling.

Two-Marvel Powder (*èr miào sǎn*): For damp-heat in the lower extremities manifesting with muscle wasting or itchy discharges from the skin or vagina.

INGREDIENTS

wine-fried Phellodendri Cortex (*jiǔ chǎo huáng bǎi*) 30g
wine-fried Anemarrhenae Rhizoma (*jiǔ chǎo zhī mǔ*) 30g
Cinnamomi Cortex (*ròu guì*) 1.5g

Preparation notes: The ingredients are ground into a powder that is made into very small pills that are then taken with warm water on an empty stomach.

Actions: clears heat • enriches the yin • opens urinary obstruction • promotes urination

Main pattern: urinary obstruction due to heat collecting in the

──────────────── **COMPOSITION** ────────────────

Chief
君

wine-fried Phellodendri Cortex
(*jiǔ chǎo huáng bǎi*)

drains fire from excess affecting the Kidneys and clears lower burner damp-heat, removing the cause of urinary obstruction

Deputy
臣

wine-fried Anemarrhenae Rhizoma (*jiǔ chǎo zhī mǔ*)

directs yin fire from the Lungs and the Stomach downward and protects the yin

Assistant
佐

Cinnamomi Cortex (*ròu guì*)

anchors the yang qi by promoting the qi dynamic in the lower burner

痛瀉要方
Important Formula for Painful Diarrhea
tòng xiè yào fāng

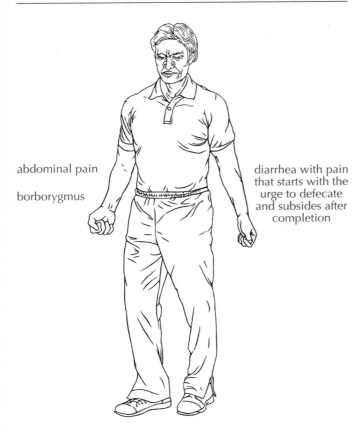

abdominal pain

borborygmus

diarrhea with pain that starts with the urge to defecate and subsides after completion

INGREDIENTS

dry-fried Atractylodis macrocephalae Rhizoma
(*chǎo bái zhú*).. 9-12g
dry-fried Paeoniae Radix alba (*chǎo bái sháo*)................. 6-24g
dry-fried Citri reticulatae Pericarpium (*chǎo chén pí*) 4.5-9g
Saposhnikoviae Radix (*fáng fēng*).................................... 3-6g

Actions: tonifies the Spleen • softens the Liver • expels dampness • stops diarrhea

Main pattern: painful diarrhea due to Spleen deficiency and an over-controlling Liver

Key symptoms: borborygmus • abdominal pain • diarrhea with pain that starts with the urge to defecate and subsides after completion

Secondary symptoms: reduced appetite • a stifling sensation or distention in the flanks • abdominal distention • fatigue • belching • flatulence

Tongue: thin and white or thin and greasy coating

Pulse: wiry and moderate or wiry and thin; or wiry on the left and moderate on the right

Abdomen: distention in flanks and around umbilicus • splashing sounds

▶ CLINICAL NOTES

• This formula can be used for diarrhea irrespective of origin and presentation as long as there are some signs of Spleen deficiency along with a wiry pulse, spasmodic abdominal pain, or other signs indicating excess Liver qi. One example is diarrhea associated with anger and irritability.

• Can be used for chronic diarrhea in the weak and elderly with the addition of Cimicifugae Rhizoma (*shēng má*) to assist the Spleen in raising the clear yang.

• Can be used in children, especially for diarrhea that is yellow and watery but unaccompanied by heat symptoms.

Contraindications: diarrhea due to food stagnation, heat, or other conditions marked by excess only

▶ FORMULAS WITH SIMILAR INDICATIONS

Ginseng, Poria, and White Atractylodes Powder (*shēn líng bái zhú săn*): For diarrhea with mucus in the stools due to Spleen deficiency and dampness, but no Liver involvement. There will be reduced appetite, weakness, a stifling sensation in the chest and epigastrium, pale tongue with white coating, and a moderate pulse.

Preserve Harmony Pill (*băo hé wán*): For diarrhea from food stagnation with abdominal pain that improves or disappears after the bowels have been evacuated. There will also be an upset stomach, aversion to food, a yellow, greasy tongue coating, and a slippery pulse.

COMPOSITION

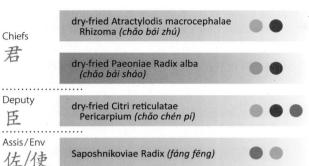

Chiefs 君	dry-fried Atractylodis macrocephalae Rhizoma *(chǎo bái zhú)*	strengthens the Spleen and dries dampness
	dry-fried Paeoniae Radix alba *(chǎo bái sháo)*	softens the overactive Liver and alleviates pain
Deputy 臣	dry-fried Citri reticulatae Pericarpium *(chǎo chén pí)*	harmonizes the functions of the middle burner and transforms dampness; also helps chief herb strengthen the Spleen and eliminate dampness
Assis/Env 佐/使	Saposhnikoviae Radix *(fáng fēng)*	enters the Liver and Spleen channels and helps relieve the overcontrol of the Spleen by the Liver, while focusing the actions of all the herbs on these two organs

托裡消毒飲（托里消毒饮）
Support the Interior and Eliminate Toxin Drink
tuō lǐ xiāo dú yǐn

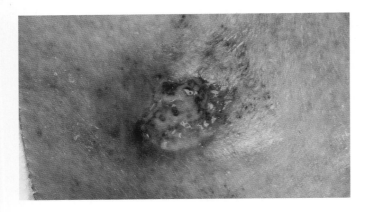

— INGREDIENTS —

Ginseng Radix (*rén shēn*)...3-5g
Chuanxiong Rhizoma (*chuān xiōng*)..............................3-4g
Paeoniae Radix alba (*bái sháo*)...................................3-6g
Astragali Radix (*huáng qí*)...5-9g
Angelicae dahuricae Radix (*bái zhǐ*)...........................2-4g
Gleditsiae Spina (*zào jiǎo cì*).......................................3-9g
Angelicae sinensis Radix (*dāng guī*)............................3-5g
Atractylodis macrocephalae Rhizoma (*bái zhú*)..........3-9g
Poria (*fú líng*)...3-9g
Lonicerae Flos (*jīn yín huā*).......................................5-15g
Glycyrrhizae Radix (*gān cǎo*)..2g
Platycodi Radix (*jié gěng*)...2-4g

Actions: tonifies the qi and blood • expels pus from the interior • draws out toxicity

Main pattern: toxic sores in those with deficient constitutions

Key symptoms: sores that do not suppurate or only slowly leak pus • sores that are slow to heal

Secondary symptoms: fever • lassitude • lusterless complexion

Tongue: pale body • thin or moderate coating

Pulse: rapid with no strength

Abdomen: no specific signs

▶ **CLINICAL NOTES**

- This formula treats qi deficient patients who present with toxic swellings in one of two states. In the first, the swelling is firm and painful, yet after several days, it fails to dissipate or progress to the stage where the flesh putrefies and transforms into pus. In the second, the sore has already suppurated but instead of closing properly, it continues to leak thin, watery pus. Both of these situations reveal a body that is too weak to properly heal the lesion.

- In modern times this formula is frequently applied to swollen and inflamed lymph nodes, boils, carbuncles, abscesses, and inflamed cysts. It is often appropriate to simultaneously treat these lesions topically with Golden-Yellow Plaster (*jīn huáng gāo*).

Contraindications: during pregnancy

▶ **FORMULAS WITH SIMILAR INDICATIONS**

Immortals' Formula for Sustaining Life (*xiān fāng huó mìng yǐn*): Treats initial stage lesions using herbs to disperse accumulations, invigorate the blood, push out pus, and resolve heat toxin. Support the Interior and Eliminate Toxin Drink (*tuō lǐ xiāo dú yǐn*) does the same, but by adding a significant number of tonifying herbs, it shifts the emphasis to treatment of deficient patients and sores that are either in their initial or final stages.

COMPOSITION

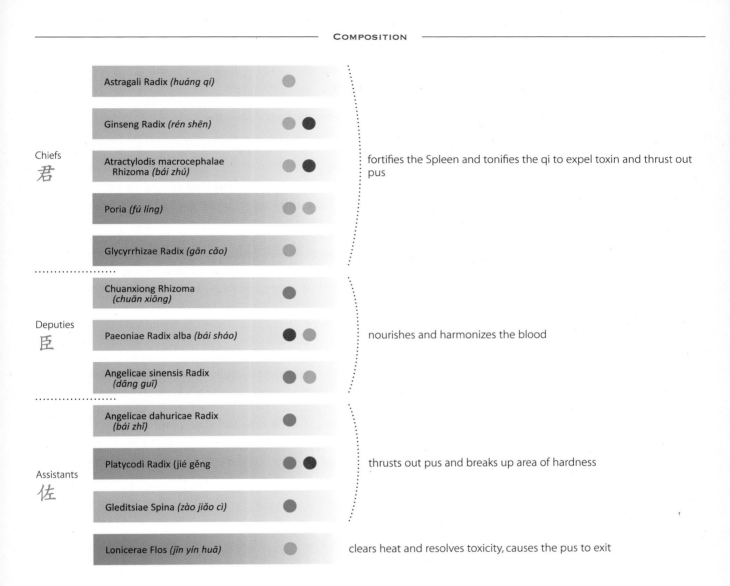

Chiefs
君

Astragali Radix (huáng qí)

Ginseng Radix (rén shēn)

Atractylodis macrocephalae Rhizoma (bái zhú)

Poria (fú líng)

Glycyrrhizae Radix (gān cǎo)

fortifies the Spleen and tonifies the qi to expel toxin and thrust out pus

Deputies
臣

Chuanxiong Rhizoma (chuān xiōng)

Paeoniae Radix alba (bái sháo)

Angelicae sinensis Radix (dāng guī)

nourishes and harmonizes the blood

Assistants
佐

Angelicae dahuricae Radix (bái zhǐ)

Platycodi Radix (jié gěng

Gleditsiae Spina (zào jiǎo cì)

thrusts out pus and breaks up area of hardness

Lonicerae Flos (jīn yín huā)

clears heat and resolves toxicity, causes the pus to exit

葦莖湯 (苇茎汤)
Reed Decoction
wěi jīng tāng

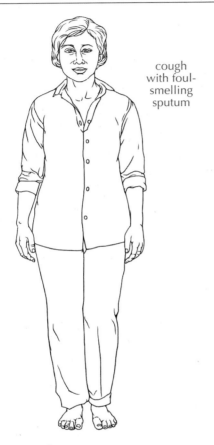

cough with foul-smelling sputum

Secondary symptoms: mild chest pain • slight fever • dry, scaly skin

Tongue: red body • yellow, greasy coating

Pulse: slippery • rapid

Abdomen: no specific signs

▶ CLINICAL NOTES

- While originally designed for treating Lung abscess, this formula is frequently applied to the tail end of heat disorders where the heat is not completely cleared and the patient presents with cough and copious phlegm. For this purpose, omit Persicae Semen (*táo rén*) and add such herbs as Houttuyniae Herba (*yú xīng cǎo*) and Trichosanthis Pericarpium (*guā lóu pí*) to increase the formula's ability to expel phlegm and resolve clumped heat.

- In the dermatology clinic this formula is modified to treat pustular skin lesions such as folliculitis, acne, and pustular psoriasis when the pattern presents with signs of Lung heat and a greasy, yellow tongue coating. Herbs such as Moutan Cortex (*mǔ dān pí*), Lonicerae Flos (*jīn yín huā*), Imperatae Rhizoma (*bái máo gēn*), and Forsythiae Fructus (*lián qiào*) may be added as appropriate.

Contraindications: during pregnancy

INGREDIENTS

Phragmititis Caulis (*wěi jīng*) 60g
Coicis Semen (*yì yǐ rén*) 30g
Benincasae Semen (*dōng guā zǐ*) 24g
Persicae Semen (*táo rén*) 9g

Actions: clears heat from the Lungs • transforms phlegm • drives out blood stasis • discharges pus

Main pattern: Lung abscess from wind-heat toxin, phlegm, and blood stasis

Key symptoms: cough with foul-smelling sputum • blood-streaked sputum

───────────────────── COMPOSITION ─────────────────────

Chief 君	Phragmititis Caulis *(wěi jīng)*	●	clears heat from the Lungs
Deputies 臣	Coicis Semen *(yì yǐ rén)*	● ●	clears heat from the Lungs, disperses pus from the upper parts of the body, and leaches out dampness
	Benincasae Semen *(dōng guā zǐ)*	●	clears and transforms phlegm-heat, resolves dampness, and eliminates pus
Assistant 佐	Persicae Semen *(táo rén)*	● ●	invigorates the blood and eliminates blood stasis, reduces clumping and breaks up the abscess

溫膽湯（温胆汤）
Warm Gallbladder Decoction
wēn dǎn tāng

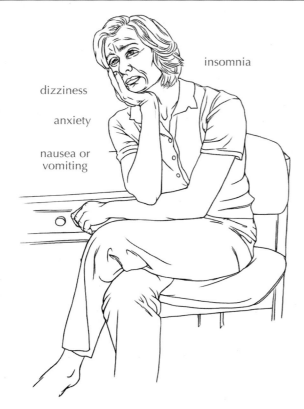

dizziness

insomnia

anxiety

nausea or vomiting

INGREDIENTS

Bambusae Caulis in taeniam (*zhú rú*) 6g

Aurantii Fructus immaturus (*zhǐ shí*) 6g

Pinelliae Rhizoma praeparatum (*zhì bàn xià*) 6g

Citri reticulatae Pericarpium (*chén pí*) 9-15g

Poria (*fú líng*) 4.5g

Glycyrrhizae Radix praeparata (*zhì gān cǎo*) 3g

Zingiberis Rhizoma recens (*shēng jiāng*) 3-9g

Jujubae Fructus (*dà zǎo*) .... 1 piece

Actions: regulates the qi • transforms phlegm • clears the Gallbladder • harmonizes the Stomach

Main pattern: disharmony between the Stomach and Gallbladder with phlegm-heat obstructing the qi dynamic

Key symptoms: nausea or vomiting • insomnia or dream-disturbed sleep with strange or unusual dreams • palpitations • dizziness • anxiety

Secondary symptoms: timid and being easily startled • indeterminate gnawing hunger • seizures accompanied by copious sputum • focal distention of the chest • bitter taste • slight thirst

Tongue: white, greasy coating

Pulse: rapid and slippery • rapid and wiry

Abdomen: splashing sounds in upper abdomen • focal distention in epigastric region • pulsations in the umbilical region

► CLINICAL NOTES

• This is the major formula for treating phlegm constraint in the middle burner and diaphragm that results in heat in the Gallbladder, Stomach, and Triple Burner. This can manifest in many different ways:

→ When wind-phlegm ascends it obstructs the orifices of the Heart and leads to insomnia, timidity, feelings of apprehension, unfounded fears, and hypersensitivity to noise, sounds, and smells. In severe cases this can present as schizophrenia, mania, or depression. Herbs such as Acori tatarinowii Rhizoma (*shí chāng pǔ*) and Arisaema cum Bile (*dǎn nán xīng*) are often included in treating this pattern.

→ Phlegm-heat in the middle burner may lead to digestive problems such as nausea and vomiting. Biomedicine may view these symptoms as functional or as involving an inflammatory response. This pattern can be seen in peptic ulcers, cholecystitis, or gallstones. For gallbladder disorders, Bupleuri Radix (*chái hú*), Curcumae Radix (*yù jīn*), and Lysimachiae Herba (*jīn qián cǎo*) are often added, and for gastric disorders, Left Metal Pill (*zuǒ jīn wán*).

→ To treat constraint-induced rebellious qi that carries phlegm upward and leads to dizziness, nausea, tinnitus, or seizures, it is often appropriate to add such substances as Gastrodiae Rhizoma (*tiān má*), Scutellariae Radix (*huáng qín*), Inulae Flos (*xuán fù huā*), and Haematitum (*dài zhě shí*).

• This formula can also be used for damp-warmth disorders at the qi level manifesting with alternating chills and fever, focal distention of the chest and flanks, distention of the abdomen, nausea, dizziness, irritability, a wiry pulse, and a greasy, yellow tongue coating.

→ For severe heat, add Coptidis Rhizoma (*huáng lián*) or Scutellariae Radix (*huáng qín*).

→ For qi constraint with palpitations and anxiety, add Cassiae Semen (*jué míng zǐ*) and Zingiberis Rhizomatis Succus (*jiāng zhī*).

Contraindications: should not be used without modification when the heat or constraint aspects of this condition are intense, as its focus is on treating phlegm

▶ FORMULAS WITH SIMILAR INDICATIONS

Lophatherum and Gypsum Decoction (*zhú yè shí gāo tāng*):

For relatively mild constraint of the qi dynamic in the chest and epigastrium due to heat in the qi aspect that has damaged the fluids and qi and produced phlegm. This may manifest with insomnia, irritability, dry mouth, thirst, a deep-red tongue with scanty coating, and a deficient, rapid pulse.

*Gardenia and Prepared Soybean Decoction (*zhī zǐ chǐ tāng*): For constraint due to heat without phlegm or deficiency leading to insomnia with tossing and turning, a stifling sensation in the chest with a soft epigastrium, and hunger with no desire to eat. There is a slightly yellow tongue coating and a pulse that is slightly rapid or strong and floating at the distal position.

*Cinnamon Twig Decoction plus Dragon Bone and Oyster Shell (*guì zhī jiā lóng gǔ mǔ lì tāng*): For timidity, excess dreaming, and insomnia due to dual deficiency of yin and yang with cold in the lower burner.

COMPOSITION

Chief 君	Pinelliae Rhizoma praeparatum (*zhì bàn xià*)	●	opens qi constraint, directs rebellious qi downward, dries dampness, transforms phlegm, and regulates the Stomach qi
Deputy 臣	Bambusae Caulis in taeniam (*zhú rú*)	●	enters the Stomach to expel heat and stop nausea, and the Gallbladder to calm the spirit, release constraint, and alleviate irritability
Assistants 佐	Aurantii Fructus immaturus (*zhǐ shí*)	● ●	focuses on reversing the flow of rebellious qi; treats focal distention
	Citri reticulatae Pericarpium (*chén pí*)	● ● ●	dries dampness and expels phlegm while regulating the qi and harmonizing its circulation in the Stomach
	Poria (*fú líng*)	● ●	strengthens the Spleen, leaches out dampness, harmonizes the functions of the middle burner, and calms the spirit
	Glycyrrhizae Radix praeparata (*zhì gān cǎo*)	●	
Envoys 使	Zingiberis Rhizoma recens (*shēng jiāng*)	●	harmonizes both the protective and nutritive levels and the functions of the Spleen and Stomach
	Jujubae Fructus (*dà zǎo*)	●	

溫經湯（温经汤）
Flow-Warming Decoction
wēn jīng tāng

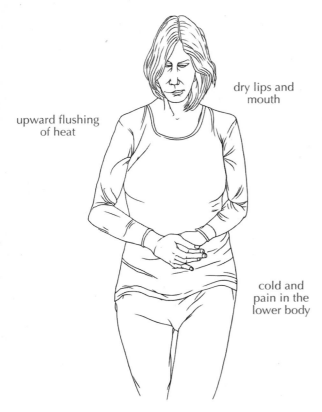

upward flushing of heat

dry lips and mouth

cold and pain in the lower body

──── INGREDIENTS ────

Evodiae Fructus (*wú zhū yú*) 9g

Cinnamomi Ramulus (*guì zhī*) 6g

Angelicae sinensis Radix (*dāng guī*) 6g

Chuanxiong Rhizoma (*chuān xiōng*) 6g

¹Paeoniae Radix (*sháo yào*) 6g

Asini Corii Colla (*ē jiāo*)

    [dissolve in the strained decoction] 6g

Ophiopogonis Radix (*mài mén dōng*) 9-12g

Moutan Cortex (*mǔ dān pí*) 6g

Ginseng Radix (*rén shēn*) 6g

_____
1. As the primary function here is to restrain, tonify, or soften, Paeoniae Radix alba *(bái sháo)* is preferred.

Glycyrrhizae Radix (*gān cǎo*) 6g
Zingiberis Rhizoma recens (*shēng jiāng*) 6g
Pinelliae Rhizoma praeparatum (*zhì bàn xià*) 6-9g

Actions: warms the vessels • dispels cold • nourishes the blood • dispels blood stasis

Main pattern: deficiency cold of the Conception and Penetrating vessels together with blood stasis and deficiency heat

Key symptoms: cold and pain in the lower body (abdomen, lower back, lower extremities) • upward flushing of heat • dry lips and mouth

Secondary symptoms: mild, persistent uterine bleeding • irregular menstruation (either early or late) • extended or continuous menstrual flow • bleeding between periods • lower abdominal distention • diarrhea during menstruation • white vaginal discharge • tendency to miscarry • warm palms and soles • palmar erythema

Tongue: dry body • scanty coating

Pulse: thin • rough • submerged

Abdomen: pain on pressure in the lower abdomen that is often worse on the left side • hypertonicity of the rectus abdominis muscle • overall soft and weak abdomen • lower abdomen cold to the touch

▶ CLINICAL NOTES

• This formula is specific for blood stasis in the lower abdomen due to deficiency cold that disrupts the fluid dynamic. This generates dryness and causes heat from deficiency to flush upward. Manifestations of blood deficiency and internal cold include a pale complexion, aversion to cold, cold lower extremities, loose stools, increased urination, a pale, puffy tongue body, and a thin, forceless pulse. The deficiency cold in this pattern will be accompanied by signs of heat or dryness such as dry and cracked lips or mucous membranes, dry mouth, hot hands and feet, hot flushes, or feverish sensations. Finally, while there are signs of stasis in this pattern, such as abdominal fullness, pain, or muscle tension, the abdomen generally remains soft.

• Historically (and continuing to the current day), this formula has been indicated for women's disorders. However, it can also be used for men who present with a similar combination of "cold below and heat above" while suffering from disorders such as infertility, impotence, urinary incontinence, or seminal insufficiency.

Contraindications: blood stasis associated with excess patterns

▶ FORMULAS WITH SIMILAR INDICATIONS

Tangkuei and Peony Powder (*dāng guī sháo yào sǎn*): For blood stasis in the lower abdomen in the context of Liver-Spleen disharmony, blood deficiency, and water buildup with no signs of heat from deficiency or dryness.

*Ass-Hide Gelatin and Mugwort Decoction (*jiāo ài tāng*): For deficiency cold in the lower abdomen without deficiency heat and dryness.

COMPOSITION

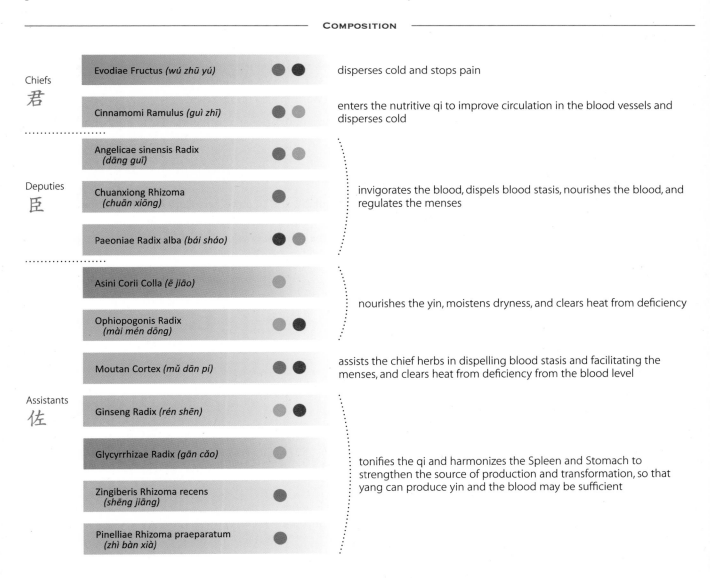

Chiefs 君	Evodiae Fructus (*wú zhū yú*)	disperses cold and stops pain
	Cinnamomi Ramulus (*guì zhī*)	enters the nutritive qi to improve circulation in the blood vessels and disperses cold
Deputies 臣	Angelicae sinensis Radix (*dāng guī*)	invigorates the blood, dispels blood stasis, nourishes the blood, and regulates the menses
	Chuanxiong Rhizoma (*chuān xiōng*)	
	Paeoniae Radix alba (*bái sháo*)	
Assistants 佐	Asini Corii Colla (*ē jiāo*)	nourishes the yin, moistens dryness, and clears heat from deficiency
	Ophiopogonis Radix (*mài mén dōng*)	
	Moutan Cortex (*mǔ dān pí*)	assists the chief herbs in dispelling blood stasis and facilitating the menses, and clears heat from deficiency from the blood level
	Ginseng Radix (*rén shēn*)	tonifies the qi and harmonizes the Spleen and Stomach to strengthen the source of production and transformation, so that yang can produce yin and the blood may be sufficient
	Glycyrrhizae Radix (*gān cǎo*)	
	Zingiberis Rhizoma recens (*shēng jiāng*)	
	Pinelliae Rhizoma praeparatum (*zhì bàn xià*)	

溫脾湯 （温脾汤）
Warm the Spleen Decoction
wēn pí tāng

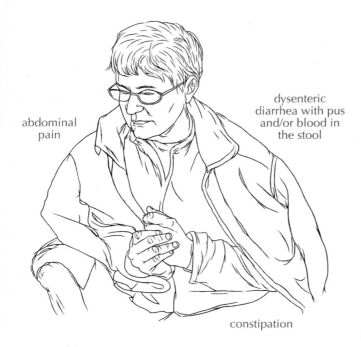

abdominal pain

dysenteric diarrhea with pus and/or blood in the stool

constipation

INGREDIENTS

Rhei Radix et Rhizoma (*dà huáng*)............ [add near end] 12g
Ginseng Radix (*rén shēn*)... 6g
Glycyrrhizae Radix (*gān cǎo*)................................. 3-6g
Zingiberis Rhizoma (*gān jiāng*).............................. 6g
¹Aconiti Radix lateralis praeparata (*zhì fù zǐ*)...................... 9g

Actions: warms and tonifies the Spleen yang • purges cold accumulation

Main pattern: Spleen cold from yang deficiency with accumulation impeding the Intestines

Key symptoms: constipation • dysenteric diarrhea with pus and/or blood in the stool • abdominal pain

Secondary symptoms: cold extremities

---

1. This herb can be difficult to obtain because of legal issues. Cinnamomi Cortex (*ròu guì*) may be substituted.

Tongue: white coating

Pulse: submerged • wiry

Abdomen: pain and distention that improves with warmth and pressure

► CLINICAL NOTES

• This formula treats long-term internal cold accumulation with residual damp-heat or heat from constraint.

• Focuses mainly on treating deficiency and only secondarily on draining excess.

• Although patients may experience a sensation of fullness in the lower abdomen, pressure relieves this sensation. Warmth also brings relief.

Contraindications: constipation due to interior heat with clumping and damage to the body fluids

► FORMULAS WITH SIMILAR INDICATIONS

Rhubarb and Aconite Accessory Root Decoction (*dà huáng fù zǐ tāng*): For cold excess accumulating below the flanks or in the abdomen with pain that increases on palpation.

COMPOSITION

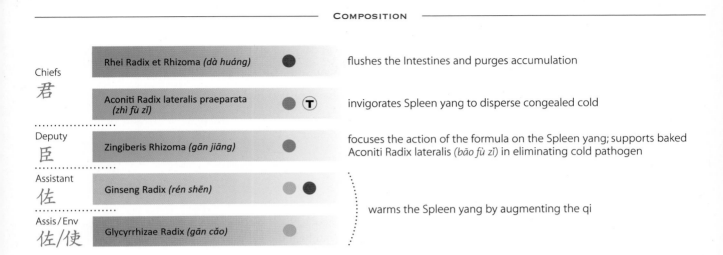

Chiefs
君

Rhei Radix et Rhizoma *(dà huáng)* — flushes the Intestines and purges accumulation

Aconiti Radix lateralis praeparata *(zhì fù zǐ)* — invigorates Spleen yang to disperse congealed cold

Deputy
臣

Zingiberis Rhizoma *(gān jiāng)* — focuses the action of the formula on the Spleen yang; supports baked Aconiti Radix lateralis *(bāo fù zǐ)* in eliminating cold pathogen

Assistant
佐

Ginseng Radix *(rén shēn)*

Assis / Env
佐/使

Glycyrrhizae Radix *(gān cǎo)* — warms the Spleen yang by augmenting the qi

五淋散
Powder for Five Types of Painful Urinary Dribbling
wǔ lín sǎn

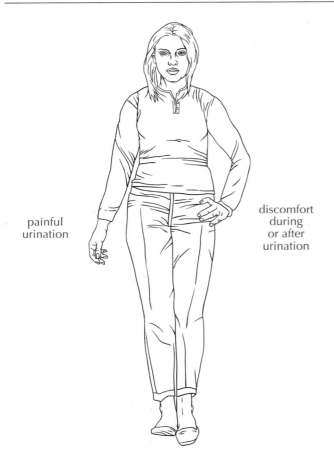

painful urination

discomfort during or after urination

Key symptoms: rough, painful urination • discomfort during or after urination

Secondary symptoms: acute lower abdominal pain

Tongue: thin coating that is either white or yellow

Pulse: slippery • rapid

Abdomen: discomfort and pain on pressure in lower abdomen

▶ CLINICAL NOTES

• This formula was originally designed for treating the acute phase of bloody urinary dribbling disorders. It can be modified to treat other manifestations of urinary dribbling patterns, specifically those from heat or those manifesting with stones. Once the acute symptoms have been relieved, switch to a formula addressing the underlying disharmony.

Contraindications: deficiency cold patterns

▶ FORMULAS WITH SIMILAR INDICATIONS

Eight-Herb Powder for Rectification (*bā zhèng sǎn*): For heat-type painful urinary dribbling disorder associated with a more pronounced damp-heat manifestation as well as signs of Heart channel heat.

INGREDIENTS

Poria rubra (*chì fú líng*)... 12-18g
Angelicae sinensis Radix (*dāng guī*) 9-15g
Glycyrrhizae Radix (*gān cǎo*)... 3-6g
Paeoniae Radix rubra (*chì sháo*) 9-18g
Gardeniae Fructus (*zhī zǐ*)... 6-15g

Actions: clears heat • cools the blood • promotes urination • unblocks painful urinary dribbling

Main pattern: damp-heat bloody painful urinary dribbling

COMPOSITION

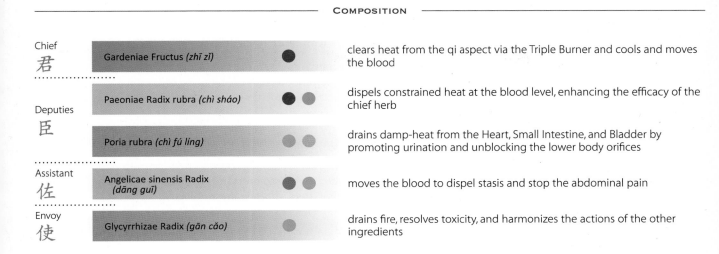

Chief
君

Gardeniae Fructus *(zhī zǐ)* — clears heat from the qi aspect via the Triple Burner and cools and moves the blood

Deputies
臣

Paeoniae Radix rubra *(chì sháo)* — dispels constrained heat at the blood level, enhancing the efficacy of the chief herb

Poria rubra *(chì fú líng)* — drains damp-heat from the Heart, Small Intestine, and Bladder by promoting urination and unblocking the lower body orifices

Assistant
佐

Angelicae sinensis Radix *(dāng guī)* — moves the blood to dispel stasis and stop the abdominal pain

Envoy
使

Glycyrrhizae Radix *(gān cǎo)* — drains fire, resolves toxicity, and harmonizes the actions of the other ingredients

五苓散
Five-Ingredient Powder with Poria
wǔ líng sǎn

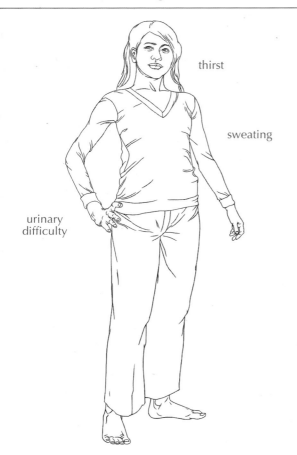

thirst

sweating

urinary difficulty

INGREDIENTS

Alismatis Rhizoma (*zé xiè*) 15g
Poria (*fú líng*) 9g
Polyporus (*zhū líng*) 9g
Atractylodis macrocephalae Rhizoma (*bái zhú*) 9g
Cinnamomi Ramulus (*guì zhī*) 6g

Actions: promotes urination • drains dampness • strengthens the Spleen • warms the yang • promotes the transforming functions of qi • unblocks the qi dynamic

Main patterns: water buildup as part of a greater yang or terminal yin warp disorder • Spleen deficiency with internal accumulation of water and dampness that overflows into the muscles and skin • thin mucus in the lower burner

Key symptoms: thirst • urinary difficulty • sweating

Secondary symptoms: headache • edema • nausea • vomiting • vertigo • generalized sensation of heaviness • diarrhea • shortness of breath • coughing

Tongue: wet, swollen body • tooth-marked

Pulse: floating • large

Abdomen: splashing sounds in epigastrium or upper abdomen • discomfort in epigastrium • throbbing pulsations just below the umbilicus

▶ CLINICAL NOTES

• This is one of the main formulas for treating dysfunction of the water metabolism. A key clinical marker is the presence of thirst or fever in combination with water excess. The excess may be in the exterior (causing headache or a generalized sensation of heaviness) as well as in any of the three burners. In the upper burner it causes coughing and shortness of breath as well as insomnia; in the middle burner, nausea, vomiting, and diarrhea; and in the lower burner, urinary dysfunction.

• Obstruction of the qi dynamic by water excess can also manifest with upward flushing of heat into the face and upper body or rebellious qi. This upward rebellion is usually only subjectively experienced by the patient. Water-excess obstruction of the qi dynamic can also lead to symptoms such as sensations of fullness or blockage in the chest, throat, or abdomen. In severe cases, there may be coughing and wheezing or pain, as in headache. The obstruction pattern can also be reflected in a superficial and large pulse.

• Where there is deficiency, combine with formulas that tonify and nourish the Spleen and Stomach such as Six-Gentlemen Decoction (*liù jūn zǐ tāng*). Where obstruction of the water pathway that leads to urinary difficulty is accompanied by yin deficiency, modify to protect the yin from further injury by combining with a formula like Two-Solstice Pill (*èr zhì wán*) or adding Anemarrhenae Rhizoma (*zhī mǔ*).

Contraindications: thirst due to excess heat or yin deficiency

▶ FORMULAS WITH SIMILAR INDICATIONS

White Tiger Decoction (*bái hǔ tāng*): For yang brightness excess heat patterns with thirst and a floating large pulse accompanied by increased sweating and a desire for cold drinks.

Minor Bluegreen Dragon Decoction (*xiǎo qīng lóng tāng*): For greater yang patterns characterized by cold obstructing the exterior with dampness in the interior. Here the symptoms of water excess are confined to the upper burner (Lungs) and to the exterior, and there is no thirst.

Stephania and Astragalus Decoction (*fáng jǐ huáng qí tāng*): For water and dampness accumulating in the exterior in patients with qi deficiency. This manifests as spontaneous sweating, swollen joints, and edema, with the latter two symptoms tending to occur in the lower body.

Polyporus Decoction (*zhū líng tāng*): For urinary dysfunction in yang brightness patterns that present with excess heat and damage to the yin.

Poria, Cinnamon Twig, Atractylodes, and Licorice Decoction (*líng guì zhú gān tāng*): For thin mucus accumulating in the epigastrium and flooding the Triple Burner. This presentation is similar to that for Five-Ingredient Powder with Poria (*wǔ líng sǎn*), but with more deficiency.

─────────── COMPOSITION ───────────

Role	Herb			Actions
Chief 君	Alismatis Rhizoma (*zé xiè*)	●	●	leaches out dampness, promotes urination and eliminates the heat constraint caused by water buildup or thin mucus obstructing the ascent of yang qi
Deputies 臣	Poria (*fú líng*)	●	●	leaches out dampness by promoting urination, strengthening the Spleen, and assisting the yang
	Polyporus (*zhū líng*)	●	●	eliminates dampness and promotes urination
Assistant 佐	Atractylodis macrocephalae Rhizoma (*bái zhú*)	●	●	strengthens the Spleen qi, aids in the transformation and transportation of fluids and the resolution of dampness
Assis / Env 佐/使	Cinnamomi Ramulus (*guì zhī*)	●	●	warms the fire at the gate of vitality, helps to dispel pathogenic influences from the exterior and release the exterior aspects of the greater yang-warp disorder

烏梅丸 （乌梅丸）
Mume Pill
wū méi wán

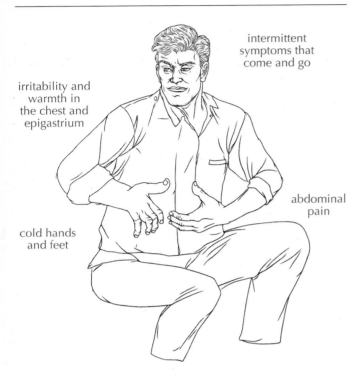

irritability and
warmth in
the chest and
epigastrium

intermittent
symptoms that
come and go

cold hands
and feet

abdominal
pain

INGREDIENTS

Mume Fructus (*wū méi*)	24-30g
Zanthoxyli Pericarpium (*huā jiāo*)	1.5-3g
[1]Asari Radix et Rhizoma (*xì xīn*)	1.5-3g
Coptidis Rhizoma (*huáng lián*)	9-12g
Phellodendri Cortex (*huáng bǎi*)	6-9g
Zingiberis Rhizoma (*gān jiāng*)	6-9g
[2]Aconiti Radix lateralis praeparata (*zhì fù zǐ*)	3-6g
Cinnamomi Ramulus (*guì zhī*)	3-6g
Ginseng Radix (*rén shēn*)	6-9g
Angelicae sinensis Radix (*dāng guī*)	3-9g

1. This herb can be difficult to obtain because of legal issues. Clematidis Radix *(wēi líng xiān)* may be substituted.

2. This ingredient can also be difficult to obtain because of legal issues. Psoraleae Fructus *(bǔ gǔ zhī)* may be substituted.

Actions: warms the yin Organs • drains heat • calms roundworms • drains the Liver • calms the Stomach

Main patterns: terminal yin disorders • chronic diarrhea or dysentery • cold below and heat above • inversion from roundworms

Key symptoms: intermittent symptoms that come and go • abdominal pain • irritability and warmth in the chest and epigastrium • cold hands and feet

Secondary symptoms: stifling sensation • vomiting after eating • unquenchable thirst • qi rushing upward toward the chest • pain and heat in the epigastrium • incessant diarrhea • discharge of small amounts of pus • abdominal pain that responds favorably to the application of pressure and heat • borborygmus • roundworms

Tongue: red body • white coating

Pulse: frail

Abdomen: tightness in the lower abdomen that responds favorably to pressure

▶ CLINICAL NOTES

• This is the main formula for terminal yin disorders. A key clinical marker is the intermittent or wind-like nature of the symptoms, which is similar to symptoms associated with lesser yang patterns, including the presence of alternating heat and cold. However, while lesser yang symptoms are due to stagnation, as reflected in a wiry excess-type pulse and fullness below the ribs on palpation, terminal yin patterns arise from yang deficiency cold in the interior, reflected in a frail pulse along with lower abdominal tightness that responds favorably to pressure or warmth. There may also be symptoms like diarrhea or pain in the lower abdomen. This will be accompanied by excess heat symptoms, typically of an intermittent or wind-like nature, such as upward gushing of qi into the chest, pain and heat in the epigastrium, stifling sensation in the chest, vomiting after eating, unquenchable thirst, hot flushes or fever. This is commonly described as cold below/heat above.

- The terminal yin Liver channel traverses the lower abdomen and groin and connects to the genitals. For this reason the formula can be used for a variety of pelvic problems in both sexes. Examples include painful periods, uterine prolapse, vaginal or penile discharge, vomiting during pregnancy, or prostatitis.
- The formula can also be used to treat headaches at the crown of the head, hypertension, and other Liver wind symptoms provided the presentation concurs with the cold below/heat above presentation that defines terminal yin patterns.
- Although this formula is traditionally indicated for the treatment of roundworms, their presence is not required for use of the formula.

Contraindications: explosive diarrhea • damp-heat dysenteric disorders

▶ FORMULAS WITH SIMILAR INDICATIONS

Regulate the Middle Pill (*lǐ zhōng wán*): For cold in the middle burner that manifests with abdominal pain, diarrhea, or cold extremities. While symptoms may be intermittent, they are aggravated by exertion and thus worsen with exercise or eating. In the pattern that this formula addresses, if there is heat, it will be 'floating yang' (i.e., false heat) and not the excess heat associated with terminal yin patterns.

Frigid Extremities Powder (*sì nì sǎn*): For cold extremities associated with lesser yang patterns. Symptoms arise from qi constraint and will often be associated with emotional stress. All symptoms are of an excess type as reflected in a wiry pulse and palpable tightness below the ribs.

True Warrior Decoction (*zhēn wǔ tāng*): For lesser yin patterns with cold in the interior and false yang floating to the exterior. The symptoms of interior cold can be similar to those of a Mume Pill (*wū méi wán*) pattern, but because this formula also drains water excess, it also addresses edema, wet tongue, or other signs of excess water. The pattern treated by True Warrior Decoction (*zhēn wǔ tāng*) may exhibit heat signs in the upper body, like headaches or a flushed face, but this heat is false (stemming from deficiency); it does not come and go, and it improves with warmth.

COMPOSITION

Chief
君

Mume Fructus *(wū méi)* ● ● — restrains, inhibits, stops, and binds up; it can thus be used for all chronic coughs, chronic dysenteric disorders, deficiency sweating, and devastated blood

Deputies
臣

Zanthoxyli Pericarpium *(huā jiāo)* ● — expels parasites and warms the Organs

Asari Herba *(xì xīn)* ●

Coptidis Rhizoma *(huáng lián)* ● — makes the worms move downward

Phellodendri Cortex *(huáng bǎi)* ●

Assistants
佐

Zingiberis Rhizoma *(gān jiāng)* ●

Aconiti Radix lateralis praeparata *(zhì fù zǐ)* ● (T) — warms the interior; very useful in dispersing internal cold

Cinnamomi Ramulus *(guì zhī)* ● ●

Ginseng Radix *(rén shēn)* ● ● — tonifies the qi and nourishes the blood to prevent further injury to the normal qi

Angelicae sinensis Radix *(dāng guī)* ● ●

[This page intentionally left blank]

五皮散
Five-Peel Powder
wǔ pí sǎn

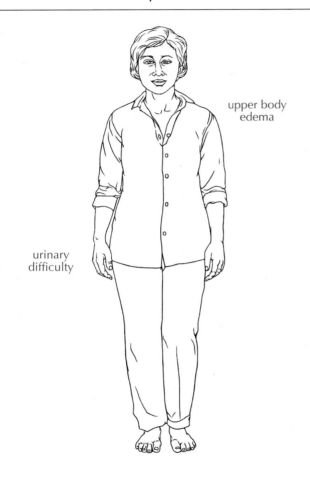

upper body edema

urinary difficulty

INGREDIENTS

Mori Cortex (*sāng bái pí*) 9-15g

Zingiberis Rhizomatis Cortex (*shēng jiāng pí*) 6-9g

Poriae Cutis (*fú líng pí*) 9-15g

Citri reticulatae Pericarpium (*chén pí*) 6-9g

Arecae Pericarpium (*dà fù pí*) 9-15g

Preparation notes: Do not cook for more than 20 minutes.

Actions: resolves dampness • reduces edema • regulates the qi • strengthens the Spleen

Main pattern: skin edema

Key symptoms: upper body edema • distention and fullness in the epigastrium and abdomen • urinary difficulty

Secondary symptoms: sensation of heaviness in the extremities and body • labored and heavy breathing • rebellious ascent of qi on walking

Tongue: white, greasy coating

Pulse: submerged • moderate

Abdomen: fullness and distention in the epigastrium and upper abdomen

▶ CLINICAL NOTES

- This formula is specific for non-pitting edema indicating excess of water-dampness in the skin. The edema typically starts or is more pronounced in the upper half of the body, though it may gradually extend to the lower extremities as well.
- Spleen-tonifying herbs should be added for cases with severe Spleen deficiency.
- This formula can be used for edema during pregnancy.
- Note that the version of this formula commercially available often includes Acanthopanacis Cortex (*wǔ jiā pí*) and Lycii Cortex (*dì gǔ pí*) instead of Citri reticulatae Pericarpium (*chén pí*) and Arecae Pericarpium (*dà fù pí*). That version focuses more on lower body edema, while the version presented here focuses more on edema of the face.

Contraindications: none noted

▶ FORMULAS WITH SIMILAR INDICATIONS

Stephania and Astragalus Decoction (*fáng jǐ huáng qí tāng*): For superficial edema from qi deficiency characterized by aversion to cold, damp skin or spontaneous sweating, and a floating pulse. This formula is often used for swelling of the joints, especially in the lower extremities.

Five-Ingredient Powder with Poria (*wǔ líng sǎn*): For water accumulation in the lower abdomen that may manifest with edema. This type of edema is usually worse in the lower extremities and accompanied by signs of water excess in the interior such as diarrhea or loose stools, vomiting of frothy saliva, dizziness, and urinary difficulty.

COMPOSITION

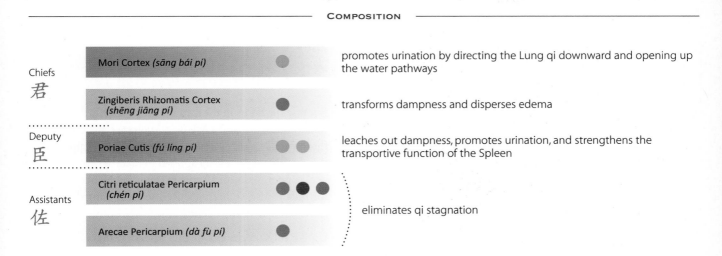

Chiefs
君

Mori Cortex *(sāng bái pí)* — promotes urination by directing the Lung qi downward and opening up the water pathways

Zingiberis Rhizomatis Cortex *(shēng jiāng pí)* — transforms dampness and disperses edema

Deputy
臣

Poriae Cutis *(fú líng pí)* — leaches out dampness, promotes urination, and strengthens the transportive function of the Spleen

Assistants
佐

Citri reticulatae Pericarpium *(chén pí)*

Arecae Pericarpium *(dà fù pí)*

eliminates qi stagnation

五味消毒飲（五味消毒饮）
Five-Ingredient Drink to Eliminate Toxin
wǔ wèi xiāo dú yǐn

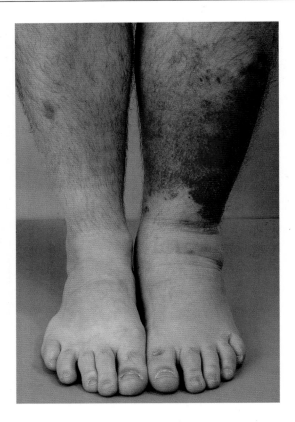

INGREDIENTS

Lonicerae Flos (*jīn yín huā*) 15-20g
Taraxaci Herba (*pú gōng yīng*)..................................... 9-15g
Violae Herba (*zǐ huā dì dīng*)....................................... 9-15g
Chrysanthemi indici Flos (*yě jú huā*).......................... 9-15g
Semiaquilegiae Radix (*tiān kuí zǐ*)............................... 9-15g

Preparation notes: Add 2-3 tablespoons of rice wine before cooking and do not cook for more than 15 minutes.

Actions: clears heat • resolves toxicity • cools the blood • reduces swelling

Main patterns: boils and carbuncles • deep-rooted and hard lesions

Key symptoms: localized erythema, swelling, heat, and pain

Secondary symptoms: fever • chills

Tongue: yellow coating

Pulse: rapid

Abdomen: no specific signs

▶ CLINICAL NOTES

• Because the herbs in the formula are primarily flowers and thus quite light, and because the intense toxic heat that this formula treats most often manifests in the upper body, this formula is primarily applied to disorders of the head, neck, upper torso, and upper extremities. Nonetheless, the formula is also sometimes used to treat damp-heat skin rashes that typically occur in the lower body.

• Unlike most formulas in this category, this one has no herbs that specifically move blood, disperse stasis, or push out pus. It primarily addresses heat toxin, and if the lesions of the heat-toxin disorder are swollen or hard, the practitioner should include herbs that move blood and qi such as Gleditsiae Spina (*zào jiǎo cì*), Paeoniae Radix rubra (*chì sháo*), Olibanum (*rǔ xiāng*), and Myrrha (*mò yào*). For disorders where the lesions are pus-forming, add herbs to push out pus such as Platycodi Radix (*jié gěng*) and Angelicae dahuricae Radix (*bái zhǐ*). If damp-heat is a factor, it is generally appropriate to add such herbs as Kochiae Fructus (*dì fū zǐ*) or Smilacis glabrae Rhizoma (*tǔ fú líng*) to resolve the dampness.

• Aside from the abscesses and rooted sores for which this formula is known, it can also be applied to a wide variety of heat-toxin related disorders manifesting as the biomedical diagnosis of herpes zoster, herpes simplex, folliculitis, erysipelas, and infections of sweat glands and lymph nodes.

• Often herbs that promote urination, such as Plantaginis Semen (*chē qián zǐ*) or Kochiae Fructus (*dì fū zǐ*), are added to help clear heat from the body via the urine.

Contraindications: yin-type swellings • use with caution in cases of Spleen deficiency

▶ FORMULAS WITH SIMILAR INDICATIONS

Support the Interior and Eliminate Toxin Drink (*tuō lǐ xiāo dú yǐn*): Much weaker at clearing heat toxin but more suitable for weak patients with sores that are slow to develop and heal.

Immortals' Formula for Sustaining Life (*xiān fāng huó mìng yǐn*): Treats initial stage lesions with herbs to disperse accumulation, invigorate the blood, and push out pus while at the same time resolving heat toxin. Five-Ingredient Drink to Eliminate Toxin (*wǔ wèi xiāo dú yǐn*) focuses almost entirely on resolving heat toxin.

COMPOSITION

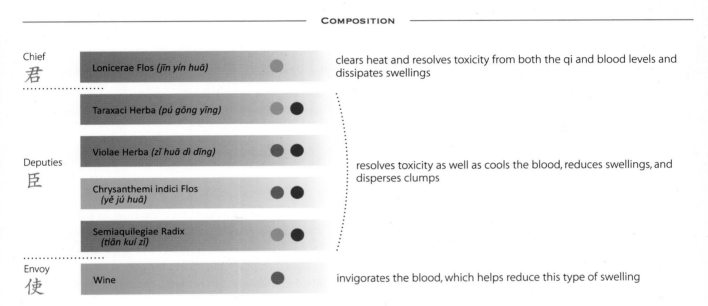

Chief 君	Lonicerae Flos (*jīn yín huā*)	clears heat and resolves toxicity from both the qi and blood levels and dissipates swellings
Deputies 臣	Taraxaci Herba (*pú gōng yīng*)	resolves toxicity as well as cools the blood, reduces swellings, and disperses clumps
	Violae Herba (*zǐ huā dì dīng*)	
	Chrysanthemi indici Flos (*yě jú huā*)	
	Semiaquilegiae Radix (*tiān kuí zǐ*)	
Envoy 使	Wine	invigorates the blood, which helps reduce this type of swelling

吳茱萸湯（吴茱萸汤）
Evodia Decoction
wú zhū yú tāng

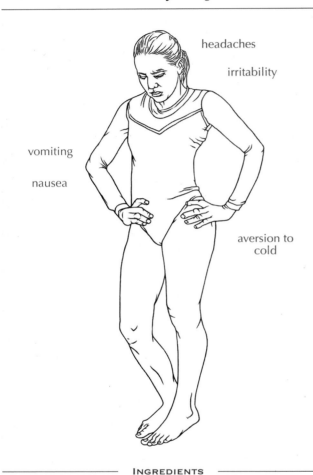

headaches

irritability

vomiting

nausea

aversion to
cold

Key symptoms: migraine-like headaches • vertex headaches
• aversion to cold (or cold as trigger) • nausea • vomiting
• irritability

Secondary symptoms: vomiting immediately after eating
• indeterminate gnawing hunger • acid reflux with or
without epigastric pain • dry heaves • spitting up of clear
fluids • diarrhea • cold hands and feet • agitation • neck pain
• backache

Tongue: white, wet, or slippery coating

Pulse: submerged and frail • submerged, thin, and wiry

Abdomen: drum-like distention or depression of
epigastrium • splashing sounds • reduced tone in abdominal
muscles

► CLINICAL NOTES

- For bouts of headaches (specifically migraines)
  accompanied by nausea and vomiting in patients who
  are sensitive to cold or where the headaches are triggered
  by cold. Can be used both to treat acute attacks and to
  resolve the underlying root in the period between attacks.
  Meniere's disease, labyrinthitis, epilepsy, or hypertension
  can also manifest with this presentation, with the presence
  of irritability helping make the diagnosis.

- The formula can also be used to treat vomiting and
  diarrhea in patients with cold extremities that presents
  together with irritability or fever. Irritability and fever,
  in this case, are not due to heat excess but floating yang
  prevented from returning to the lower burner by turbid
  yin excess.

- A third area of use are conditions presenting with
  epigastric discomfort, fullness, or distention but with a
  submerged and frail pulse, distinguishing this pattern
  from those involving heat or stasis. This includes a variety
  of chronic inflammatory conditions of the digestive
  system.

- Evodiae Fructus (*wú zhū yú*), the main herb in this formula,
  is slightly toxic, especially if used in the large dosage
  indicated here. This can lead to transitory sensation of
  discomfort in the chest, dizziness, and aggravation of

INGREDIENTS

Evodiae Fructus (*wú zhū yú*) 3-9g
Zingiberis Rhizoma recens (*shēng jiāng*) 18g
Ginseng Radix (*rén shēn*) 6-9g
Jujubae Fructus (*dà zǎo*) .... 4 pieces

Actions: warms and tonifies the Liver and Stomach • directs
rebellious qi downward • stops vomiting

Main pattern: deficiency cold in the middle burner with
upward rebellion of turbid yin that, in some cases, prevents the
yang from returning to its source in the lower burner

the headache after taking the decoction. These side effects are more likely to occur in old and weak patients but are generally transitory in nature. In such cases, the patient should lie down for 30 minutes after which these symptoms should have passed. For particularly severe vomiting, the decoction will be easier to keep down if taken cool and swallowed in small sips.

Contraindications: vomiting or acid reflux due to heat • during pregnancy or while breastfeeding

▶ FORMULAS WITH SIMILAR INDICATIONS

*Clove and Persimmon Calyx Decoction (*dīng xiāng shì dì tāng*): For hiccup due to cold from deficiency in the Stomach. Focuses on warming and tonifying the Stomach rather than eliminating turbid dampness and guiding false yang back to the lower burner.

*Cinnamon Twig and Ginseng Decoction (*guì zhī rén shēn tāng*): For similar symptoms due to Spleen deficiency in the interior accompanied by cold in the exterior as reflected by pain in the muscles and joints.

*Frigid Extremities plus Evodia and Fresh Ginger (*dāng guī sì nì jiā wú zhū yú shēng jiāng tāng*): For interior cold and blood deficiency manifesting primarily with symptoms involving the micro-circulation such as cold extremities and chilblains.

Regulate the Middle Pill (*lǐ zhōng wán*): For middle burner deficiency-cold diarrhea that comes and goes in relation to factors such as food intake, climate, or physical and mental exhaustion without more pronounced lesser yin warp signs.

Frigid Extremities Decoction (*sì nì tāng*): For unrelenting diarrhea resulting from the yang of the middle burner having been cut off from its source in the gate of vitality. This is indicated by systemic signs of deficiency cold such as cold extremities and fatigue that are symptomatic of lesser yin warp disorders.

――――――――――― COMPOSITION ―――――――――――

Chief 君	Evodiae Fructus (*wú zhū yú*)	● ●	warms the middle, disperses cold, promotes the movement of qi, and directs rebellious qi downward
Deputy 臣	Zingiberis Rhizoma recens (*shēng jiāng*)	●	warms the Stomach and directs its qi downward
Assistant 佐	Ginseng Radix (*rén shēn*)	● ●	strengthens the middle burner, promotes the generation of fluids, and calms the spirit
Envoy 使	Jujubae Fructus (*dà zǎo*)	●	moderates the acrid, drying properties of the chief and deputy ingredients, supports the qi-tonifying action of the assistant ingredient

仙方活命飲（仙方活命饮）
Immortals' Formula for Sustaining Life
xiān fāng huó mìng yǐn

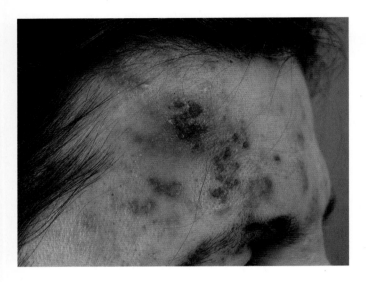

INGREDIENTS

Lonicerae Flos (*jīn yín huā*) .... 9-27 g
Glycyrrhizae Radix (*gān cǎo*)...................................... 3g
Fritillariae thunbergii Bulbus (*zhè bèi mǔ*) 6-9g
Trichosanthis Radix (*tiān huā fěn*)................................. 6-12g
Angelicae sinensis radicis Cauda (*dāng guī wěi*)............... 6-12g
Paeoniae Radix rubra (*chì sháo*) 9g
Olibanum (*rǔ xiāng*) 6g
Myrrha (*mò yào*)... 6g
Saposhnikoviae Radix (*fáng fēng*).................................. 9g
Angelicae dahuricae Radix (*bái zhǐ*) 6g
Vaccariae Semen (*wáng bù liú xíng*) 10g
Gleditsiae Spina (*zào jiǎo cì*).. 6g
Citri reticulatae Pericarpium (*chén pí*)............................ 9g

Actions: clears heat and resolves fire toxicity • reduces swelling and promotes the discharge of pus • invigorates the blood • alleviates pain

Main pattern: early-stage sores and carbuncles

Key symptoms: red, swollen, hot, and painful skin lesions

Secondary symptoms: fever • mild chills • headache

Tongue: thin and white or yellow coating

Pulse: rapid • forceful

Abdomen: no specific signs

▶ CLINICAL NOTES

• This formula can treat any type of acute, hot, red swelling. If the core of the lesion is hard (and has not yet developed pus), it helps disperse it internally. If the core is soft (suppurated), it will help it drain.

• The scope of this formula has expanded in modern times beyond external sores to include internal disorders such as tonsillitis, ulcerative colitis, bursitis, and acute appendicitis.

• In the dermatology department this formula has become a staple for all manner of toxic heat accumulation and thus addresses manifestations that present as disorders as varied as post-herpetic neuralgia, pustular psoriasis, suppurating infections of the fingernails or toenails, and folliculitis.

• This formula treats the acute manifestations of toxic heat accumulation. It is inappropriate for long-term use.

Contraindications: Without modification, this formula should not be used for yin sores or those that have begun to discharge pus. Use with caution in weak patients.

▶ FORMULAS WITH SIMILAR INDICATIONS

Five-Ingredient Drink to Eliminate Toxin (*wǔ wèi xiāo dú yǐn*): Focuses much more on clearing heat and resolving toxicity, particularly for upper body lesions. For acute hot sores, one may combine important elements of these two formulas.

Support the Interior and Eliminate Toxin Drink (*tuō lǐ xiāo dú yǐn*): Focuses on tonifying the body's qi and blood to help patients with qi deficiency overcome toxic swellings. Since much of its attention is spent on tonification, its ability to clear heat, resolve toxicity, and disperse swellings is much weaker than Immortals' Formula for Sustaining Life (*xiān fāng huó mìng yǐn*).

COMPOSITION

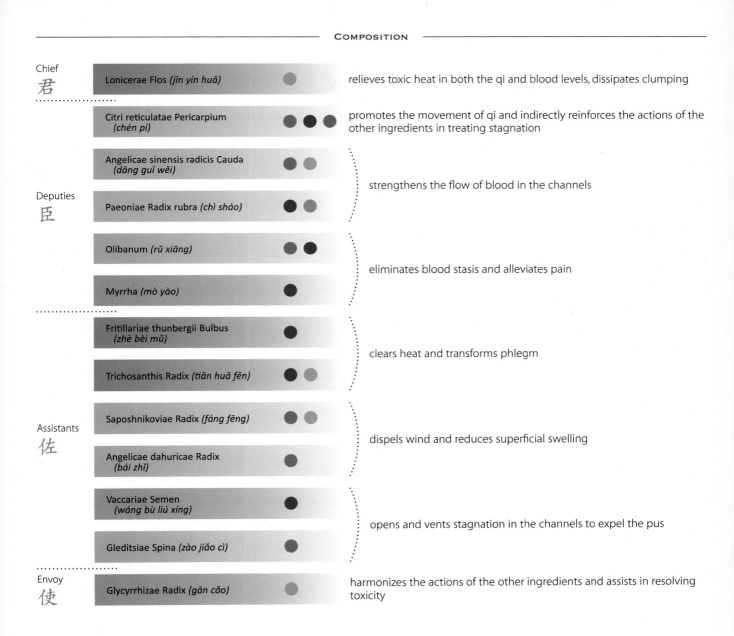

Chief
君

Lonicerae Flos (jīn yín huā) — relieves toxic heat in both the qi and blood levels, dissipates clumping

Citri reticulatae Pericarpium (chén pí) — promotes the movement of qi and indirectly reinforces the actions of the other ingredients in treating stagnation

Deputies
臣

Angelicae sinensis radicis Cauda (dāng guī wěi)

Paeoniae Radix rubra (chì sháo)

strengthens the flow of blood in the channels

Olibanum (rǔ xiāng)

Myrrha (mò yào)

eliminates blood stasis and alleviates pain

Fritillariae thunbergii Bulbus (zhè bèi mǔ)

Trichosanthis Radix (tiān huā fěn)

clears heat and transforms phlegm

Assistants
佐

Saposhnikoviae Radix (fáng fēng)

Angelicae dahuricae Radix (bái zhǐ)

dispels wind and reduces superficial swelling

Vaccariae Semen (wáng bù liú xíng)

Gleditsiae Spina (zào jiǎo cì)

opens and vents stagnation in the channels to expel the pus

Envoy
使

Glycyrrhizae Radix (gān cǎo) — harmonizes the actions of the other ingredients and assists in resolving toxicity

香砂六君子湯（香砂六君子汤）
Six-Gentlemen Decoction with Aucklandia and Amomum
xiāng shā liù jūn zǐ tāng

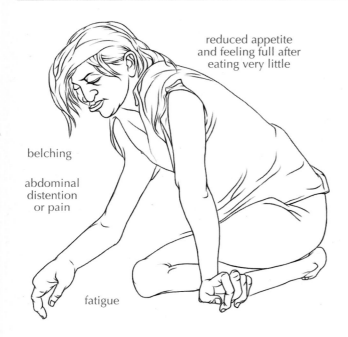

reduced appetite and feeling full after eating very little

belching

abdominal distention or pain

fatigue

INGREDIENTS

Ginseng Radix (*rén shēn*).. 3g
Atractylodis macrocephalae Rhizoma (*bái zhú*) 6g
Poria (*fú líng*) 6g
Glycyrrhizae Radix praeparata (*zhì gān cǎo*) 2g
Citri reticulatae Pericarpium (*chén pí*)........................... 2.5g
Pinelliae Rhizoma praeparatum (*zhì bàn xià*) 3g
Amomi Fructus (*shā rén*)... 2.5g
Aucklandiae Radix (*mù xiāng*) 2g
Zingiberis Rhizoma recens (*shēng jiāng*)........................... 6g

Actions: strengthens the Spleen • harmonizes the Stomach • regulates the qi • transforms phlegm • alleviates pain

Main pattern: Spleen and Stomach qi deficiency with damp-cold stagnating in the middle burner

Key symptoms: reduced appetite and feeling full after eating very little • belching • abdominal distention or pain • fatigue

Secondary symptoms: vomiting • diarrhea

Tongue: pale body • greasy coating

Pulse: slippery • weak

Abdomen: epigastric tenderness • superficial tenderness with weakness on deeper palpation

▶ CLINICAL NOTES

- Qi stagnation in the middle burner in the context of long-standing deficiency means that the symptoms are often chronic and related to dietary intemperance. Distention after eating, belching, and poor appetite in a generally weak and tired person are the main indications for this formula.

- Once the symptoms of qi stagnation have been resolved, it is advised to switch to a more tonifying formula such as Four-Gentlemen Decoction (*sì jūn zǐ tāng*) or Six-Gentlemen Decoction (*liù jūn zǐ tāng*). The patient should also be asked to modify their diet by avoiding greasy, rich and cold foods, as this will greatly aid recovery.

- With the appropriate presentation, this formula can treat morning sickness.

Contraindications: excess patterns

▶ FORMULAS WITH SIMILAR INDICATIONS

Four-Gentlemen Decoction (*sì jūn zǐ tāng*): For simple deficiency of the middle burner with no signs of qi stagnation or phlegm.

Calm the Stomach Powder (*píng wèi sǎn*): For excess dampness obstructing the middle burner causing qi stagnation marked by abdominal distention and fullness, loss of appetite, and loose stools with a thick, white, and greasy tongue coating.

Preserve Harmony Pill (*bǎo hé wán*): For food stagnation as reflected in nausea, abdominal distention, foul-smelling diarrhea, or belching with a fetid odor.

COMPOSITION

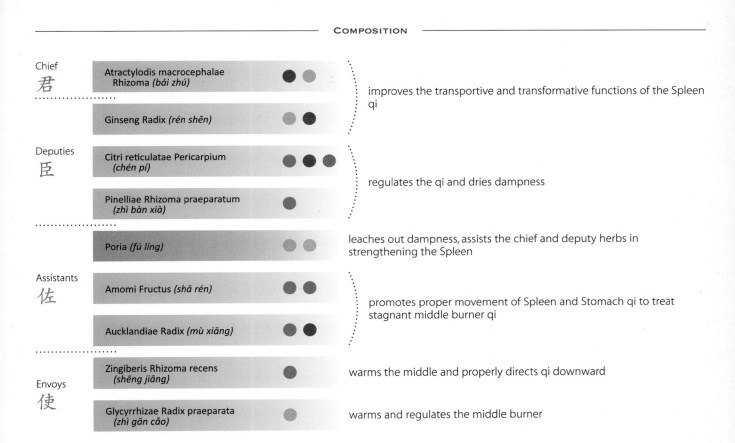

Chief 君

Atractylodis macrocephalae Rhizoma (bái zhú)

Ginseng Radix (rén shēn)

improves the transportive and transformative functions of the Spleen qi

Deputies 臣

Citri reticulatae Pericarpium (chén pí)

Pinelliae Rhizoma praeparatum (zhì bàn xià)

regulates the qi and dries dampness

Poria (fú líng)

leaches out dampness, assists the chief and deputy herbs in strengthening the Spleen

Assistants 佐

Amomi Fructus (shā rén)

Aucklandiae Radix (mù xiāng)

promotes proper movement of Spleen and Stomach qi to treat stagnant middle burner qi

Envoys 使

Zingiberis Rhizoma recens (shēng jiāng)

warms the middle and properly directs qi downward

Glycyrrhizae Radix praeparata (zhì gān cǎo)

warms and regulates the middle burner

小柴胡湯（小柴胡汤）
Minor Bupleurum Decoction
xiǎo chái hú tāng

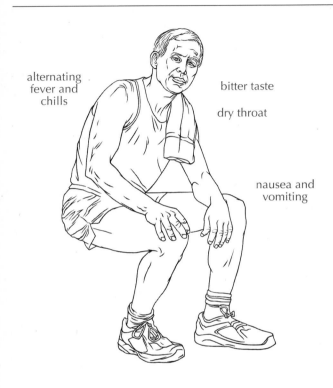

alternating fever and chills

bitter taste

dry throat

nausea and vomiting

Key symptoms: alternating fever and chills • fever of unknown origin • pain and distention in chest and flanks • fullness in chest and pain in flanks • abdominal pain • irritability and restlessness • feeling downcast • frequent sighing or difficulty taking deep breaths • reduced intake of food and drink • disinterest in food • nausea and vomiting • dry retching • bitter taste • dry throat

Secondary symptoms: dizziness • tinnitus • thirst • focal distention in the epigastrium • heartburn • palpitations • coughing • urinary dysfunction • constipation

Tongue: thin, white, or greasy coating

Pulse: wiry

Abdomen: tension in the hypochondrium (particularly on left) • discomfort or focal distention in epigastrium

► CLINICAL NOTES

- Harmonizes the lesser yang warp and resolves its constraint, but can equally be used as a base formula for joint disorders involving the lesser yang and any of the other yang warps. A wiry pulse, a white and perhaps slightly greasy tongue coating, a bitter taste or dry throat together with any one of the other signs and symptoms listed above is considered sufficient to prescribe this formula.

- Dredges and unblocks qi constraint in the Triple Burner characterized by fullness in the epigastrium, disinterest in food, constipation, sweating from the head only, slight chills, cold extremities, and a thin or deep and tight pulse.

- Frequently used for nervous system and emotional disorders with a lesser yang presentation including insomnia, anxiety, headache, and nerve pain as well as for so-called 'strange disorders' that manifest with unusual symptoms or with presentations that are difficult to match with common patterns or disorders.

- Can be used to dredge the Liver and regulate the menses when qi constraint causes clumping and blood stasis. Particularly indicated for heat entering the blood palace characterized by chills and fevers occurring regularly around menstruation and diurnal normality with nocturnal restlessness "as if one had encountered a ghost."

―――― INGREDIENTS ――――

Bupleuri Radix (*chái hú*) 12-24g
Scutellariae Radix (*huáng qín*) 9g
Pinelliae Rhizoma praeparatum (*zhì bàn xià*) 9g
Zingiberis Rhizoma recens (*shēng jiāng*) 9g
Ginseng Radix (*rén shēn*) 6-9g
Glycyrrhizae Radix praeparata (*zhì gān cǎo*) 5-9g
Jujubae Fructus (*dà zǎo*) .... 4 pieces

Actions: harmonizes the lesser yang • supports normal qi • dispels pathogens

Main patterns: cold pathogen constraining the lesser yang warp causing it to lose its ability to direct ascent of the clear and descent of the turbid • qi constraint of the Liver and Gallbladder with Gallbladder heat accosting the Stomach and Liver qi invading the Spleen

- Supports the normal qi and dispels pathogenic qi in both acute and chronic conditions ranging from common colds to disorders characterized by compromised or disordered immune function, inflammation, or fevers of unknown origin.
- Although the formula can be modified to match presenting signs and symptoms, the relative dosage of Bupleuri Radix (*chái hú*) to that of Scutellariae Radix (*huáng qín*) should stay around 8:3, and the dosage of these herbs should always exceed the total combined dosage of Ginseng Radix (*rén shēn*) and Glycyrrhizae Radix (*gān cǎo*) in order to allow the formula to focus on resolving constraint, opening obstruction, and eliminating pathogenic qi.
- Patients with relatively weak normal qi may experience fever and chills as the pathogenic influence is vented from the lesser yang warp via the greater yang.

Contraindications: patients with excess above and deficiency below, Liver fire, or bleeding of the gums • use with caution in cases of ascendant Liver yang, hypertension, or vomiting of blood due to yin deficiency

► FORMULAS WITH SIMILAR INDICATIONS

Major Bupleurum Decoction (*dà chái hú tāng*): For combined lesser yang and yang brightness disorders with heat marked by abdominal distention and tension that is aggravated by pressure, and either constipation or diarrhea.

Sweet Wormwood and Scutellaria Decoction to Clear the Gallbladder (*hāo qín qīng dǎn tāng*): For damp-heat in the lesser yang with fever more pronounced than chills and more prominent signs of phlegm-dampness.

--- COMPOSITION ---

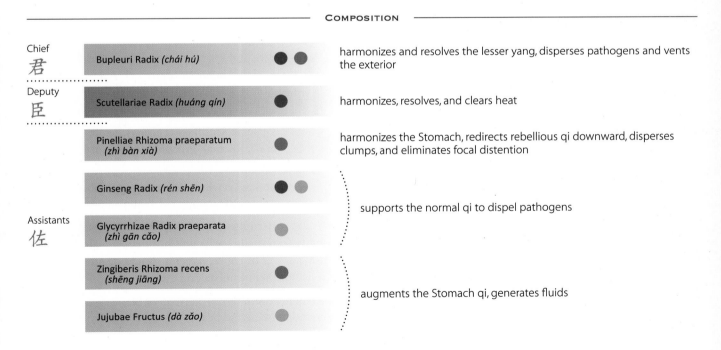

Chief 君	Bupleuri Radix (*chái hú*) ●●	harmonizes and resolves the lesser yang, disperses pathogens and vents the exterior
Deputy 臣	Scutellariae Radix (*huáng qín*) ●	harmonizes, resolves, and clears heat
Assistants 佐	Pinelliae Rhizoma praeparatum (*zhì bàn xià*) ●	harmonizes the Stomach, redirects rebellious qi downward, disperses clumps, and eliminates focal distention
	Ginseng Radix (*rén shēn*) ●●	supports the normal qi to dispel pathogens
	Glycyrrhizae Radix praeparata (*zhì gān cǎo*) ●	
	Zingiberis Rhizoma recens (*shēng jiāng*) ●	augments the Stomach qi, generates fluids
	Jujubae Fructus (*dà zǎo*) ●	

消風散 (消风散)
Eliminate Wind Powder from
Orthodox Lineage
xiāo fēng sǎn

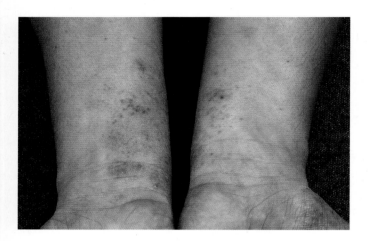

INGREDIENTS

Schizonepetae Herba (*jīng jiè*) 3-9g
Saposhnikoviae Radix (*fáng fēng*) 3-9g
Arctii Fructus (*niú bàng zǐ*) 3-9g
Cicadae Periostracum (*chán tuì*) 3-9g
Atractylodis Rhizoma (*cāng zhú*) 3-9g
Sophorae flavescentis Radix (*kǔ shēn*) 3-9g
Akebiae Caulis (*mù tōng*) 1.5-3g
Gypsum fibrosum (*shí gāo*) 3-9g
Anemarrhenae Rhizoma (*zhī mǔ*) 3-9g
Rehmanniae Radix (*shēng dì huáng*) 3-9g
Angelicae sinensis Radix (*dāng guī*) 3-9g
Sesami Semen nigrum (*hēi zhī má*) 3-9g
Glycyrrhizae Radix (*gān cǎo*) 1.5-3g

Actions: disperses wind • eliminates dampness • clears heat • cools the blood

Main patterns: wind rash • damp rash

Key symptoms: weepy, itchy, red skin lesions that may occur all over the body

Tongue: yellow or white coating

Pulse: floating • forceful • rapid

Abdomen: no specific signs

▶ CLINICAL NOTES

- Suitable as a base formula for treating all types of rashes due to wind, heat, and dampness including urticaria, eczema, psoriasis, drug rash, contact dermatitis, Schönlein-Henoch purpura, tinea infection, and diaper rash. Modify according to specific presentations and the precise combination of various pathogens at the qi and blood levels.

- This formula is seldom used without modifications:
  → For severe qi aspect heat when the patient is hot and thirsty, increase the dosage of Gypsum fibrosum (*shí gāo*) and Anemarrhenae Rhizoma (*zhī mǔ*). For toxic heat with rapidly spreading rashes, add Lonicerae Flos (*jīn yín huā*), Forsythiae Fructus (*lián qiào*), and Taraxaci Herba (*pú gōng yīng*).
  → For heat in the blood aspect with rashes that are raised, red, and bleed when scratched, add Paeoniae Radix rubra (*chì sháo*), Moutan Cortex (*mǔ dān pí*), and Arnebiae Radix/Lithospermi Radix (*zǐ cǎo*).
  → For pronounced dampness with sticky discharge, add Smilacis glabrae Rhizoma (*tǔ fú líng*), Plantaginis Semen (*chē qián zǐ*), Kochiae Fructus (*dì fū zǐ*), or Dioscoreae hypoglaucae Rhizoma (*bì xiè*).
  → For pronounced wind with strong or stubborn itching, add Zaocys (*wū shāo shé*) and Scolopendra (*wú gōng*).

- As the pattern this formula treats is aggravated by spicy foods (especially garlic and hot pepper), alcohol, shell fish, and tea or coffee, patients should be advised not to consume them while taking this formula.

Contraindications: rashes due to qi or blood deficiency without dampness and heat

▶ FORMULAS WITH SIMILAR INDICATIONS

*Tangkuei Drink (*dāng guī yǐn zi*): Based on Four-Substance Decoction (*sì wù tāng*) and Tangkuei Decoction to Tonify the Blood (*dāng guī bǔ xuè tāng*), this formula addresses chronic skin disorders where blood deficiency is the main issue.

COMPOSITION

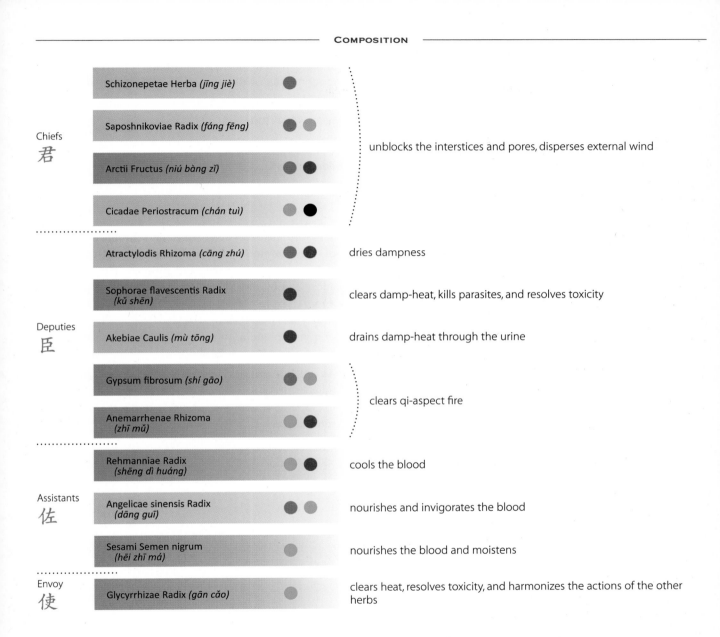

Chiefs
君

Schizonepetae Herba (*jīng jiè*)

Saposhnikoviae Radix (*fáng fēng*)

Arctii Fructus (*niú bàng zǐ*)

Cicadae Periostracum (*chán tuì*)

unblocks the interstices and pores, disperses external wind

Deputies
臣

Atractylodis Rhizoma (*cāng zhú*) — dries dampness

Sophorae flavescentis Radix (*kǔ shēn*) — clears damp-heat, kills parasites, and resolves toxicity

Akebiae Caulis (*mù tōng*) — drains damp-heat through the urine

Gypsum fibrosum (*shí gāo*)

Anemarrhenae Rhizoma (*zhī mǔ*)

clears qi-aspect fire

Assistants
佐

Rehmanniae Radix (*shēng dì huáng*) — cools the blood

Angelicae sinensis Radix (*dāng guī*) — nourishes and invigorates the blood

Sesami Semen nigrum (*hēi zhī má*) — nourishes the blood and moistens

Envoy
使

Glycyrrhizae Radix (*gān cǎo*) — clears heat, resolves toxicity, and harmonizes the actions of the other herbs

小活絡丹（小活络丹）
Minor Invigorate the Collaterals Special Pill
xiǎo huó luò dān

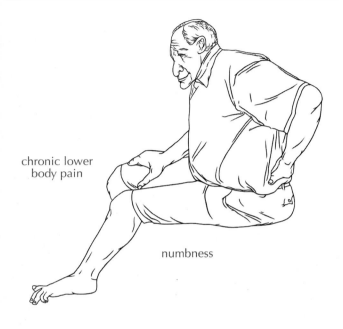

chronic lower
body pain

numbness

———— INGREDIENTS ————

[1]Aconiti kusnezoffii Radix praeparata (*zhì cǎo wū*) 180g
[1]Aconiti Radix praeparata (*zhì chuān wū*)......................... 180g
Arisaematis Rhizoma praeparatum (*zhì tiān nán xīng*)...... 180g
Myrrha (*mò yào*).. 66g
Olibanum (*rǔ xiāng*) 66g
Pheretima (*dì lóng*) 180g

Preparation notes: This formula is always taken in prepared
form, usually as pills with a dosage of 3g once or twice daily,
taken with either warm water or wine.

Actions: dispels wind • eliminates dampness • transforms
phlegm • invigorates the blood • unblocks the collaterals
• alleviates pain

Main pattern: obstruction of the channels and collaterals by
wind-cold-dampness, blood stasis, and phlegm

———

1. These ingredients can be difficult to obtain because of legal issues. No
useful substitutes are available.

Key symptoms: chronic pain, weakness, and numbness
(especially in the lower extremities) due to wind-stroke
• migrating pain in the bones and joints with reduced
range of motion when due to wind-cold-damp painful
obstruction

Tongue: white • wet

Pulse: rough or jumpy

Abdomen: no specific signs

► CLINICAL NOTES

• This formula treats deep-seated and chronic obstruction
of the channels and collaterals by wind-cold-damp
pathogens, blood stasis, and phlegm. The symptoms
addressed by this formula are aggravated by cold. It is
a more severe condition than painful obstruction due
simply to wind, dampness, and cold where the movement
of qi and blood are impeded but no phlegm or lifeless
blood have yet accumulated.

• As this is a very strong formula it should be used carefully. In patients with weak constitutions it may be best
to combine it with formulas that tonify the underlying
root conditions.

Contraindications: yin deficiency • pregnancy

COMPOSITION

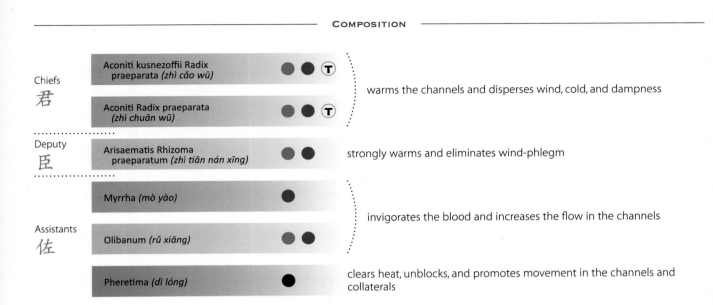

Chiefs
君

Aconiti kusnezoffii Radix praeparata *(zhì cǎo wū)*

Aconiti Radix praeparata *(zhì chuān wū)*

warms the channels and disperses wind, cold, and dampness

Deputy
臣

Arisaematis Rhizoma praeparatum *(zhì tiān nán xīng)*

strongly warms and eliminates wind-phlegm

Assistants
佐

Myrrha *(mò yào)*

Olibanum *(rǔ xiāng)*

invigorates the blood and increases the flow in the channels

Pheretima *(dì lóng)*

clears heat, unblocks, and promotes movement in the channels and collaterals

小建中湯（小建中汤）
Minor Construct the Middle Decoction
xiǎo jiàn zhōng tāng

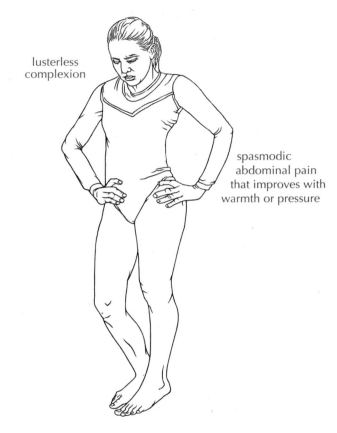

lusterless complexion

spasmodic abdominal pain that improves with warmth or pressure

Main patterns: interior deficiency with cold damage • consumptive deficiency

Key symptoms: spasmodic abdominal pain (often focused in either the epigastrium or around the umbilicus) that improves with local application of warmth and pressure • lusterless complexion

Secondary symptoms: low-grade fever • spontaneous sweating • night sweats • palpitations • irritability • aversion to cold • cold and sore extremities with nonspecific discomfort • reduced appetite • alternating diarrhea and constipation • dry mouth and throat • increased urination • bedwetting in children

Tongue: normal or slightly pale color • little coating

Pulse: thin, wiry, and moderate • large and deficient

Abdomen: distended but with weak muscle tone • visible peristaltic movements • hypertonicity of rectus abdominis muscle • pencil line of tension above and below the umbilicus

▶ CLINICAL NOTES

- An important formula for treating all types of abdominal pain in patients with a weak constitution. The pain typically comes and goes and responds favorably to warmth and pressure. These symptoms indicate that both blood and qi have been damaged.

- The formula is also used to treat deficiency conditions characterized by fatigue and exhaustion such as the type seen in recovery from a severe illness, surgery, or parturition. It can be used as long as the abdominal signs are present. Exhaustion from yin deficiency may present with many similar symptoms and must be carefully excluded as the underlying cause.

- The mild action of this formula makes it particularly suitable for children. It is often used in the treatment of bedwetting and for treatment of weak, cold children who have abdominal pain and a poor appetite.

- This formula is frequently combined with either Angelicae sinensis Radix (*dāng guī*) or Astragali Radix (*huáng qí*) or both to enhance its blood and/or qi tonifying properties.

━━━━━━━━━ INGREDIENTS ━━━━━━━━━

Maltosum (*yí táng*) .... [add to strained decoction] 30g
Cinnamomi Ramulus (*guì zhī*)... 9g
¹Paeoniae Radix (*sháo yào*).. 18g
Glycyrrhizae Radix praeparata (*zhì gān cǎo*) 6g
Zingiberis Rhizoma recens (*shēng jiāng*).............................. 9g
Jujubae Fructus (*dà zǎo*).. 4 pieces

Actions: warms and tonifies the middle burner • moderates spasmodic abdominal pain

━━━━━━━━━━

1. As the primary function here is to restrain, tonify, or soften, Paeoniae Radix alba (*bái sháo*) is preferred.

• It is important that you *not* replace Maltosum (*yí táng*) with white sugar, which is considered cooling in nature and might further damage the middle in these patterns. Cinnamomi Ramulus (*guì zhī*) may be replaced by or used in combination with Cinnamomi Cortex (*ròu guì*) for patients with more severe internal cold.

Contraindications: heat from yin deficiency • abdominal distention from excess patterns

▶ FORMULAS WITH SIMILAR INDICATIONS

Tonify the Middle to Augment the Qi Decoction (*bǔ zhōng yì qì tāng*): Focuses on tonifying and raising the qi rather than harmonizing the yin and yang and is thus better for conditions that manifest as sinking of Spleen qi instead of pain. These patterns often include heat that follows exertion but improves with rest, whereas patterns for which Minor Construct the Middle Decoction (*xiǎo jiàn zhōng tāng*) is indicated are marked by aggravation from cold.

*Major Construct the Middle Decoction (*dà jiàn zhōng tāng*): For very acute presentations of middle burner yang qi deficiency characterized by severe pain, a strong sensation of cold in the abdomen, and upsurging of qi manifested in nausea and vomiting.

COMPOSITION

Chiefs 君	Maltosum *(yí táng)*	tonifies both the qi and blood, generates fluids, alleviates thirst, and moderates spasmodic abdominal pain
	Cinnamomi Ramulus *(guì zhī)*	harmonizes the nutritive and protective qi
Deputy 臣	Paeoniae Radix alba *(bái sháo)*	
Assistant 佐	Glycyrrhizae Radix praeparata *(zhì gān cǎo)*	works with the deputy to stop spasmodic abdominal pain
Envoys 使	Zingiberis Rhizoma recens *(shēng jiāng)*	tonifies both the nutritive and protective while strengthening the middle burner
	Jujubae Fructus *(dà zǎo)*	

小青龍湯（小青龙汤）
Minor Bluegreen Dragon Decoction
xiǎo qīng lóng tāng

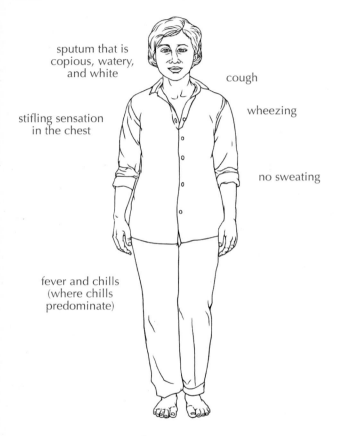

sputum that is copious, watery, and white

cough

wheezing

stifling sensation in the chest

no sweating

fever and chills (where chills predominate)

INGREDIENTS

[1]Ephedrae Herba (*má huáng*)... 9g
Cinnamomi Ramulus (*guì zhī*).. 6-9g
Zingiberis Rhizoma (*gān jiāng*)... 3-6g
[2]Asari Herba (*xì xīn*) 3-6g
Schisandrae Fructus (*wǔ wèi zǐ*).. 3g
Paeoniae Radix alba (*bái sháo*).. 9g
Pinelliae Rhizoma praeparatum (*zhì bàn xià*)......................... 9g

1. This herb can be difficult to obtain because of legal issues. Perillae Folium (*zǐ sū yè*) may be substituted.

2. This herb can also be difficult to obtain because of legal issues. Clematidis Radix (*wēi líng xiān*) may be substituted.

Glycyrrhizae Radix praeparata (*zhì gān cǎo*).................... 6g

Actions: releases wind-cold from the exterior • transforms thin mucus • warms the Lungs • directs rebellious qi downward

Main patterns: externally-contracted wind-cold accompanied by internal accumulation of thin mucus • thin mucus accumulating in the epigastrium

Key symptoms: fever and chills (where chills predominate) without sweating • cough • wheezing • sputum that is copious, watery, and white • stifling sensation in the chest • generalized sensation of heaviness or body aches

Secondary symptoms: thirst • diarrhea • urinary difficulty • superficial edema (in severe cases) • difficulty breathing when lying down • lower abdominal fullness

Tongue: wet body with a thin, white coating

Pulse: floating or wiry and tight

Abdomen: tight rectus abdominis muscle • splashing sound in epigastrium

▶ CLINICAL NOTES

• For patients with chronic cold-dampness who contract greater yang exterior wind-cold. Pathogenic water and cold mutually exacerbate each other making it more difficult for cold to be dispelled and for water to be transformed, hence the pattern becomes chronic.

• Pathogenic thin mucus may accumulate in different areas such as the upper respiratory tract, lungs, face, lower abdomen, bowels, or skin; thus this formula can treat a wide variety of presentations.

• Visible mucus is thin, watery, and bubbly. Sputum may resemble uncooked egg white in consistency and will be transparent.

• Once acute symptoms have abated it is advisable to switch to a milder formula to promote the transformation of qi and water. The subsequent step would be to tonify and warm the Spleen.

Contraindications: Should not be used long term, nor for conditions with heat, coughing of blood, or cough due to yin deficiency. Use with caution in patients with hypertension.

► FORMULAS WITH SIMILAR INDICATIONS

Five-Ingredient Powder with Poria (*wǔ líng sǎn*): For water ac-cumulation, especially in the lower burner, with inhibited urination, thirst, and sweating. By tonifying earth and promoting urination, this formula treats both root and branch.

───── COMPOSITION ─────

Chiefs 君	Ephedrae Herba *(má huáng)*	●●	releases the exterior, arrests wheezing, and promotes urination
	Cinnamomi Ramulus *(guì zhī)*	●●	releases the exterior, opens blood vessels, and promotes qi transformation
Deputies 臣	Zingiberis Rhizoma *(gān jiāng)*	●	warms the interior, transforms thin mucus, and helps the chief herbs release the exterior
	Asari Herba *(xì xīn)*	●	
Assistants 佐	Schisandrae Fructus *(wǔ wèi zǐ)*	●●	prevents the chief and deputy herbs from injuring the qi and fluids while preserving proper Lung functions
	Paeoniae Radix alba *(bái sháo)*	●●	
	Pinelliae Rhizoma praeparatum *(zhì bàn xià)*	●	transforms thin mucus and harmonizes the Stomach
Envoy 使	Glycyrrhizae Radix praeparata *(zhì gān cǎo)*	●	augments qi and harmonizes the effects of other ingredients

小陷胸湯（小陷胸汤）
Minor Decoction [for Pathogens] Stuck in the Chest
xiǎo xiàn xiōng tāng

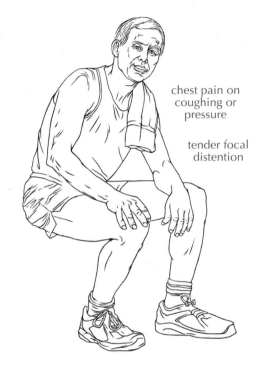

chest pain on coughing or pressure

tender focal distention

INGREDIENTS

Trichosanthis Fructus (*guā lóu*).................................... 15-30g
Coptidis Rhizoma (*huáng lián*)....................................... 6-9g
Pinelliae Rhizoma praeparatum (*zhì bàn xià*)............... 12-15g

Actions: clears heat • transforms phlegm • expands the chest • dissipates clumping

Main pattern: clumping of phlegm and heat in the chest

Key symptoms: focal distention (with or without nodules) in the chest and epigastrium that is painful when pressed

Secondary symptoms: expectoration of yellow and viscous sputum • chest pain on coughing • nausea • bitter taste • constipation

Tongue: white, gray, or yellow, greasy coating

Pulse: slippery and rapid • slippery and floating

Abdomen: fullness and distention in epigastric area with tenderness on pressure

▶ CLINICAL NOTES

• The key marker for this formula is focal distention in the epigastrium, flanks, and chest with tenderness when pressed. The pattern this formula addresses can manifest as disorders that may involve the Lungs, Heart, and Stomach.

• Typical indications are:
  → Coughing with yellow-green, sticky sputum that is difficult to expectorate, chest tightness, and a greasy, yellow tongue coating for which one might add such herbs as Aurantii Fructus (*zhǐ ké*), Curcumae Radix (*yù jīn*), Benincasae Semen (*dōng guā zǐ*), Scutellariae Radix (*huáng qín*), Armeniacae Semen (*xìng rén*), and Fritillariae thunbergii Bulbus (*zhè bèi mǔ*); for violent cough that has damaged the blood vessels in the Lungs and lead to blood stasis, add Armeniacae Semen (*xìng rén*) and Persicae Semen (*táo rén*);
  → Digestive problems accompanied by feelings of distention or pain, nausea and vomiting, acid regurgitation, and constipation which would require additions such as Bambusae Caulis in taeniam (*zhú rú*), Zingiberis Rhizoma recens (*shēng jiāng*), Aurantii Fructus immaturus (*zhǐ shí*), and Rhei Radix et Rhizoma (*dà huáng*);
  → Damp-heat type soft stools, a tongue with a sticky, yellow coating at the root and a wiry, slippery pulse which would benefit from the addition of herbs like Atractylodis Rhizoma (*cāng zhú*), Poria (*fú líng*), and Aucklandiae Radix (*mù xiāng*).

• It is important to remember that while the heat aspect of the pathology treated by this formula can arise from constraint occurring in the course of the invasion of an external pathogen, it can also originate from internally-generated heat excess, specifically from excess Liver yang.

Contraindications: pronounced Spleen deficiency

▶ FORMULAS WITH SIMILAR INDICATIONS

Pinellia Decoction to Drain the Epigastrium (*bàn xià xiè xīn tāng*): For a pattern of Spleen and Stomach deficiency cold with damp-heat obstructing the middle burner. This presents with symptoms such as epigastric focal distention that is soft when pressed, a stifling sensation, and nausea or vomiting.

Clear the Qi and Transform Phlegm Pill (*qīng qì huà tán wán*): Treats a very similar pattern of phlegm-heat in the Lungs but with more emphasis on treating the cough and the sticky, yellow phlegm and less on the focal distention in the epigastrium, flanks, and chest.

──────── COMPOSITION ────────

Chief 君	Trichosanthis Fructus *(guā lóu)*	●	cools and transforms phlegm-heat, moistens the Intestines, and directs the turbid phlegm downward
Deputy 臣	Coptidis Rhizoma *(huáng lián)*	●	helps the chief herb drain heat and turbidity from the upper and middle burners
Assistant 佐	Pinelliae Rhizoma praeparatum *(zhì bàn xià)*	●	directs the rebellious qi downward, harmonizes the Stomach, transforms phlegm, eliminates focal distention, and dissipates clumps

小續命湯 （小续命汤）
Minor Extend Life Decoction
xiǎo xù mìng tāng

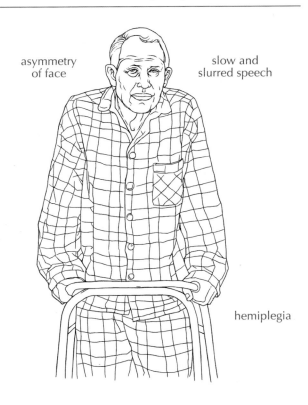

asymmetry of face

slow and slurred speech

hemiplegia

─── INGREDIENTS ───

[1]Ephedrae Herba (*má huáng*)........................... 3-6g
Chuanxiong Rhizoma (*chuān xiōng*) 3-6g
Stephaniae tetrandrae Radix (*hàn fáng jǐ*) 6-12g
Armeniacae Semen (*xìng rén*) 9-12g
Saposhnikoviae Radix (*fáng fēng*) 9-12g
Zingiberis Rhizoma recens (*shēng jiāng*)................. 9-12 slices
Ginseng Radix (*rén shēn*) 3-6g
[2]Aconiti Radix lateralis praeparata (*zhì fù zǐ*) 9-15g
Cinnamomi Cortex (*ròu guì*) 3-6g

1. This herb may be difficult to obtain because of legal issues. Notopterygii Rhizoma seu Radix *(qiāng huó)* may be substituted.

2. This ingredient may also be difficult to obtain because of legal issues.

[3]Paeoniae Radix (*sháo yào*)........................6-12g
Scutellariae Radix (*huáng qín*)................4.5-9g
Glycyrrhizae Radix (*gān cǎo*)................ 3-6g

Actions: warms the channels • unblocks the yang qi • dispels wind • supports the normal qi

Main patterns: wind-stroke due to invasion of wind from the exterior into the channels • pain from wind-damp painful obstruction

Key symptoms: hemiplegia • asymmetry of the face • slow and slurred speech • fever and chills

Secondary symptoms: none noted

Tongue: pale body • white coating

Pulse: deficient • floating

Abdomen: no specific signs

▶ CLINICAL NOTES

• This formula treats patterns of acute wind-stroke in the channels and collaterals. It relies on the dispersing method to dispel pathogenic wind to the exterior. Thus it is inappropriate for wind-stroke due to internal wind (with or without phlegm-heat) or blood stasis (with or without qi deficiency).

• Some physicians suggest that the formula be altered based on which of the six main channel systems is affected topographically:

→ For greater yang channel symptoms without sweating, double the dosage of Ephedrae Herba (*má huáng*), Armeniacae Semen (*xìng rén*), and Saposhnikoviae Radix (*fáng fēng*).

→ For greater yang channel symptoms with sweating and aversion to wind, double the dosage of Cinnamomi Ramulus (*guì zhī*), Paeoniae Radix alba (*bái sháo*), and Armeniacae Semen (*xìng rén*).

→ For yang brightness channel symptoms without sweating, add Puerariae Radix (*gé gēn*) and double the dosage of Scutellariae Radix (*huáng qín*).

→ For yang brightness channel symptoms with sweating and no internal cold, substitute Aconiti Radix lateralis praeparata (*zhì fù zǐ*) with Gypsum fibrosum (*shí gāo*) and Anemarrhenae Rhizoma (*zhī mǔ*).

3. As the primary function here is to restrain, tonify, or soften, Paeoniae Radix alba *(bái sháo)* is preferred.

→ For greater yin channel wind-stroke, double the dosage of Aconiti Radix lateralis praeparata (*zhì fù zǐ*) and Glycyrrhizae Radix (*gān cǎo*), and add Zingiberis Rhizoma (*gān jiāng*).

→ For lesser yin channel wind-stroke without sweating or fever, double the dosage of Aconiti Radix lateralis praeparata (*zhì fù zǐ*), Cinnamomi Ramulus (*guì zhī*), and Glycyrrhizae Radix (*gān cǎo*).

• When the symptoms are less clearly associated with any of the six channels but are related to the lesser yang and terminal yin warps with symptoms that come and go or there is numbness and spasms of the extremities, add Notopterygii Rhizoma seu Radix (*qiāng huó*) and Forsythiae Fructus (*lián qiào*).

• In current practice, this formula is also used for the pain associated with wind-damp painful obstruction.

Contraindications: wind-stroke due to internal stirring of Liver wind • hot painful obstruction

▶ FORMULAS WITH SIMILAR INDICATIONS

Major Large Gentian Decoction (*dà qín jiāo tāng*): For wind-stroke in the channels and collaterals in the context of qi and blood deficiency. This formula is thus suitable for more chronic patterns.

COMPOSITION

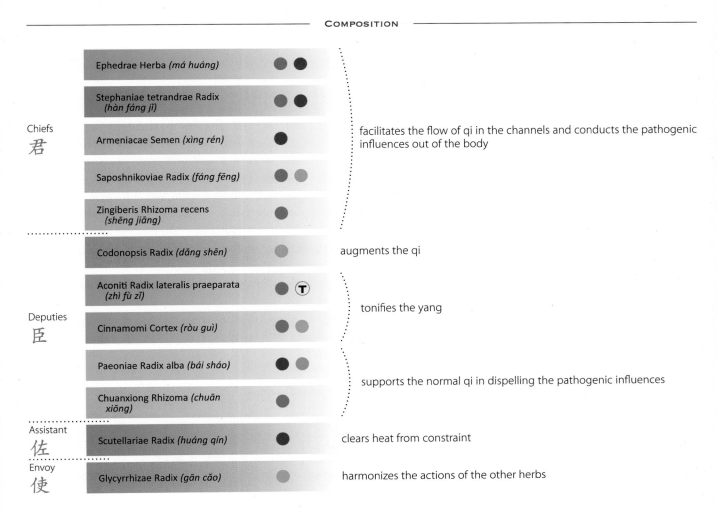

Chiefs 君

Ephedrae Herba (*má huáng*)
Stephaniae tetrandrae Radix (*hàn fáng jǐ*)
Armeniacae Semen (*xìng rén*)
Saposhnikoviae Radix (*fáng fēng*)
Zingiberis Rhizoma recens (*shēng jiāng*)
— facilitates the flow of qi in the channels and conducts the pathogenic influences out of the body

Codonopsis Radix (*dǎng shēn*) — augments the qi

Deputies 臣

Aconiti Radix lateralis praeparata (*zhì fù zǐ*)
Cinnamomi Cortex (*ròu guì*)
— tonifies the yang

Paeoniae Radix alba (*bái sháo*)
Chuanxiong Rhizoma (*chuān xiōng*)
— supports the normal qi in dispelling the pathogenic influences

Assistant 佐

Scutellariae Radix (*huáng qín*) — clears heat from constraint

Envoy 使

Glycyrrhizae Radix (*gān cǎo*) — harmonizes the actions of the other herbs

逍遥散
Rambling Powder
xiāo yáo sǎn

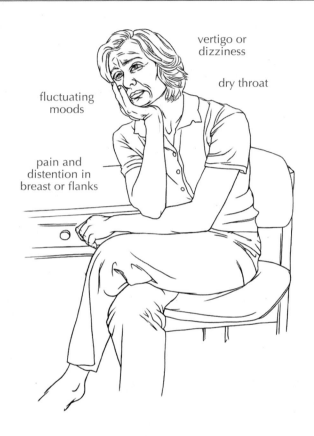

vertigo or dizziness

dry throat

fluctuating moods

pain and distention in breast or flanks

INGREDIENTS

Bupleuri Radix (*chái hú*)...9g

Angelicae sinensis Radix (*dāng guī*)..............................9g

Paeoniae Radix alba (*bái sháo*)....................................30g

Atractylodis macrocephalae Rhizoma (*bái zhú*)..................9g

Poria (*fú líng*)...15g

Glycyrrhizae Radix praeparata (*zhì gān cǎo*)....................9g

roasted Zingiberis Rhizoma recens (*wēi jiāng*)............1 slice

Menthae haplocalycis Herba (*bò hé*)...............................2g

Actions: spreads the Liver qi • strengthens the Spleen • nourishes the blood

Main pattern: Liver constraint with blood deficiency and a frail Spleen

Key symptoms: vertigo or dizziness • pain and distention in breast or flanks • dry throat • fluctuating moods

Secondary symptoms: alternating fever and chills • bitter taste • headache • tension in the shoulders and neck • abdominal distention • reduced appetite • soft or incomplete and difficult bowel movements • irregular menstruation • insomnia • anxiety

Tongue: pale red

Pulse: wiry • deficient

Abdomen: hypochondriac distention (right > left) • pain on palpation of lower abdomen • splashing sound in epigastrium • palpable periumbilical pulsations

▶ CLINICAL NOTES

• An important formula in the treatment of psycho-emotional symptoms such as irritability, restlessness, depression, and anxiety, particularly where these symptoms are associated with the menstrual cycle or menopause. There should be signs of heat constraint.

• Dredges the Liver and builds the Spleen in patterns characterized by fatigue, pain, and chronic inflammation such as cholecystitis, stomach or duodenal ulcers, pelvic, or inflammatory disease.

• Can also be used to vent pathogens in a patient who also has significant underlying deficiency. This can be seen in such problems as hepatitis and fevers of unexplained origin.

• Used for many disorders involving stagnation of Liver qi and deficiency of Liver blood including irregular menstruation, infertility, and a variety of ophthalmological disorders.

Contraindications: purely deficient disorders

▶ FORMULAS WITH SIMILAR INDICATIONS

Escape Restraint Pill (*yuè jū wán*): For an excess pattern marked by constraint in the chest and abdomen manifesting with distention and pain.

Frigid Extremities Powder (*sì nì săn*): For excess patterns with frigid extremities, diarrhea or constipation, and excess-type abdominal pain.

Tangkuei and Peony Powder (*dāng guī sháo yào săn*): For mixed pattern of Liver and Spleen deficiency complicated by blood stasis and dampness marked by pain (usually aching or cramping), a tendency to feel cold, and fluid accumulation.

*Restrain the Liver Powder (*yì gān săn*): Similar presentation but with more signs of wind such as spasms, headache, and dizziness.

─── COMPOSITION ───

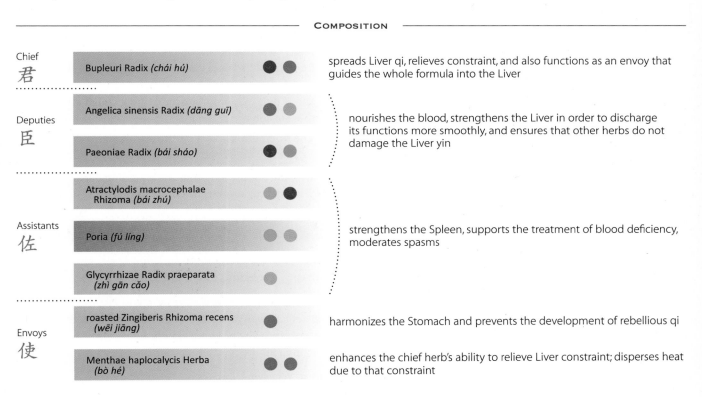

Chief 君	Bupleuri Radix (*chái hú*)	spreads Liver qi, relieves constraint, and also functions as an envoy that guides the whole formula into the Liver
Deputies 臣	Angelica sinensis Radix (*dāng guī*) / Paeoniae Radix (*bái sháo*)	nourishes the blood, strengthens the Liver in order to discharge its functions more smoothly, and ensures that other herbs do not damage the Liver yin
Assistants 佐	Atractylodis macrocephalae Rhizoma (*bái zhú*) / Poria (*fú líng*) / Glycyrrhizae Radix praeparata (*zhì gān căo*)	strengthens the Spleen, supports the treatment of blood deficiency, moderates spasms
Envoys 使	roasted Zingiberis Rhizoma recens (*wēi jiāng*)	harmonizes the Stomach and prevents the development of rebellious qi
	Menthae haplocalycis Herba (*bò hé*)	enhances the chief herb's ability to relieve Liver constraint; disperses heat due to that constraint

瀉白散（泻白散）
Drain the White Powder from
Craft of Medicinal Treatment
for Childhood Disease Patterns
xiè bái săn

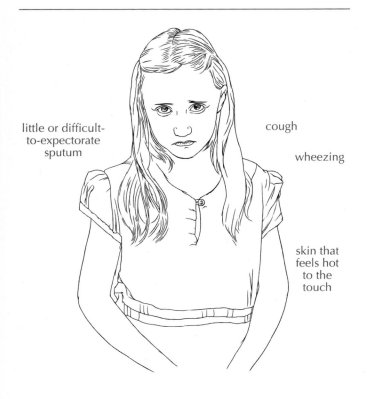

little or difficult-to-expectorate sputum

cough

wheezing

skin that feels hot to the touch

--- INGREDIENTS ---

dry-fried Mori Cortex (*chǎo sāng bái pí*)...................... 15-30g
Lycii Cortex (*dì gǔ pí*)... 15-30g
Glycyrrhizae Radix praeparata (*zhì gān cǎo*) 3g
Nonglutinous rice (*jīng mǐ*) 15-30g

Actions: drains heat from the Lungs • calms wheezing

Main pattern: lurking fire due to constrained heat in the Lungs

Key symptoms: cough • wheezing • little or difficult-to-expectorate sputum

Secondary symptoms: fever • skin that feels hot to the touch • dry mouth

Tongue: red body • yellow coating

Pulse: thin • rapid

Abdomen: no specific signs

▶ CLINICAL NOTES

• This formula is specific for Lung fire as indicated by a high, clear-sounding cough with scanty sputum and forearms that are dry and hot to the touch. It does not dispel external pathogens or resolve constraint of Lung qi and is thus inappropriate for treating cough arising from these origins.

• The formula is very mild and balanced and thus particularly indicated for the treatment of children.

Contraindications: coughing and wheezing due to wind-cold, wind-heat, or phlegm-dampness

▶ FORMULAS WITH SIMILAR INDICATIONS

White Tiger Decoction (*bāi hú tāng*): For heat in the chest with strong sweating, thirst, and irritability.

Ephedra, Apricot Kernel, Gypsum, and Licorice Decoction (*má xìng shí gān tāng*): For coughing and wheezing due to heat constraint in the Lungs as indicated by bronchial spasms. Coughing fits are typically accompanied by sweating.

Arrest Wheezing Decoction (*dìng chuǎn tāng*): For wind-cold patterns complicated by phlegm-heat in the Lungs with thick, sticky phlegm.

COMPOSITION

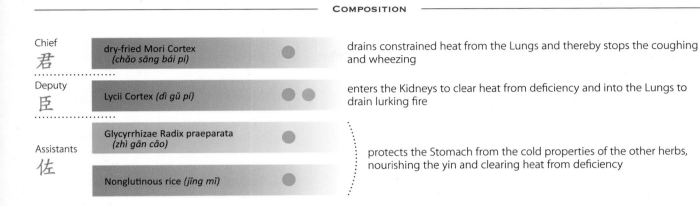

Chief 君	dry-fried Mori Cortex *(chǎo sāng bái pí)*	drains constrained heat from the Lungs and thereby stops the coughing and wheezing
Deputy 臣	Lycii Cortex *(dì gǔ pí)*	enters the Kidneys to clear heat from deficiency and into the Lungs to drain lurking fire
Assistants 佐	Glycyrrhizae Radix praeparata *(zhì gān cǎo)*	protects the Stomach from the cold properties of the other herbs, nourishing the yin and clearing heat from deficiency
	Nonglutinous rice *(jīng mǐ)*	

瀉黃散 （泻黄散）
Drain the Yellow Powder
xiè huáng săn

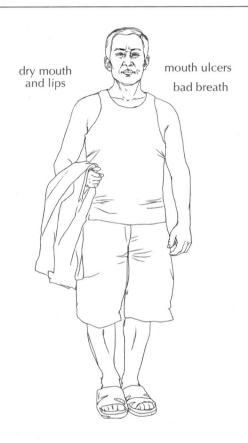

dry mouth and lips

mouth ulcers

bad breath

Key symptoms: mouth ulcers • bad breath • dry mouth and lips

Secondary symptoms: tongue thrusting • leaking of saliva from the corners of the mouth • frequent hunger

Tongue: red

Pulse: rapid

Abdomen: epigastric focal distention

▶ CLINICAL NOTES

• The formula treats fire constraint in the Spleen. Fire excess arises from the Stomach but fails to be discharged due to the presence of dampness in the Spleen. Compared with Stomach fire patterns, the heat is therefore less strong and there is no damage to the yin. The diagnosis can be made by the presence of apparently contradictory symptoms such as dry lips but leaking of saliva from the corners of the mouth, or tongue thrusting indicating constraint.

Contraindications: Stomach yin deficiency • qi deficiency

▶ FORMULAS WITH SIMILAR INDICATIONS

Clear the Stomach Powder (*qīng wèi săn*): For blazing fire in the Stomach with heat entering into the nutritive aspect and damaging the yin, fluids, and blood as reflected in bleeding gums and putrefaction.

─────── INGREDIENTS ───────

Gypsum fibrosum (*shí gāo*).. 15-20g
Gardeniae Fructus (*zhī zǐ*)....................................... 6-12g
dry-fried Saposhnikoviae Radix (*chǎo fáng fēng*)............ 9-15g
Pogostemonis/Agastaches Herba (*huò xiāng*)................. 9-15g
Glycyrrhizae Radix (*gān cǎo*).. 3-6g

Preparation notes: Originally, very different relative amounts of the ingredients were fried with honey and wine and then ground up; 3-6g were decocted in one cup of water.

Actions: clears lurking fire from the Spleen and Stomach

Main pattern: lurking fire in the Spleen

COMPOSITION

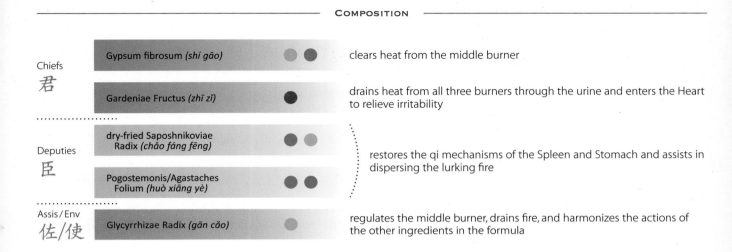

Chiefs
君

Gypsum fibrosum *(shí gāo)* — clears heat from the middle burner

Gardeniae Fructus *(zhī zǐ)* — drains heat from all three burners through the urine and enters the Heart to relieve irritability

Deputies
臣

dry-fried Saposhnikoviae Radix *(chǎo fáng fēng)*

Pogostemonis/Agastaches Folium *(huò xiāng yè)*

restores the qi mechanisms of the Spleen and Stomach and assists in dispersing the lurking fire

Assis / Env
佐/使

Glycyrrhizae Radix *(gān cǎo)* — regulates the middle burner, drains fire, and harmonizes the actions of the other ingredients in the formula

辛夷清肺飲（辛夷清肺饮）
Magnolia Flower Drink to Clear the Lungs
xīn yí qīng fèi yǐn

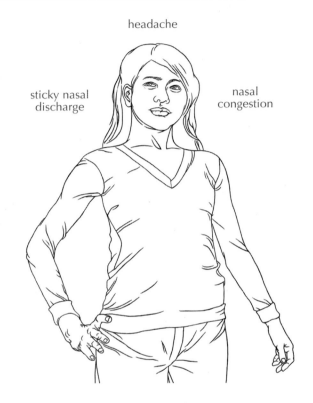

headache

sticky nasal discharge

nasal congestion

Main pattern: Lung heat leading to nasal congestion

Key symptoms: nasal congestion • sticky nasal discharge • headache

Secondary symptoms: thirst • throat pain

Tongue: red, dry body • yellow coating

Pulse: rapid

Abdomen: no specific signs

▶ CLINICAL NOTES

- This formula treats heat excess in the Lungs that impedes the Lung qi from reaching the nose, which in turn prevents the dispersing of wind and dampness resulting in the gradual formation of nasal congestion.
- This formula was originally used for the treatment of nasal polyps, but in contemporary practice it is more commonly used for nasal congestion related to disorders such as atrophic rhinitis, allergic rhinitis, or sinusitis.

Contraindications: Lung heat arising from fettering of the exterior by wind-cold or from yin deficiency

▶ FORMULAS WITH SIMILAR INDICATIONS

*Kudzu Decoction (*gé gēn tāng*) **plus Chuanxiong Rhizoma** (*chuān xiōng*) **and Magnoliae Flos** (*xīn yí*): For nasal congestion due to wind-cold fettering the exterior leading to heat constraint in the yang brightness channel as characterized by neck pain or stiffness, fever, aversion to cold, and a superficial pulse.

*Schizonepeta and Forsythia Decoction (*jīng jiè lián qiào tang*): For wind-heat attacking the upper body leading to nasal congestion due to constraint in the Kidney and Gallbladder channels.

INGREDIENTS

Magnoliae Flos (*xīn yí*) 2.5g

Scutellariae Radix (*huáng qín*) 3g

Gardeniae Fructus (*zhī zǐ*) 3g

Ophiopogonis Radix (*mài mén dōng*) 3g

Lilii Bulbus (*bǎi hé*) 3g

Gypsum fibrosum (*shí gāo*) 3g

Glycyrrhizae Radix (*gān cǎo*) 1.5g

Eriobotryae Folium (*pí pá yè*) 3g

Anemarrhenae Rhizoma (*zhī mǔ*) 3g

Cimicifugae Rhizoma (*shēng má*) 1g

Actions: disseminates Lung qi • clears heat • unblocks the orifices (specifically the nose)

COMPOSITION

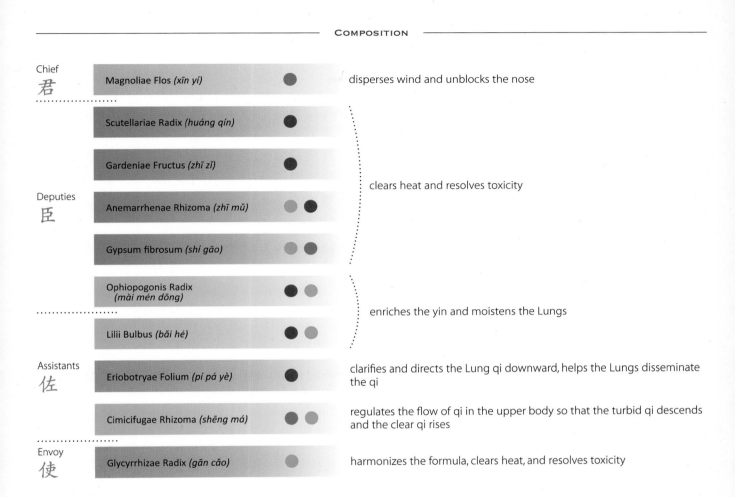

Chief 君	Magnoliae Flos *(xīn yí)*	disperses wind and unblocks the nose
Deputies 臣	Scutellariae Radix *(huáng qín)*	
	Gardeniae Fructus *(zhī zǐ)*	clears heat and resolves toxicity
	Anemarrhenae Rhizoma *(zhī mǔ)*	
	Gypsum fibrosum *(shí gāo)*	
	Ophiopogonis Radix *(mài mén dōng)*	enriches the yin and moistens the Lungs
	Lilii Bulbus *(bǎi hé)*	
Assistants 佐	Eriobotryae Folium *(pí pá yè)*	clarifies and directs the Lung qi downward, helps the Lungs disseminate the qi
	Cimicifugae Rhizoma *(shēng má)*	regulates the flow of qi in the upper body so that the turbid qi descends and the clear qi rises
Envoy 使	Glycyrrhizae Radix *(gān cǎo)*	harmonizes the formula, clears heat, and resolves toxicity

杏蘇散（杏苏散）
Apricot Kernel and Perilla Leaf Powder
xìng sū săn

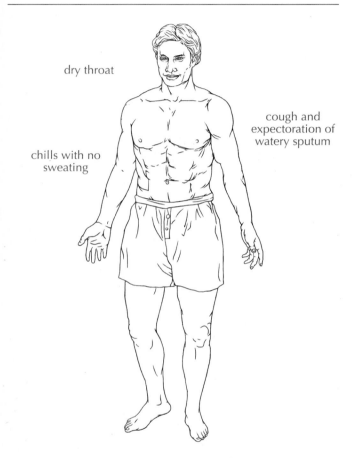

dry throat

cough and
expectoration of
watery sputum

chills with no
sweating

INGREDIENTS

Perillae Folium (*zǐ sū yè*) 6-9g
Peucedani Radix (*qián hú*) 6-9g
Armeniacae Semen (*xìng rén*) 6-9g
Platycodi Radix (*jié gěng*) 6g
Aurantii Fructus (*zhǐ ké*) 6g
Citri reticulatae Pericarpium (*chén pí*) 6g
Poria (*fú líng*) 6-9g
Pinelliae Rhizoma praeparatum (*zhì bàn xià*) 6-9g
Zingiberis Rhizoma recens (*shēng jiāng*) .... 2-3 pieces
Jujubae Fructus (*dà zǎo*) .... 2-3 pieces

Glycyrrhizae Radix (*gān cǎo*) 3g

Actions: gently disperses cool-dryness • disseminates Lung qi • transforms thin mucus

Main pattern: externally-contracted cool-dryness

Key symptoms: chills with no sweating • cough and expectoration of watery sputum • dry throat

Secondary symptoms: slight headache • stuffy nose

Tongue: dry body • white coating

Pulse: wiry

Abdomen: no specific signs

► CLINICAL NOTES

• This formula resolves cool-dryness fettering the exterior and constraining the downward-directing function of the Lungs. Thus the key markers of this pattern are the seemingly contradictory signs of dry throat and cough with expectoration of watery sputum. This comes about as cold and dryness amplify each other's effect in constraining the qi dynamic of the Lungs.

• This formula can be used to treat both acute and chronic conditions, such as common colds and upper respiratory infections throughout the year, as long as the indications match those associated with externally-contracted cool-dryness.

Contraindications: cough due to warm-dryness

► FORMULAS WITH SIMILAR INDICATIONS

Mulberry Leaf and Apricot Kernel Decoction (*sāng xìng tāng*): For warm-dryness at the protective level characterized by moderate fever, a dry cough or one with scanty, thick, and sticky sputum, irritability, and a floating, rough pulse.

Stop Coughing Powder (*zhǐ sòu săn*): For cough due to wind-cold where the original pathogen has been essentially resolved but the Lung qi remains constrained. This pattern is characterized by cough with phlegm that is difficult to expectorate and an aversion to drafts that is minimal or entirely absent.

COMPOSITION

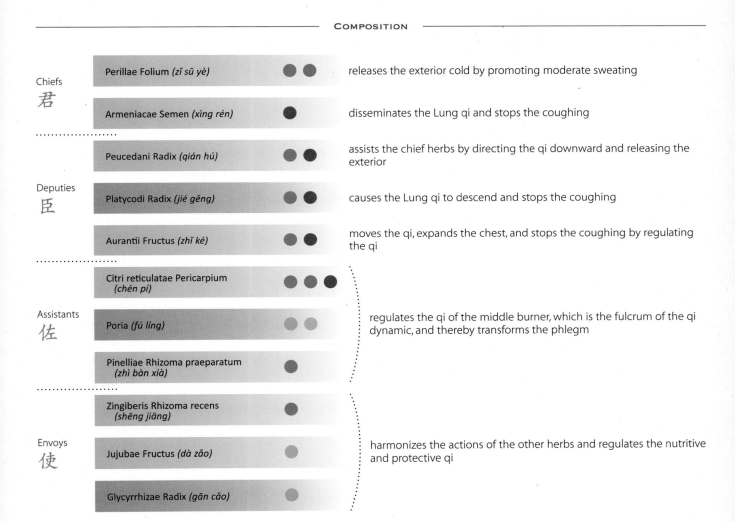

Chiefs
君

Perillae Folium (zǐ sū yè) — releases the exterior cold by promoting moderate sweating

Armeniacae Semen (xìng rén) — disseminates the Lung qi and stops the coughing

Deputies
臣

Peucedani Radix (qián hú) — assists the chief herbs by directing the qi downward and releasing the exterior

Platycodi Radix (jié gěng) — causes the Lung qi to descend and stops the coughing

Aurantii Fructus (zhǐ ké) — moves the qi, expands the chest, and stops the coughing by regulating the qi

Assistants
佐

Citri reticulatae Pericarpium (chén pí)

Poria (fú líng)

regulates the qi of the middle burner, which is the fulcrum of the qi dynamic, and thereby transforms the phlegm

Pinelliae Rhizoma praeparatum (zhì bàn xià)

Envoys
使

Zingiberis Rhizoma recens (shēng jiāng)

Jujubae Fructus (dà zǎo)

harmonizes the actions of the other herbs and regulates the nutritive and protective qi

Glycyrrhizae Radix (gān cǎo)

宣痹湯（宣痹汤）
Disband Painful Obstruction Decoction
xuān bì tāng

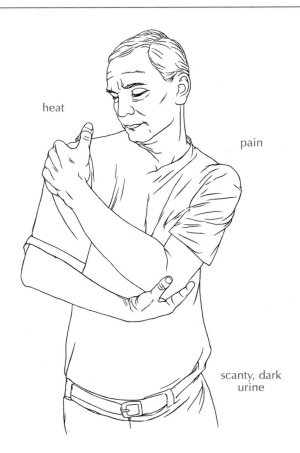

heat

pain

scanty, dark urine

INGREDIENTS

Stephaniae tetrandrae Radix (*hàn fáng jǐ*) 15g

Armeniacae Semen (*xìng rén*) 15g

Talcum (*huá shí*) 15g

Forsythiae Fructus (*lián qiào*) 9g

Gardeniae Fructus (*zhī zǐ*) 9g

Coicis Semen (*yì yǐ rén*) 15g

Pinelliae Rhizoma praeparatum (*zhì bàn xià*) 9g

Bombycis Faeces (*cán shā*) 9g

Phaseoli Semen (*chì xiǎo dòu*) 9g

Actions: clears and resolves damp-heat • unblocks the channels

• disbands painful obstruction

Main pattern: painful obstruction due to damp-heat in the channels and collaterals

Key symptoms: heat and pain in the joints • reduced mobility

Secondary symptoms: fever and shaking chills • a lusterless, yellow complexion • scanty, dark urine • focal distention in the chest and upper abdomen

Tongue: yellow or gray, greasy coating

Pulse: soft • soggy

Abdomen: no specific signs

► CLINICAL NOTES

• For damp-heat painful obstruction of the Triple Bruner qi dynamic that manifests predominantly with painful obstruction of the channels and collaterals. Heat and dampness are equally pronounced. In addition to stiffness, pain, and a sensation of heat in the joints that may be subjective or palpable (sometimes only on prolonged or deep pressure), reduced urination with dark urine, focal distention in the chest and upper abdomen, a soggy or soft pulse, and a greasy tongue coating also point to the pattern for which this formula is indicated.

Contraindications: wind-damp-cold painful obstruction

► FORMULAS WITH SIMILAR INDICATIONS

Tangkuei Decoction to Pry Out Pain (*dāng guī niān tòng tāng*): For damp-heat painful obstruction accompanied by manifestations of externally-contracted wind. This formula also deals with a more complex presentation that includes both blood stasis and blood and qi deficiency.

──────────────────────── **COMPOSITION** ────────────────────────

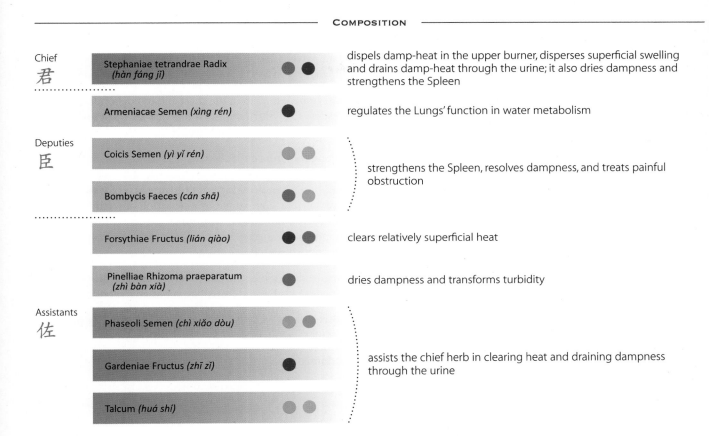

Chief
君

Stephaniae tetrandrae Radix
(hàn fáng jǐ)

dispels damp-heat in the upper burner, disperses superficial swelling and drains damp-heat through the urine; it also dries dampness and strengthens the Spleen

Armeniacae Semen (xìng rén)

regulates the Lungs' function in water metabolism

Deputies
臣

Coicis Semen (yì yǐ rén)

Bombycis Faeces (cán shā)

strengthens the Spleen, resolves dampness, and treats painful obstruction

Forsythiae Fructus (lián qiào)

clears relatively superficial heat

Pinelliae Rhizoma praeparatum
(zhì bàn xià)

dries dampness and transforms turbidity

Assistants
佐

Phaseoli Semen (chì xiǎo dòu)

Gardeniae Fructus (zhī zǐ)

assists the chief herb in clearing heat and draining dampness through the urine

Talcum (huá shí)

血府逐瘀湯 (血府逐瘀汤)
Drive Out Stasis from the Mansion of Blood Decoction
xuè fǔ zhú yū tāng

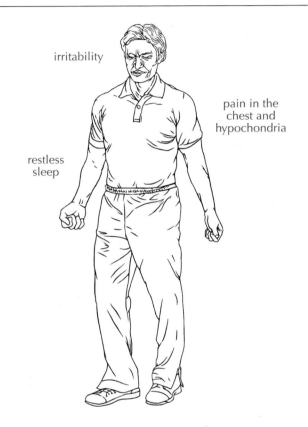

irritability

pain in the chest and hypochondria

restless sleep

Actions: invigorates the blood • dispels blood stasis • spreads the Liver qi • unblocks the channels

Main pattern: blood and qi stasis in the chest with impairment of blood flow in the area above the diaphragm

Key symptoms: pain in the chest and hypochondria • restless sleep • irritability • fevers that are most severe in early night and disappear by morning

Secondary symptoms: chronic, stubborn headache with a fixed, piercing quality • chronic, incessant hiccup • choking sensation when drinking • dry heaves • loss of visual acuity • low spirits accompanied by a sensation of warmth in the chest • palpitations • insomnia • excessive dreaming • unprovoked anger • extreme mood swings • evening tidal fever • purplish lips, complexion, or sclera

Tongue: dark red or purplish body • dark purplish spots on the sides • visible and distended sublingual blood vessels

Pulse: choppy • wiry and tight • may also be racing or irregular

Abdomen: no specific signs

▶ CLINICAL NOTES

- This formula treats blood stasis in the chest and diaphragmatic region that leads to, or is combined with, qi constraint. Because this affects the systemic circulation of qi and blood, it can produce the very wide range of symptoms listed above. Key clinical markers are as follows: pain, if present, will be fixed in location and stabbing in nature; symptoms will often worsen toward evening and early in the night. In fact, Wang Qing-Ren, the author of this formula, identified feverishness in the latter half of the day that becomes more severe in the first half of the night and disappears by morning to be the main clinical marker.

- Because all chronic and unexplained symptoms can be related to blood stasis, this formula is used to treat stubborn problems that have not responded to other treatment, or so-called 'strange' symptoms that defy explanation by common pathophysiological mechanisms.

Contraindications: blood stasis associated with deficiency

INGREDIENTS

Persicae Semen (*táo rén*)... 12g
Carthami Flos (*hóng huā*).. 9g
Angelicae sinensis Radix (*dāng guī*) 9g
Chuanxiong Rhizoma (*chuān xiōng*) 4.5g
Paeoniae Radix rubra (*chì sháo*)... 6g
Achyranthis bidentatae Radix (*niú xī*).................................. 9g
Bupleuri Radix (*chái hú*) 3g
Platycodi Radix (*jié gěng*) 4.5g
Aurantii Fructus (*zhǐ ké*).. 6g
Rehmanniae Radix (*shēng dì huáng*).................................... 9g
Glycyrrhizae Radix (*gān cǎo*) 6g

▶ FORMULAS WITH SIMILAR INDICATIONS

Peach Pit Decoction to Order the Qi (*táo hé chéng qì tāng*): For blood stasis in the lower abdomen with upward flushing of heat.

Salvia Drink (*dān shēn yǐn*): For blood stasis and qi stagnation that gives rise to pain in the chest and epigastrium accompanied by heat signs. This formula is specific for the chest, flanks, and epigastric region.

COMPOSITION

Chiefs
君

Persicae Semen (*táo rén*)

Carthami Flos (*hóng huā*)

Chuanxiong Rhizoma (*chuān xiōng*)

invigorates the blood and dispels blood stasis, particularly in the upper part of the body

Deputies
臣

Angelicae sinensis Radix (*dāng guī*)

Paeoniae Radix rubra (*chì sháo*)

Rehmanniae Radix (*shēng dì huáng*)

enables the formula to dispel blood stasis without injuring the yin and blood

Achyranthis bidentatae Radix (*niú xī*)

improves the circulation by eliminating blood stasis and inducing the downward movement of blood

Assistants
佐

Bupleuri Radix (*chái hú*)

smooths the flow of Liver qi, relieves constraint, and raises the clear yang

Platycodi Radix (*jié gěng*)

Aurantii Fructus (*zhǐ ké*)

expands the chest and promotes the movement of qi

Envoy
使

Glycyrrhizae Radix (*gān cǎo*)

regulates and harmonizes the actions of the other herbs

一貫煎（一贯煎）
Linking Decoction
yī guàn jiān

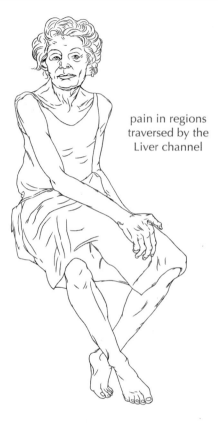

indistinct or faint burning pain in the epigastrium

pain in regions traversed by the Liver channel

INGREDIENTS

Rehmanniae Radix (*shēng dì huáng*)............................. 15-30g
Lycii Fructus (*gǒu qǐ zǐ*)... 9-18g
Glehniae Radix (*běi shā shēn*).................................... 9g
Ophiopogonis Radix (*mài mén dōng*) 9g
Angelicae sinensis Radix (*dāng guī*) 9g
Toosendan Fructus (*chuān liàn zǐ*).............................. 4.5g

Actions: enriches the yin • spreads the Liver qi

Main pattern: yin deficiency of the Liver and Kidneys with qi stagnation in the Liver channel

Key symptoms: pain in regions traversed by the Liver channel (epigastric pain, hypochondriac pain, chest pain, menstrual pain, pain in the groin and lower abdomen) • indistinct or faint burning pain in the epigastrium • dry and parched mouth and throat

Secondary symptoms: acid regurgitation • amenorrhea

Tongue: red and dry body

Pulse: thin and frail or deficient and wiry

Abdomen: tense rectus abdominis muscle

▶ CLINICAL NOTES

• This is the primary formula for Liver constraint due to blood and yin deficiency. The main symptom is pain in any area traversed by the Liver channel. Headaches are generally due to Liver wind or Liver yang and thus not a primary indication. Also, Liver qi constraint readily moves horizontally into the Stomach generating secondary symptoms of acid regurgitation, bitter taste, or epigastric pain.

• The pulse will vary depending on the relative intensity of the yin deficiency and constraint. When yin deficiency predominates, the pulse will be thin and frail, but when constraint is more significant, the pulse will be deficient and wiry.

Contraindications: pain involving dampness, phlegm, and thin mucus

▶ FORMULAS WITH SIMILAR INDICATIONS

Frigid Extremities Powder (*sì nì sǎn*): For Liver constraint with heat in the interior and cold extremities and no signs of yin deficiency.

Rambling Powder (*xiāo yáo sǎn*): For Liver constraint associated with blood and qi deficiency that affects the Spleen.

COMPOSITION

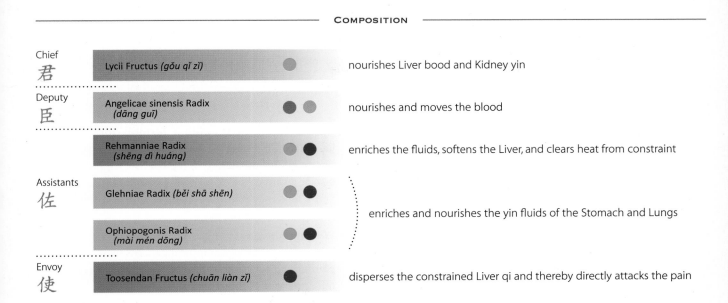

Chief 君	Lycii Fructus *(gǒu qǐ zǐ)*		nourishes Liver bood and Kidney yin
Deputy 臣	Angelicae sinensis Radix *(dāng guī)*		nourishes and moves the blood
	Rehmanniae Radix *(shēng dì huáng)*		enriches the fluids, softens the Liver, and clears heat from constraint
Assistants 佐	Glehniae Radix *(běi shā shēn)*		enriches and nourishes the yin fluids of the Stomach and Lungs
	Ophiopogonis Radix *(mài mén dōng)*		
Envoy 使	Toosendan Fructus *(chuān liàn zǐ)*		disperses the constrained Liver qi and thereby directly attacks the pain

茵陳蒿湯 (茵陈蒿汤)
Virgate Wormwood Decoction
yīn chén hāo tāng

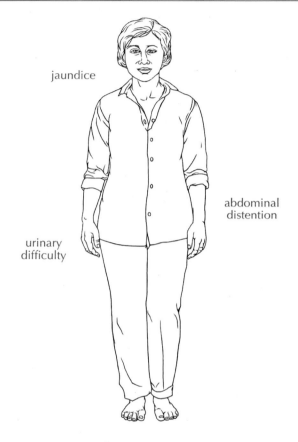

jaundice

urinary difficulty

abdominal distention

Tongue: yellow, greasy coating

Pulse: slippery, rapid, forceful • deep and rapid

Abdomen: slight abdominal distention

▶ CLINICAL NOTES

- This is the most important formula for yang-type jaundice. This type of jaundice has more heat than dampness, as manifested in the relative brightness of the discoloration of the skin and eyes. Abdominal distention and a tendency towards constipation reveal the internal nature of the dampness.

- With appropriate additions, the formula can also be used to treat lower burner damp-heat patterns manifesting with painful urinary dribbling, acute, itchy skin disorders, or inflammation of the oral cavity.

Contraindications: yin-type jaundice or jaundice in which dampness predominates • use with extreme caution during pregnancy

▶ FORMULAS WITH SIMILAR INDICATIONS

*Gardenia and Phellodendron Decoction (*zhī zǐ bǎi pí tāng*): Focuses on jaundice due to heat arising from constraint in the muscle layer without heat stasis in the interior. There will be palpitations and reduced urination, but no abdominal distention.

▬ INGREDIENTS ▬

Artemisiae scopariae Herba (*yīn chén*) 18g
Gardeniae Fructus (*zhī zǐ*).. 9-12g
Rhei Radix et Rhizoma (*dà huáng*)...................................... 6g

Actions: clears heat • resolves dampness • reduces jaundice

Main pattern: yang-type jaundice

Key symptoms: whole-body jaundice with a color that resembles a 'fresh tangerine' • slight abdominal distention • urinary difficulty

Secondary symptoms: no sweating or sweating only from the head • thirst • tendency towards constipation

────────── COMPOSITION ──────────

Chief 君	Artemisiae scopariae Herba *(yīn chén)*	● ●	treats all types of jaundice, especially due to damp-heat
Deputy 臣	Gardeniae Fructus *(zhī zǐ)*	●	clears heat from the three burners, and more specifically, drains damp-heat through the urine
Assistant 佐	Rhei Radix et Rhizoma *(dà huáng)*	●	purges heat, eliminates stasis heat, directs downward, and facilitates the expression of pathogenic toxin retained by the clogging of the qi dynamic by damp-heat

銀翹散（银翘散）
Honeysuckle and Forsythia Powder
yín qiáo sǎn

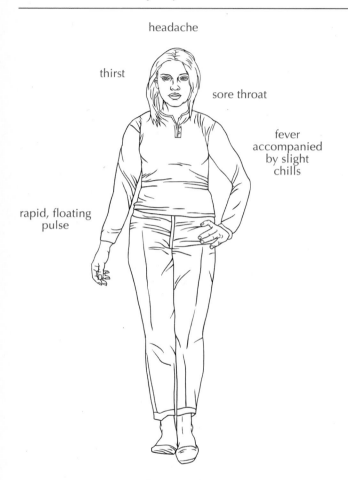

headache

thirst

sore throat

fever
accompanied
by slight
chills

rapid, floating
pulse

INGREDIENTS

Lonicerae Flos (*jīn yín huā*) 9g
Forsythiae Fructus (*lián qiào*) 9g
Platycodi Radix (*jié gěng*)... 6g
Arctii Fructus (*niú bàng zǐ*) 9g
Menthae haplocalycis Herba (*bò hé*)............ [add near end] 6g
Sojae Semen praeparatum (*dàn dòu chǐ*) 5g
Schizonepetae Herba (*jīng jiè*) 5g
Lophatheri Herba (*dàn zhú yè*)... 4g
Phragmitis Rhizoma recens (*xiān lú gēn*) 15-30g

Glycyrrhizae Radix (*gān cǎo*)...5g

Preparation notes: Do not cook for more than 20 minutes.

Actions: disperses wind-heat • clears heat • resolves toxicity

Main patterns: early stage warm pathogen disorders • wind-heat toxins invading the Lungs and upper burner protective qi

Key symptoms: fever accompanied by slight chills, or chills only for a very brief period before aversion to heat develops • thirst • sore throat

Secondary symptoms: mild or no sweating • headache • cough

Tongue: red tip with a thin, white or thin, yellow coating

Pulse: rapid • floating (particularly in the right distal position)

Abdomen: no specific signs

► CLINICAL NOTES

• For early stage wind-heat pathogen disorders due to heat toxin. This is characterized by a distinctive subjective feeling of coming down with something, as opposed to just having a sore throat.

• Slight chills are not a contraindication for this formula as they can indicate that the pathogen is located in the protective qi aspect.

• Combines acrid, cool, light, and aromatic herbs to treat foul turbidity and toxic heat at the protective level. Should be given frequently in relatively high dosage (especially true for the chief herbs that resolve heat toxin).

• For best results the source text recommends the following modifications: for a stifling sensation in the chest, add Pogostemonis/Agastaches Herba (*huò xiāng*); for severe thirst, add Trichosanthis Radix (*tiān huā fěn*); for severe sore throat, add Lasiosphaera/Calvatia (*mǎ bó*) and Scrophulariae Radix (*xuán shēn*); for pronounced cough, add Armeniacae Semen (*xìng rén*); for heat entering the interior accompanied by scant urine, add Rehmanniae Radix (*shēng dì huáng*), Ophiopogonis Radix (*mài mén dōng*), Scutellariae Radix (*huáng qín*), Anemarrhenae Rhizoma (*zhī mǔ*), and Gardeniae Fructus (*zhī zǐ*); for nosebleed, remove Schizonepetae Herba (*jīng jiè*) and Sojae Semen praeparatum (*dàn dòu chǐ*) and add Imperatae Rhizoma (*bái máo gēn*) and Gardeniae Fructus (*zhī zǐ*).

Contraindications: similar presentations of early stage damp-heat or wind-cold patterns

▶ FORMULAS WITH SIMILAR INDICATIONS

Mulberry Leaf and Chrysanthemum Drink (*sāng jú yǐn*): Focuses on venting the Lungs rather than on resolving toxicity, and is indicated for less severe cases marked by coughing.

Sweet Dew Special Pill to Eliminate Toxin (*gān lù xiāo dú dān*): For damp-heat toxin obstructing the upper burner where the throat is swollen in addition to being painful, accompanied by a heavy head and aching muscles.

COMPOSITION

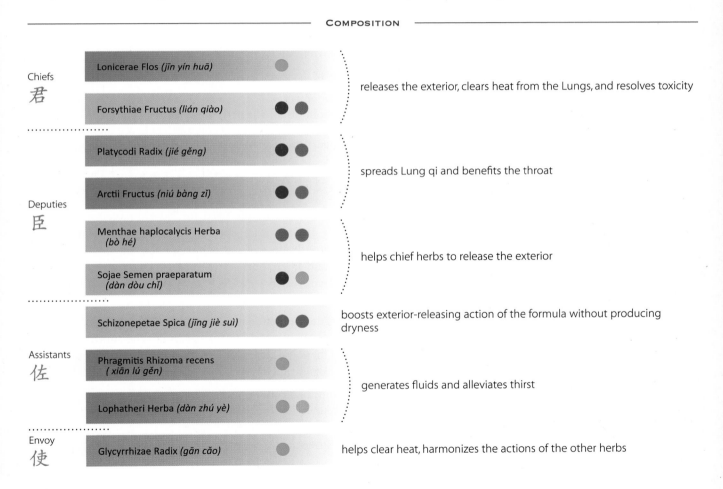

Chiefs 君

Lonicerae Flos (*jīn yín huā*) ● — releases the exterior, clears heat from the Lungs, and resolves toxicity

Forsythiae Fructus (*lián qiào*) ● ●

Deputies 臣

Platycodi Radix (*jié gěng*) ● ● — spreads Lung qi and benefits the throat

Arctii Fructus (*niú bàng zǐ*) ● ●

Menthae haplocalycis Herba (*bò hé*) ● ● — helps chief herbs to release the exterior

Sojae Semen praeparatum (*dàn dòu chǐ*) ● ●

Assistants 佐

Schizonepetae Spica (*jīng jiè suì*) ● ● — boosts exterior-releasing action of the formula without producing dryness

Phragmitis Rhizoma recens (*xiān lú gěn*) ● — generates fluids and alleviates thirst

Lophatheri Herba (*dàn zhú yè*) ● ●

Envoy 使

Glycyrrhizae Radix (*gān cǎo*) ● — helps clear heat, harmonizes the actions of the other herbs

右歸丸（右归丸）
Restore the Right [Kidney] Pill
yòu guī wán

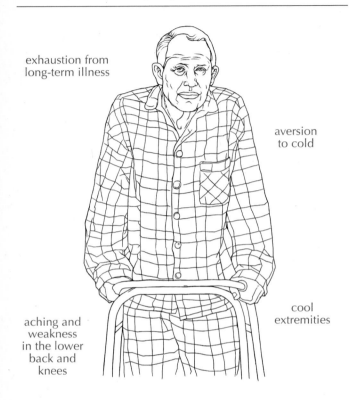

exhaustion from long-term illness

aversion to cold

aching and weakness in the lower back and knees

cool extremities

INGREDIENTS
---

[1]Aconiti Radix lateralis praeparata (*zhì fù zǐ*) 6g
Cinnamomi Cortex (*ròu guì*) 6g
Cervi Cornus Colla (*lù jiǎo jiāo*) 9g
Rehmanniae Radix praeparata (*shú dì huáng*) 15g
Corni Fructus (*shān zhū yú*)... 9g
Dioscoreae Rhizoma (*shān yào*) 9g
Lycii Fructus (*gǒu qǐ zǐ*)... 9g
Cuscutae Semen (*tù sī zǐ*) 9g
Eucommiae Cortex (*dù zhòng*)... 9g

---

1. This ingredient may be difficult to obtain because of legal issues. Psoraleae Fructus (*bǔ gǔ zhī*), Alpiniae oxyphyllae Fructus (*yì zhì rén*), Cynomorii Herba (*suǒ yáng*), or Epimedii Herba (*yín yáng huò*) may be substituted.

Angelicae sinensis Radix (*dāng guī*) 9g

Actions: warms and tonifies the Kidney yang • replenishes the essence • tonifies the blood

Main pattern: Kidney yang deficiency with waning of the fire at the gate of vitality

Key symptoms: exhaustion from long-term illness • aversion to cold • cool extremities • aching and weakness in the lower back and knees

Secondary symptoms: impotence • spermatorrhea • infertility • loose stools with undigested food particles • incontinence

Tongue: pale, scanty coating without luster

Pulse: deep and frail in the proximal positions

Abdomen: weak abdomen • hypertonicity of rectus abdominis muscle in the lower abdomen accompanied by a palpable weakness in the area between these muscles • pencil-line tightness of linea alba below the umbilicus

▶ CLINICAL NOTES

• Most commonly used for elderly patients and those suffering from chronic diseases with symptoms of insufficiency of source yang in both the middle (Spleen) and lower burners (Kidneys). This root insufficiency is revealed by a deep and frail pulse in the proximal positions.

• Many practitioners like to add Ginseng Radix (*rén shēn*) to this formula to further tonify the source qi. Unless there are clear signs contraindicating such usage (e.g., significant hypertension), this can be a useful addition.

Contraindications: Kidney deficiency accompanied by dampness or the presence of external pathogens

▶ FORMULAS WITH SIMILAR INDICATIONS

Kidney Qi Pill (*shèn qì wán*): For Kidney qi deficiency patterns with signs of floating yang in the upper body or water accumulation in the lower body.

──────────────── COMPOSITION ────────────────

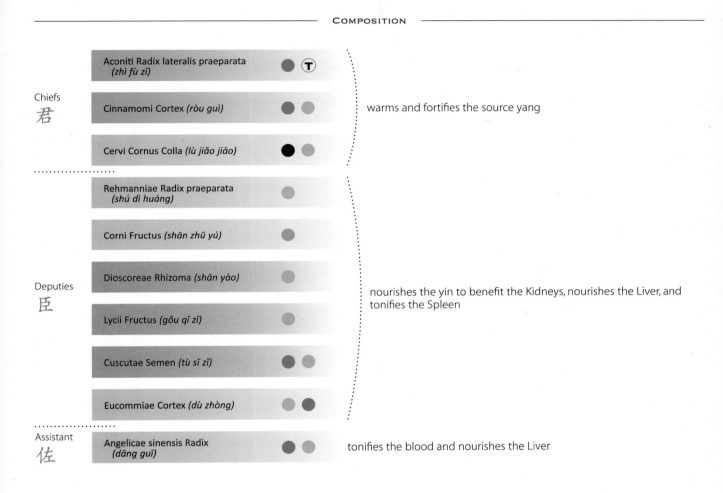

Chiefs
君

Aconiti Radix lateralis praeparata
(zhì fù zǐ)

Cinnamomi Cortex *(ròu guì)*

Cervi Cornus Colla *(lù jiǎo jiāo)*

warms and fortifies the source yang

Deputies
臣

Rehmanniae Radix praeparata
(shú dì huáng)

Corni Fructus *(shān zhū yú)*

Dioscoreae Rhizoma *(shān yào)*

Lycii Fructus *(gǒu qǐ zǐ)*

Cuscutae Semen *(tù sī zǐ)*

Eucommiae Cortex *(dù zhòng)*

nourishes the yin to benefit the Kidneys, nourishes the Liver, and tonifies the Spleen

Assistant
佐

Angelicae sinensis Radix
(dāng guī)

tonifies the blood and nourishes the Liver

玉屏風散 （玉屏风散）
Jade Windscreen Powder
yù píng fēng sǎn

shiny, pale complexion

aversion to drafts

spontaneous sweating

Secondary symptoms: recurrent colds

Tongue: pale body • white coating

Pulse: floating • deficient • soft

Abdomen: may be damp on palpation • lack of tonus of abdominal muscles • splashing sounds

▶ CLINICAL NOTES

• This is the primary formula for spontaneous sweating from qi deficiency. It is also very useful for patients who have a weak and inappropriate protective response to external invasions. This may manifest as a tendency to catch colds or as allergies, specifically allergies involving the upper respiratory system or skin (such as allergic rhinitis, hay fever, or allergic urticaria).

• By increasing the dosage of Saposhnikoviae Radix (*fáng fēng*) in relation to the qi-tonifying components of the formula by as much as 2:1:1, the formula can also be used to treat lingering colds in weak patients. This modification should not, however, be used to treat patients in whom the presence of an exterior pathogen is pronounced.

▶ FORMULAS WITH SIMILAR INDICATIONS

Cinnamon Twig Decoction (*guì zhī tāng*): For a similar presentation, but one due to disharmony between the nutritive and protective qi in the exterior of the body with more pronounced symptoms of cold, hypertonicity, and rebellious qi and less severe qi deficiency.

── INGREDIENTS ──

Astragali Radix (*huáng qí*)..12g

Atractylodis macrocephalae Rhizoma (*bái zhú*) 12g

Saposhnikoviae Radix (*fáng fēng*)......................................6g

Jujubae Fructus (*dà zǎo*).. 1 piece

Actions: augments the qi • stabilizes the exterior • stops sweating

Main pattern: deficiency of the exterior with weak and unstable protective qi

Key symptoms: aversion to drafts • spontaneous sweating • shiny, pale complexion

---
COMPOSITION

Chief
君
Astragali Radix *(huáng qí)*   ●   strengthens the qi and stabilizes the exterior

....

Deputy
臣
Atractylodis macrocephalae
   Rhizoma *(bái zhú)*   ● ●   strengthens the Spleen and augments the qi

....

Assistant
佐
Saposhnikoviae Radix *(fáng fēng)*   ● ●   expels wind

....

Envoy
使
Jujubae Fructus *(dà zǎo)*   ●   tonifies qi and generates fluids

玉泉丸
Jade Spring Pill
yù quán wán

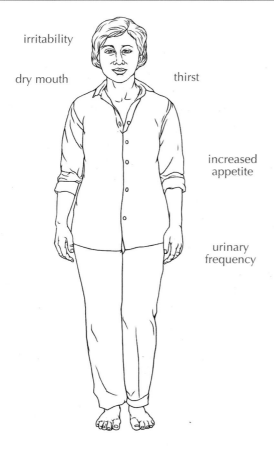

irritability

dry mouth

thirst

increased appetite

urinary frequency

Actions: augments the qi • nourishes the yin • clears heat • generates yang fluids

Main pattern: wasting and thirsting disorder (消渴 *xiāo kě*)

Key symptoms: irritability • thirst • urinary frequency • dry mouth • increased appetite

Secondary symptoms: weight loss • fatigue

Tongue: red and dry body

Pulse: large • deficient • rapid

Abdomen: no specific signs

▶ CLINICAL NOTES

- This is a specific formula for deficiency of the Spleen and Lungs, which fail to transport fluids, leading to a pattern that combines deficiency of fluids with heat constraint.
- Although the formula is specific for wasting and thirsting disorder, which overlaps to some extent with the biomedical disease category of diabetes, it should only be prescribed after careful pattern differentiation.

Contraindications: wasting and thirsting disorder involving damp-heat, phlegm, or constipation

▶ FORMULAS WITH SIMILAR INDICATIONS

*White Tiger plus Ginseng Decoction (*bái hǔ jiā rén shēn tāng*): For upper burner wasting and thirsting disorders with significant heat excess and less deficiency.

INGREDIENTS

Ophiopogonis Radix (*mài mén dōng*) ..... [remove center] 37.5g

Ginseng Radix (*rén shēn*)....................................37.5g

Poria (*fú líng*)....................................37.5g

Astragali Radix (*huáng qí*)
..........................[half honey-fried and half untreated] 37.5g

Mume Fructus (*wū méi*)................................[roasted] 37.5g

Glycyrrhizae Radix (*gān cǎo*)....................................37.5g

Trichosanthis Radix (*tiān huā fěn*)....................................56g

Puerariae Radix (*gé gēn*)....................................56g

Preparation notes: Taken as a prepared medicine.

COMPOSITION

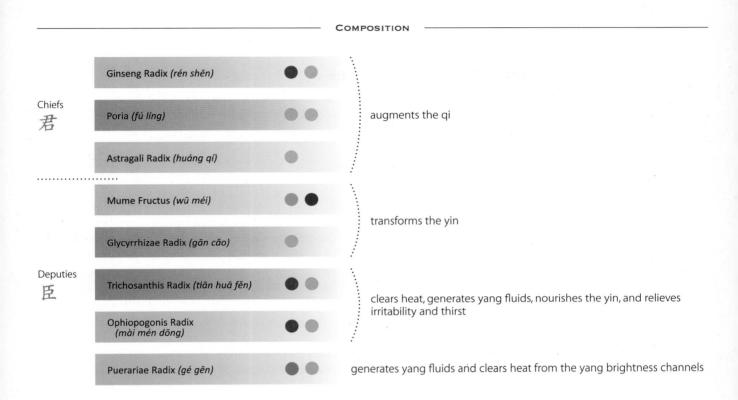

Chiefs
君

Ginseng Radix *(rén shēn)*

Poria *(fú líng)*

Astragali Radix *(huáng qí)*

augments the qi

Mume Fructus *(wū méi)*

Glycyrrhizae Radix *(gān cǎo)*

transforms the yin

Deputies
臣

Trichosanthis Radix *(tiān huā fěn)*

Ophiopogonis Radix
(mài mén dōng)

clears heat, generates yang fluids, nourishes the yin, and relieves irritability and thirst

Puerariae Radix *(gé gēn)*

generates yang fluids and clears heat from the yang brightness channels

越鞠丸
Escape Restraint Pill
yuè jū wán

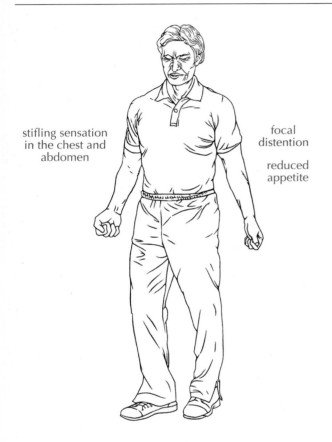

stifling sensation in the chest and abdomen

focal distention

reduced appetite

INGREDIENTS

Atractylodis Rhizoma (*cāng zhú*) 6g
Chuanxiong Rhizoma (*chuān xiōng*) 6g
Cyperi Rhizoma (*xiāng fù*) 6g
Gardeniae Fructus (*zhī zǐ*) 6g
Massa medicata fermentata (*shén qū*) 9g

Actions: promotes the movement of qi • releases constraint

Main pattern: qi constraint that may involve dampness, phlegm, fire, blood stasis, or food stagnation

Key symptoms: focal distention • stifling sensation in the chest and abdomen

Secondary symptoms: fixed pain in the hypochondria • belching • vomiting • acid reflux • mild coughing with copious sputum • reduced appetite • indigestion

Tongue: greasy coating

Pulse: varies depending on the type of stagnation, but should not be deficient or soft

Abdomen: focal distention in the epigastrium

▶ CLINICAL NOTES

- This is a core formula for treating any type of qi constraint in the middle burner and its consequences, including the presence and formation of dampness, phlegm, fire, blood stasis, or food stagnation. Any of these secondary pathologies may arise from qi constraint or may, in turn, lead to its formation. It therefore has a very wide range of indications including not just digestive problems with distention, pain, and difficulty in digesting certain foods, but also angina and diseases of the arterial circulation, gynecological conditions such as pelvic inflammatory disease, irregular or painful menstruation, and infertility in women who exhibit accumulation of dampness and phlegm.

- In light of the above, it is best to view this formula not as a ready-made prescription but as a model that can be flexibly applied in clinical practice, including or omitting ingredients as required, and adapting their dosage to the presenting pattern.

- If qi stagnation is pronounced, one may increase the dosage of Cyperi Rhizoma (*xiāng fù*) and add Linderae Radix (*wū yào*) or Aucklandiae Radix (*mù xiāng*). If blood stasis is pronounced, increase the dosage of Chuanxiong Rhizoma (*chuān xiōng*) and add Persicae Semen (*táo rén*) and Carthami Flos (*hóng huā*). If dampness is pronounced, increase the dosage of Atractylodis Rhizoma (*cāng zhú*) and add Poria (*fú líng*) and Angelicae dahuricae Radix (*bái zhǐ*). If food stagnation is pronounced, increase the dosage of Massa medicata fermentata (*shén qū*) and add Crataegi Fructus (*shān zhā*) and Hordei Fructus germinatus (*mài yá*). If fire constraint is pronounced, increase the dosage of Gardeniae Fructus (*zhī zǐ*) and add Scutellariae Radix (*huáng qín*) and Indigo naturalis (*qīng dài*). If phlegm is pronounced, add Pinelliae Rhizoma praeparatum (*zhì bàn xià*) and Trichosanthis Fructus (*guā lóu*).

- Although qi constraint often has emotional causes, such issues are not a necessary condition for the use of this formula.

Contraindications: stagnation or constraint due to deficiency

► FORMULAS WITH SIMILAR INDICATIONS

Rambling Powder (*xiāo yáo sǎn*): Specific for Liver qi con-straint, which has blood and qi deficiency at its root. This pattern is marked by lack of appetite and fatigue.

Pinellia and Magnolia Bark Decoction (*bàn xià hòu pò tāng*): For stagnation of qi and phlegm manifesting as plum-pit qi or other symptoms indicating an obstruction of the body's function of directing qi and fluids downward.

Six-Gentlemen Decoction with Aucklandia and Amomum (*xiāng shā liù jūn zǐ tāng*): For qi stagnation in the middle burner in the presence of Stomach and Spleen qi deficiency marked by fatigue and loose stools.

───── COMPOSITION ─────

Chiefs 君	Atractylodis Rhizoma (*cāng zhú*)	● ●	promotes the ascending functions of the middle burner, dries dampness, and transforms phlegm
	Chuanxiong Rhizoma (*chuān xiōng*)	●	releases constrained blood and thus resolves the fixed pain
Deputy 臣	Cyperi Rhizoma (*xiāng fù*)	● ● ●	resolves constrained qi and unblocks qi dynamics
Assistants 佐	Gardeniae Fructus (*zhī zǐ*)	●	clears heat from all three burners and resolves the fire from constraint
	Massa medicata fermentata (*shén qū*)	● ●	relieves constraint caused by food stagnation and harmonizes the Stomach

再造散
Renewal Powder
zài zào săn

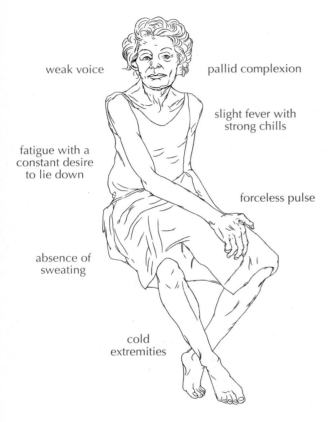

weak voice

pallid complexion

slight fever with strong chills

fatigue with a constant desire to lie down

forceless pulse

absence of sweating

cold extremities

INGREDIENTS

Astragali Radix (*huáng qí*) 6g
Ginseng Radix (*rén shēn*) 3g
[1]Aconiti Radix lateralis praeparata (*zhì fù zǐ*) 3g
Cinnamomi Ramulus (*guì zhī*) 3g
[2]Asari Radix et Rhizoma (*xì xīn*) 2g
Notopterygii Rhizoma seu Radix (*qiāng huó*) 3g
Chuanxiong Rhizoma (*chuān xiōng*) 3g

---

1. This herb can be difficult to obtain because of legal issues. Psoraleae Fructus *(bŭ gŭ zhī)* may be substituted.

2. This herb can also be difficult to obtain because of legal issues. Clematidis Radix *(wēi líng xiān)* may be substituted.

Saposhnikoviae Radix (*fáng fēng*) 3g
dry-fried Paeoniae Radix alba (*chǎo bái sháo*) 3g
Glycyrrhizae Radix (*gān cǎo*) 1.5g
roasted Zingiberis Rhizoma recens (*wēi shēng jiāng*) 3g
Jujubae Fructus (*dà zǎo*) .... 2 pieces

Actions: tonifies the yang • augments the qi • induces sweating • releases wind-cold pathogens from the exterior

Main pattern: externally-contracted wind-cold with preexisting qi and yang deficiency

Key symptoms: slight fever with strong chills • fatigue with a constant desire to lie down • pallid complexion • weak voice

Secondary symptoms: absence of sweating • cold extremities • headache

Tongue: pale body • white coating

Pulse: submerged and forceless or floating, large, and forceless

Abdomen: no specific signs

▶ CLINICAL NOTES

• This formula is a good choice to promote sweating in those who we fear will not sweat out a pathogen because of a deficiency of qi and yang. It is also useful for those who fail to sweat after taking formulas that strongly induce sweating.

Contraindications: exterior patterns without qi deficiency

▶ FORMULAS WITH SIMILAR INDICATIONS

Ephedra, Asarum, and Aconite Accessory Root Decoction (*má huáng xì xīn fù zǐ tāng*): For yang deficiency without signs of qi deficiency, such as a submerged and forceless pulse. It is stronger at opening channels blocked by cold and thus excels in the treatment of pain.

COMPOSITION

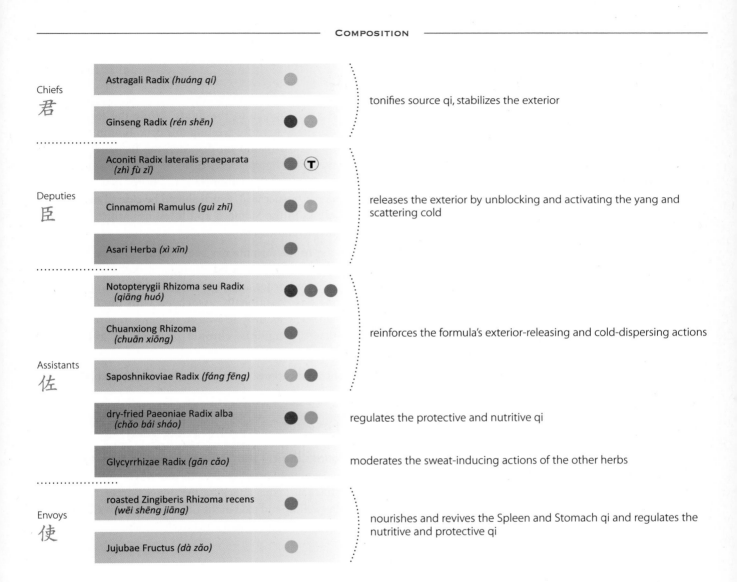

Chiefs
君

- Astragali Radix *(huáng qí)*
- Ginseng Radix *(rén shēn)*

tonifies source qi, stabilizes the exterior

Deputies
臣

- Aconiti Radix lateralis praeparata *(zhì fù zǐ)*
- Cinnamomi Ramulus *(guì zhī)*
- Asari Herba *(xì xīn)*

releases the exterior by unblocking and activating the yang and scattering cold

Assistants
佐

- Notopterygii Rhizoma seu Radix *(qiāng huó)*
- Chuanxiong Rhizoma *(chuān xiōng)*

reinforces the formula's exterior-releasing and cold-dispersing actions

- Saposhnikoviae Radix *(fáng fēng)*
- dry-fried Paeoniae Radix alba *(chǎo bái sháo)*

regulates the protective and nutritive qi

- Glycyrrhizae Radix *(gān cǎo)*

moderates the sweat-inducing actions of the other herbs

Envoys
使

- roasted Zingiberis Rhizoma recens *(wēi shēng jiāng)*
- Jujubae Fructus *(dà zǎo)*

nourishes and revives the Spleen and Stomach qi and regulates the nutritive and protective qi

增液湯（增液汤）
Increase the Fluids Decoction
zēng yè tāng

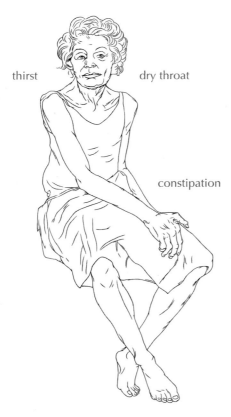

thirst   dry throat

constipation

INGREDIENTS

Scrophulariae Radix (*xuán shēn*) 30g
Ophiopogonis Radix (*mài mén dōng*) 24g
Rehmanniae Radix (*shēng dì huáng*) 24g

Actions: generates fluids • moistens dryness • unblocks the bowels

Main pattern: constipation due to exhaustion of the fluids

Key symptoms: constipation • thirst • dry throat

Secondary symptoms: none noted

Tongue: dry • red

Pulse: thin and slightly rapid • weak and forceless

Abdomen: no specific signs

► CLINICAL NOTES

• This formula is indicated for constipation with dry stools due to damage to the fluids. While the formula was originally used for treating this condition in the course of a warm-pathogen disorder, the formula is equally useful for habitual constipation. If the formula is used unmodified, it is important to ensure that there is no upper burner heat, which should be cleared first, or heat excess in the Stomach and Intestines, which should be drained downward.

• Use of the formula has been extended to the treatment of nutritive-level heat with signs of both dryness in the middle burner and signs of inflammation in the body regions traditionally associated with the Spleen and Stomach, as may be seen in diabetes, recurrent mouth ulcers, gingivitis, chronic pharyngitis, and allergic enteritis.

Contraindications: constipation due to heat or cold excess or qi deficiency

► FORMULAS WITH SIMILAR INDICATIONS

*Nourish the Yin and Clear the Lungs Decoction (*yǎng yīn qīng fèi tāng*): For Lung dryness due to yin deficiency with pestilential toxins attacking the upper burner manifesting with swelling and pain in the throat, dry mouth and lips, and a rapid and thin or rapid and forceless pulse.

──────────────────────── COMPOSITION ────────────────────────

Chief
君

Scrophulariae Radix *(xuán shēn)*   ● ● ●   nourishes the yin and generates fluids, while moistening what is dried and softening what is hard

Deputies
臣

Ophiopogonis Radix
(mài mén dōng)   ● ●   assists in enriching and moistening the yin, especially of the Stomach and Intestines

Rehmanniae Radix
(shēng dì huáng)   ● ●   nourishes the yin, clears heat, and cools the blood

鎮肝熄風湯 （鎮肝熄风汤）
Sedate the Liver and Extinguish Wind Decoction
zhèn gān xī fēng tāng

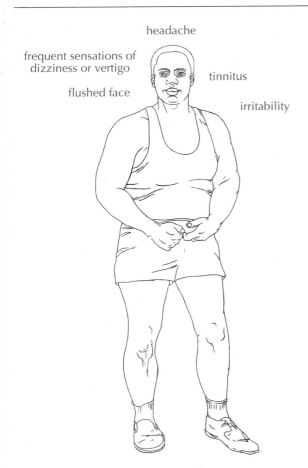

headache

frequent sensations of dizziness or vertigo

tinnitus

flushed face

irritability

INGREDIENTS

Achyranthis bidentatae Radix (*niú xī*) 30g
Haematitum (*dài zhě shí*) 30g
Fossilia Ossis Mastodi (*lóng gǔ*) 15g
Ostreae Concha (*mǔ lì*) 15g
Testudinis Plastrum (*guī bǎn*) 15g
Scrophulariae Radix (*xuán shēn*) 15g
Asparagi Radix (*tiān mén dōng*) 15g
Paeoniae Radix alba (*bái sháo*) 15g

Artemisiae scopariae Herba (*yīn chén*) 6g
Toosendan Fructus (*chuān liàn zǐ*) 6g
Hordei Fructus germinatus (*mài yá*) 6g
Glycyrrhizae Radix (*gān cǎo*) 4.5g

Actions: sedates the Liver • extinguishes wind • nourishes the yin • anchors the yang

Main pattern: wind-type stroke caused by excessive surging upward of qi, which in turn leads to congestion of blood in the brain

Key symptoms: frequent sensations of dizziness or vertigo • tinnitus • headache • irritability • flushed face (as if intoxicated) • sudden loss of consciousness

Secondary symptoms: feverish sensation in the head • feeling of distention in the eyes • frequent belching • progressive motor dysfunction of the body or development of facial asymmetry that occurs over a period of a few hours to a few days • mental confusion with moments of clarity • inability to fully recover after loss of consciousness

Tongue: red body • thin, dry coating

Pulse: wiry • long • forceful

Abdomen: palpable muscle tension extending from the left ribcage toward the umbilicus • lax muscle tone in lower abdomen close to the pelvic bones

▶ CLINICAL NOTES

• This formula is specific for hyperactivity of Liver yang in the context of yin deficiency. Key markers:

→ Wiry and forceful pulse that is also long, extending toward the thenar eminence, or excessive above and deficient below.

→ Signs indicating an upward surge of qi, often along the course of the Penetrating vessel and yang brightness channels such as facial flushing, hiccup, palpitations, dizziness, and disorientation.

• If Liver heat is severe, it is best to add herbs that clear heat such as Scutellariae Radix (*huáng qín*), Prunellae Spica (*xià kū cǎo*), and Gardeniae Fructus (*zhī zǐ*).

- Once the acute symptoms have abated, one should switch to a formula that nourishes and smooths the Liver qi and thus address the root of the disorder.

Contraindications: hypertension due to qi or yang deficiency • wind-cold fettering the exterior • yin excess

▶ FORMULAS WITH SIMILAR INDICATIONS

Antelope Horn and Uncaria Decoction (*líng jiǎo gōu téng tāng*): For Liver wind caused by heat in the nutritive and blood aspects.

Gastrodia and Uncaria Drink (*tiān má gōu téng yǐn*): For Liver yang hyperactivity in the context of yin deficiency with signs of hypertension.

— COMPOSITION —

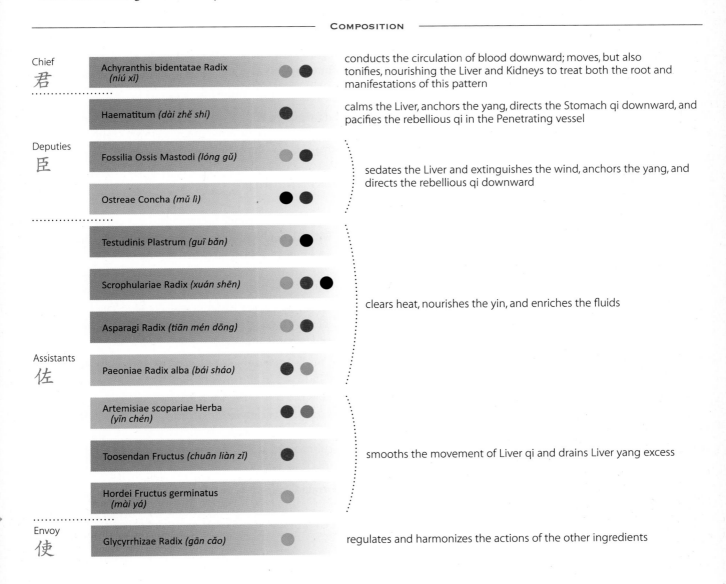

Chief 君	Achyranthis bidentatae Radix (*niú xī*)	conducts the circulation of blood downward; moves, but also tonifies, nourishing the Liver and Kidneys to treat both the root and manifestations of this pattern
	Haematitum (*dài zhě shí*)	calms the Liver, anchors the yang, directs the Stomach qi downward, and pacifies the rebellious qi in the Penetrating vessel
Deputies 臣	Fossilia Ossis Mastodi (*lóng gǔ*)	sedates the Liver and extinguishes the wind, anchors the yang, and directs the rebellious qi downward
	Ostreae Concha (*mǔ lì*)	
	Testudinis Plastrum (*guī bǎn*)	
	Scrophulariae Radix (*xuán shēn*)	clears heat, nourishes the yin, and enriches the fluids
	Asparagi Radix (*tiān mén dōng*)	
Assistants 佐	Paeoniae Radix alba (*bái sháo*)	
	Artemisiae scopariae Herba (*yīn chén*)	
	Toosendan Fructus (*chuān liàn zǐ*)	smooths the movement of Liver qi and drains Liver yang excess
	Hordei Fructus germinatus (*mài yá*)	
Envoy 使	Glycyrrhizae Radix (*gān cǎo*)	regulates and harmonizes the actions of the other ingredients

真武湯（真武汤）
True Warrior Decoction
zhēn wǔ tāng

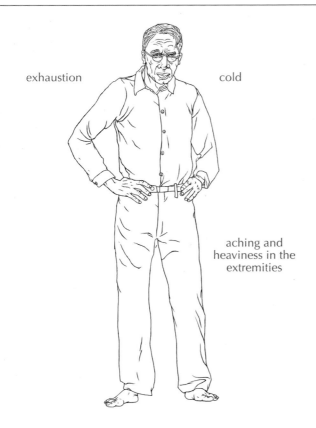

exhaustion

cold

aching and heaviness in the extremities

INGREDIENTS

¹Aconiti Radix lateralis praeparata (*zhì fù zǐ*) 9g

Atractylodis macrocephalae Rhizoma (*bái zhú*) 6g

Poria (*fú líng*).. 9g

Zingiberis Rhizoma recens (*shēng jiāng*) 9g

²Paeoniae Radix (*sháo yào*) 9g

Actions: warms the yang • promotes urination

Main patterns: Kidney yang deficiency or Spleen and Kidney

---

1. This ingredient can be difficult to obtain because of legal issues. No substitute is useful in this context.

2. As the primary function here is to restrain, tonify, or soften, Paeoniae Radix alba *(bái sháo)* is preferred.

---

yang deficiency with retention of pathogenic water • lesser yin warp patterns with water excess • externally-contracted wind-cold in the greater yang warp

Key symptoms: sensations of internal cold or cold extremities • exhaustion • deep aching and heaviness in the extremities

Secondary symptoms: dizziness • palpitations • coughing and vomiting • abdominal pain that is aggravated by cold • edema • loose stools • urinary difficulty • generalized twitching

Tongue: pale or dark body • swollen, tooth-marked body • white, slippery coating

Pulse: submerged • thin • forceless

Abdomen: splashing sounds in abdomen • pulsations in upper abdomen or around umbilicus • pencil-line tension above or below the umbilicus

► CLINICAL NOTES

- This is a key formula for treating water excess in patients with deficiency cold in the interior. The water can accumulate almost anywhere in the body including the exterior, the vessels, the upper burner Lungs and Heart, the middle burner Spleen and Stomach, the Liver, and the lower burner Kidneys and Bladder. The key clinical markers are a submerged, thin, and forceless pulse, fatigue and lethargy, and the presence of edema.

- This formula can also be used for externally-contracted wind-cold in the greater yang warp with sweating that does not reduce the fever, palpitations in the epigastrium, dizziness, generalized twitching, and physical instability. In these cases a white, slippery tongue coating and a submerged, thin, and forceless pulse help differentiate this from an excess cold pattern.

Contraindications: none noted

► FORMULAS WITH SIMILAR INDICATIONS

Poria, Cinnamon Twig, Atractylodes, and Licorice Decoction (*líng guì zhú gān tāng*): For thin mucus in the epigastrium or a thin mucus pattern that affects any of the three burners when it is associated with middle burner deficiency as opposed to the more severe Kidney-Spleen deficiency addressed by True Warrior Decoction (*zhēn wǔ tāng*).

Kidney Qi Pill (*shèn qì wán*): For thin mucus or other types of water accumulation in the context of Kidney qi deficiency. In this pattern there is typically no diarrhea and interior cold symptoms are less pronounced. Instead, there may be urinary difficulty as well as back and knee ache and other signs of Kidney deficiency.

Frigid Extremities Decoction (*sì nì tāng*): For lesser yin warp internal deficiency cold patterns without water accumulation.

─────────────────────── COMPOSITION ───────────────────────

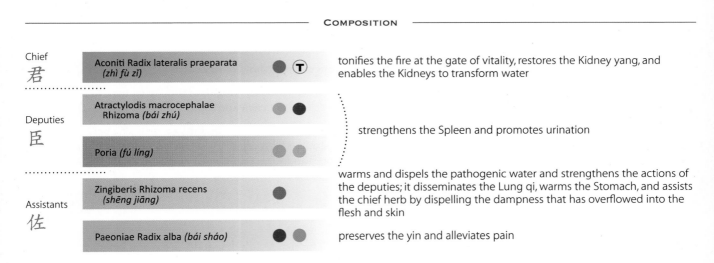

Chief 君	Aconiti Radix lateralis praeparata (*zhì fù zǐ*) ● Ⓣ	tonifies the fire at the gate of vitality, restores the Kidney yang, and enables the Kidneys to transform water
Deputies 臣	Atractylodis macrocephalae Rhizoma (*bái zhú*) ● ●	strengthens the Spleen and promotes urination
	Poria (*fú líng*) ● ●	
Assistants 佐	Zingiberis Rhizoma recens (*shēng jiāng*) ●	warms and dispels the pathogenic water and strengthens the actions of the deputies; it disseminates the Lung qi, warms the Stomach, and assists the chief herb by dispelling the dampness that has overflowed into the flesh and skin
	Paeoniae Radix alba (*bái sháo*) ● ●	preserves the yin and alleviates pain

炙甘草湯 (炙甘草汤)
Prepared Licorice Decoction
zhì gān cǎo tāng

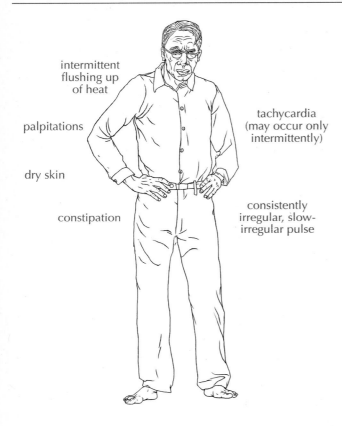

intermittent flushing up of heat

palpitations

dry skin

constipation

tachycardia (may occur only intermittently)

consistently irregular, slow-irregular pulse

Main pattern: consumptive condition with qi and blood deficiency manifesting primarily with functional disorders of the Heart system

Key symptoms: palpitations • tachycardia (may occur only intermittently) • intermittent flushing up of heat • dry skin • constipation

Secondary symptoms: anxiety • insomnia • irritability • emaciation • shortness of breath • dry mouth and throat • spontaneous sweating or night sweats • dry throat and tongue • chronic cough

Tongue: pale, shiny, or dry

Pulse: consistently irregular • slow-irregular • thin, faint, and forceless • deficient and rapid

Abdomen: epigastric discomfort • palpable periumbilical pulsations • hypertonicity of rectus abdominis muscle in upper abdomen • numbness or lack of sensation below umbilicus

▶ **CLINICAL NOTES**

• This is an important formula for Heart qi and yin deficiency presenting with a slow or consistently irregular pulse. It is not indicated for a rapid, irregular pulse. The type of Heart deficiency addressed by this formula may present in other ways, too, but always combines symptoms of dryness (constipation, dry throat, dry skin, dry eyes) and qi deficiency (fatigue, shortness of breath) with loss of control over the Heart yang (palpitations, sweating, insomnia, anxiety, irritability). Often, these excess symptoms occur in a paroxysmal fashion, that is, they have a wind-like nature.

• The indications of this formula have been extended to encompass Lung deficiency patterns involving chronic cough with dry or scanty phlegm in addition to the symptoms outlined above.

Contraindications: yin deficiency • diarrhea

▶ **FORMULAS WITH SIMILAR INDICATIONS**

Generate the Pulse Powder (*shēng mài sǎn*): For deficiency of qi and fluids of the Lungs and Heart. Although both formulas

─── **INGREDIENTS** ───

Glycyrrhizae Radix praeparata (*zhì gān cǎo*) 12g
Ginseng Radix (*rén shēn*) 6g
Cinnamomi Ramulus (*guì zhī*) 9g
Rehmanniae Radix (*shēng dì huáng*) 30-50g
Ophiopogonis Radix (*mài mén dōng*) 9g
Asini Corii Colla (*ē jiāo*) ..... [dissolve in strained decoction] 6g
Cannabis Semen (*huǒ má rén*) .... [crushed] 9g
Zingiberis Rhizoma recens (*shēng jiāng*) 9g
Jujubae Fructus (*dà zǎo*) .... 5-10 pieces

Actions: augments the qi • nourishes the blood • enriches the yin • restores the pulse

treat similar patterns, this formula acts more directly on the yang fluids, both producing them as well as binding them, in order to increase the fluids inside the vessels. Prepared Licorice Decoction (*zhì gān cǎo tāng*) acts more strongly on the yin fluids and blood, thus the symptoms of dryness of the tissues themselves.

──────────────── **COMPOSITION** ────────────────

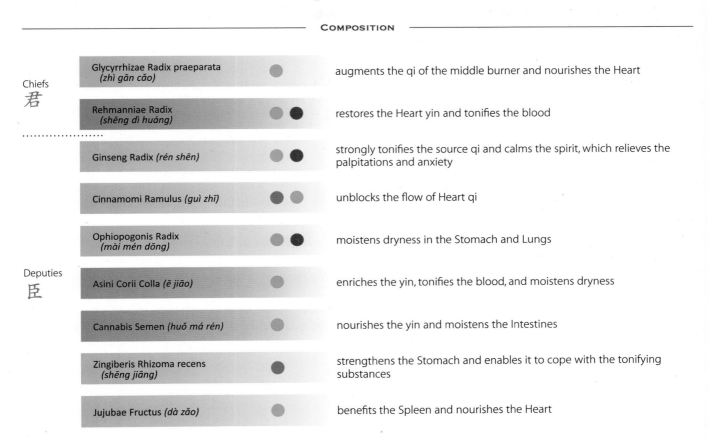

Chiefs
君

Glycyrrhizae Radix praeparata
(*zhì gān cǎo*) — augments the qi of the middle burner and nourishes the Heart

Rehmanniae Radix
(*shēng dì huáng*) — restores the Heart yin and tonifies the blood

Ginseng Radix (*rén shēn*) — strongly tonifies the source qi and calms the spirit, which relieves the palpitations and anxiety

Cinnamomi Ramulus (*guì zhī*) — unblocks the flow of Heart qi

Ophiopogonis Radix
(*mài mén dōng*) — moistens dryness in the Stomach and Lungs

Deputies
臣

Asini Corii Colla (*ē jiāo*) — enriches the yin, tonifies the blood, and moistens dryness

Cannabis Semen (*huǒ má rén*) — nourishes the yin and moistens the Intestines

Zingiberis Rhizoma recens
(*shēng jiāng*) — strengthens the Stomach and enables it to cope with the tonifying substances

Jujubae Fructus (*dà zǎo*) — benefits the Spleen and nourishes the Heart

枳實導滯丸（枳实导滞丸）
Unripe Bitter Orange Pill to Guide Out Stagnation
zhǐ shí dǎo zhì wán

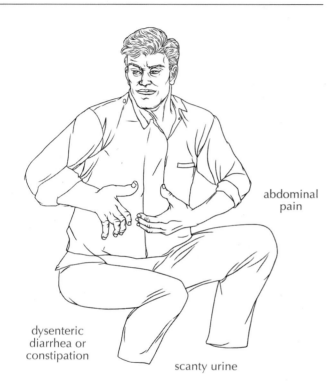

abdominal pain

dysenteric diarrhea or constipation

scanty urine

Key symptoms: pain and distention in the epigastrium and abdomen • dysenteric diarrhea or constipation • scanty, dark urine

Secondary symptoms: none noted

Tongue: greasy, yellow coating

Pulse: submerged • forceful

Abdomen: distention of the epigastrium or abdomen • pain that increases with pressure

► CLINICAL NOTES

• This formula treats relatively severe food stagnation arising from damp-heat excess. Depending on the degree of obstruction, this can manifest either as dysenteric diarrhea or as constipation.

Contraindications: deficiency conditions

► FORMULAS WITH SIMILAR INDICATIONS

Aucklandia and Betel Nut Pill (*mù xiāng bīng láng wán*): For stagnation of food and qi transforming into heat with more pronounced symptoms of qi stagnation, specifically pain, in the abdomen.

────── INGREDIENTS ──────

dry-fried Aurantii Fructus immaturus (*chǎo zhǐ shí*)........... 15g
Rhei Radix et Rhizoma (*dà huáng*)...................................... 9g
dry-fried Massa medicata fermentata (*chǎo shén qū*) 12-15g
Poria (*fú líng*).. 9g
Scutellariae Radix (*huáng qín*) 9g
Coptidis Rhizoma (*huáng lián*) 9g
Atractylodis macrocephalae Rhizoma (*bái zhú*) 9g
Alismatis Rhizoma (*zé xiè*) 6-15g

Actions: reduces and guides out stagnation and accumulation • drains heat • dispels dampness

Main pattern: damp-heat food stagnation obstructing the Stomach and Intestines

COMPOSITION

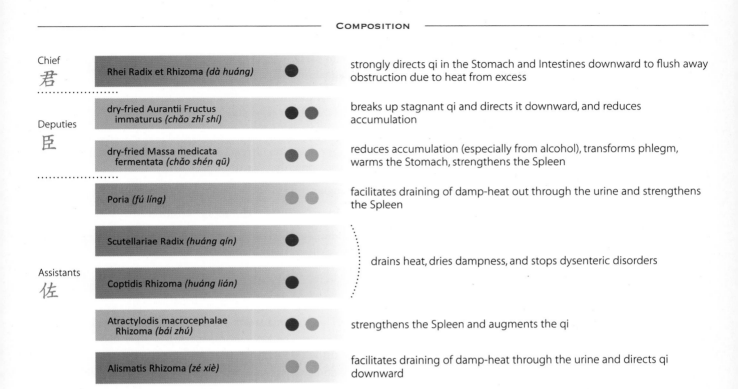

Chief 君		
Rhei Radix et Rhizoma *(dà huáng)*	●	strongly directs qi in the Stomach and Intestines downward to flush away obstruction due to heat from excess

Deputies 臣		
dry-fried Aurantii Fructus immaturus *(chǎo zhǐ shí)*	● ●	breaks up stagnant qi and directs it downward, and reduces accumulation
dry-fried Massa medicata fermentata *(chǎo shén qū)*	● ●	reduces accumulation (especially from alcohol), transforms phlegm, warms the Stomach, strengthens the Spleen

Assistants 佐		
Poria *(fú líng)*	● ●	facilitates draining of damp-heat out through the urine and strengthens the Spleen
Scutellariae Radix *(huáng qín)*	●	drains heat, dries dampness, and stops dysenteric disorders
Coptidis Rhizoma *(huáng lián)*	●	
Atractylodis macrocephalae Rhizoma *(bái zhú)*	● ●	strengthens the Spleen and augments the qi
Alismatis Rhizoma *(zé xiè)*	● ●	facilitates draining of damp-heat through the urine and directs qi downward

枳實消痞丸（枳实消痞丸）
Unripe Bitter Orange Pill to Reduce Focal Distention
zhǐ shí xiāo pǐ wán

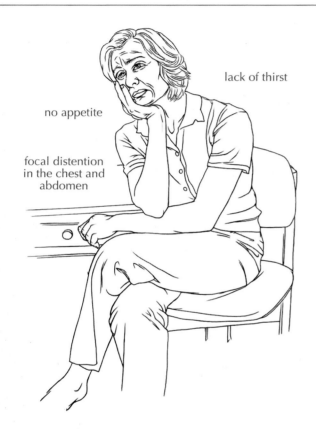

no appetite

lack of thirst

focal distention in the chest and abdomen

Actions: reduces focal distention • eliminates fullness • strengthens the Spleen • harmonizes the Stomach

Main pattern: Spleen deficiency with accumulation and stagnation

Key symptoms: focal distention in the chest and abdomen • lack of thirst • no appetite

Secondary symptoms: fatigue • weakness • wan complexion • poor digestion • irregular bowel movements (sometimes loose, sometimes hard)

Tongue: thin, greasy coating that may be yellow

Pulse: wiry at the right middle position

Abdomen: focal distention and fullness in the epigastrium • weakness around the umbilicus

▶ **CLINICAL NOTES**

• This formula treats a mixed pattern of excess and deficiency. The key clinical marker is focal distention (i.e., distention without pain) in the epigastrium or upper abdomen combined with a wiry pulse in the right middle position. To treat a condition with more pronounced signs of Spleen deficiency it is important to increase the relative dosage of the tonifying herbs and to reduce the dosage of Coptidis Rhizoma (*huáng lián*).

Contraindications: Spleen deficiency without excess

▶ **FORMULAS WITH SIMILAR INDICATIONS**

Strengthen the Spleen Pill (*jiàn pí wán*): For Spleen deficiency leading to food stagnation with bloating and focal distention but a deficient and frail pulse.

Pinellia Decoction to Drain the Epigastrium (*bàn xià xiè xīn tāng*): For a pattern of Spleen and Stomach deficiency cold with damp-heat obstructing the middle burner. This pattern manifests with focal distention, vomiting, or other signs of upper body heat and diarrhea or other signs of lower body cold.

—————— **INGREDIENTS** ——————

Aurantii Fructus immaturus (*zhǐ shí*)..............................9-15g
prepared Magnoliae officinalis Cortex (*zhì hòu pò*)..........9-12g
Coptidis Rhizoma (*huáng lián*)....................................6-9g
Pinelliae Rhizoma praeparatum (*zhì bàn xià*).....................9g
Ginseng Radix (*rén shēn*)..6-9g
Atractylodis macrocephalae Rhizoma (*bái zhú*)...............6-9g
Poria (*fú líng*)..6-9g
Hordei Fructus germinatus (*mài yá*)..............................6-9g
Zingiberis Rhizoma (*gān jiāng*)...................................3-6g
Glycyrrhizae Radix praeparata (*zhì gān cǎo*)...................3-6g

COMPOSITION

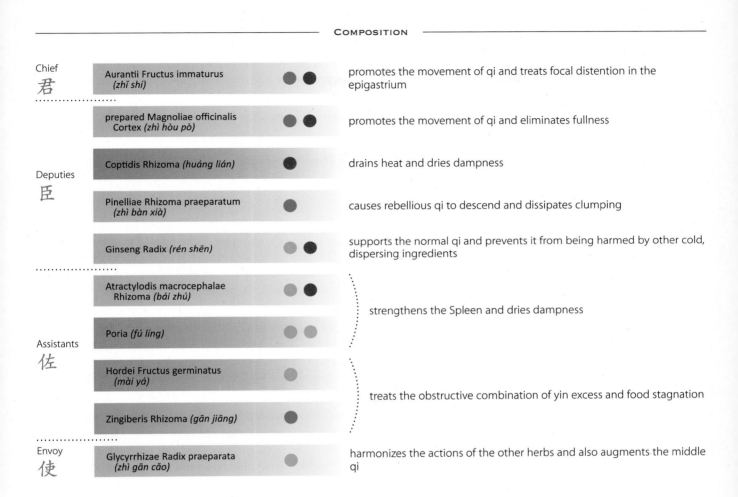

Chief
君

Aurantii Fructus immaturus
(zhǐ shí)

promotes the movement of qi and treats focal distention in the epigastrium

prepared Magnoliae officinalis
Cortex *(zhì hòu pò)*

promotes the movement of qi and eliminates fullness

Deputies
臣

Coptidis Rhizoma *(huáng lián)*

drains heat and dries dampness

Pinelliae Rhizoma praeparatum
(zhì bàn xià)

causes rebellious qi to descend and dissipates clumping

Ginseng Radix *(rén shēn)*

supports the normal qi and prevents it from being harmed by other cold, dispersing ingredients

Atractylodis macrocephalae
Rhizoma *(bái zhú)*

strengthens the Spleen and dries dampness

Assistants
佐

Poria *(fú líng)*

Hordei Fructus germinatus
(mài yá)

treats the obstructive combination of yin excess and food stagnation

Zingiberis Rhizoma *(gān jiāng)*

Envoy
使

Glycyrrhizae Radix praeparata
(zhì gān cǎo)

harmonizes the actions of the other herbs and also augments the middle qi

枳實薤白桂枝湯（枳实薤白桂枝汤）
Unripe Bitter Orange, Chinese Garlic, and Cinnamon Twig Decoction
zhǐ shí xiè bái guì zhī tāng

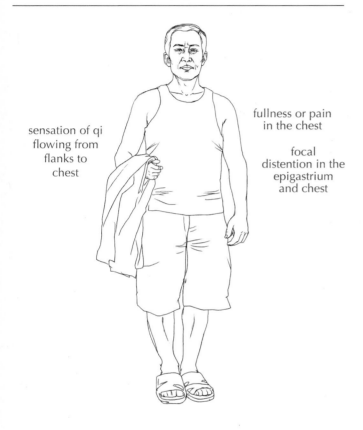

sensation of qi flowing from flanks to chest

fullness or pain in the chest

focal distention in the epigastrium and chest

INGREDIENTS

Aurantii Fructus immaturus (*zhǐ shí*).............................. 12g
Magnoliae officinalis Cortex (*hòu pò*) 12g
Allii macrostemi Bulbus (*xiè bái*) 9g
Cinnamomi Ramulus (*guì zhī*) 6g
Trichosanthis Fructus (*guā lóu*)..................................... 12g

Actions: unblocks the yang • promotes the movement of qi • expels phlegm • directs the qi downward

Main pattern: painful obstruction of the chest

Key symptoms: fullness or pain in the chest • focal distention in the epigastrium and chest • sensation of qi flowing from the

flanks to the area around the heart

Secondary symptoms: stabbing pain in the chest that can radiate from the chest to the back • shortness of breath • wheezing • cough with thick sputum • abdominal distention • constipation

Tongue: greasy, white coating

Pulse: submerged and wiry • tight

Abdomen: no specific signs

▶ **CLINICAL NOTES**

• This is a core formula for unblocking painful obstruction of the chest with severe clumping of qi that results in focal distention and pain. Many physicians therefore think that the pulse described above need be found only in the distal positions, which represent the upper burner.

• If the qi dynamic in the chest and upper burner is blocked, the qi fails to descend. This is often reflected in symptoms in the lower burner such as constipation, difficulty in emptying the bowels properly, or lower abdominal distention. This formula can be used to address these problems.

• This formula focuses on the manifestations, not the root. Once the acute symptoms have abated, a formula should be chosen that addresses the root problem. This may be yang deficiency, dampness and phlegm, or a combination of the two.

• This formula is not indicated for painful obstruction of the chest due to internal cold characterized by very severe pain radiating to the back, cold extremities, and bluish lips and nails. In such cases a formula based on Aconiti Radix lateralis praeparata (*zhì fù zǐ*) is indicated. If there is pronounced blood stasis, one should add herbs like Salviae miltiorrhizae Radix (*dān shēn*), Chuanxiong Rhizoma (*chuān xiōng*), and Carthami Flos (*hóng huā*).

Contraindications: chest pain due to deficiency • phlegm-heat

▶ **FORMULAS WITH SIMILAR INDICATIONS**

*Coix and Aconite Powder (*yì yǐ fù zǐ sǎn*): For painful obstruction of the chest due to cold with severe pain extending to the back that is sometimes mild and sometimes more severe, a sensation of obstruction in the chest, cold extremities, and bluish lips and nails.

COMPOSITION

Chiefs
君

Trichosanthis Fructus *(guā lóu)* — expels phlegm and unbinds the chest

Allii macrostemi Bulbus *(xiè bái)* — warms and unblocks the yang to promote the movement of qi and alleviate pain

Deputies
臣

Aurantii Fructus immaturus *(zhǐ shí)* — directs the qi downward, breaks up clumping, gets rid of focal distention, and eliminates fullness

Magnoliae officinalis Cortex *(hòu pò)* — directs the qi downward and eliminates fullness, dries dampness and transforms phlegm

Assistant
佐

Cinnamomi Ramulus *(guì zhī)* — unblocks the yang, disperses cold, directs rebellious qi downward, and calms flushing

止嗽散
Stop Coughing Powder
zhǐ sòu sǎn

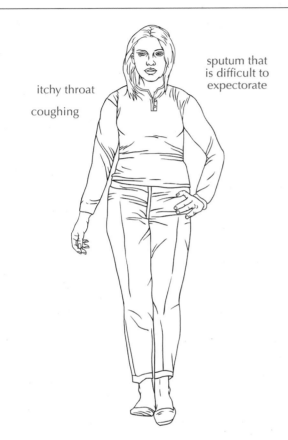

itchy throat

coughing

sputum that is difficult to expectorate

Key symptoms: coughing • itchy throat • sputum that is difficult to expectorate

Secondary symptoms: slight chills and fever

Tongue: thin, white coating

Pulse: moderate • floating

Abdomen: no specific signs

▶ CLINICAL NOTES

• This is a useful base formula to treat cough due to wind-cold with only mild symptoms of cold fettering the exterior. With appropriate modifications it can also be used where exterior symptoms are entirely absent.

→ For thick, sticky sputum, add Pinelliae Rhizoma praeparatum (*zhì bàn xià*), Poria (*fú líng*), Mori Cortex (*sāng bái pí*), Zingiberis Rhizoma recens (*shēng jiāng*), and Jujubae Fructus (*dà zǎo*).

→ For a dry, nonproductive cough, omit Schizonepetae Herba (*jīng jiè*) and Citri reticulatae Pericarpium (*chén pí*) and add Trichosanthis Fructus (*guā lóu*), Fritillariae cirrhosae Bulbus (*chuān bèi mǔ*), Anemarrhenae Rhizoma (*zhī mǔ*), and Platycladi Semen (*bǎi zǐ rén*).

→ For copious sputum, reduced appetite, stifling sensation in the chest, and white, greasy tongue coating, take with Two-Aged Herb Decoction (*èr chén tāng*).

Contraindications: yin deficiency • heat in the Lungs

▶ FORMULAS WITH SIMILAR INDICATIONS

Apricot Kernel and Perilla Leaf Powder (*xìng sū sǎn*): For cough due to cold-dryness in the exterior that has disrupted the qi dynamic and results in the internal accumulation of fluids and produces a type of thin mucus characterized by cough with watery sputum that is difficult to expectorate, stuffy nose, dry throat, and a dry, white tongue coating.

──── INGREDIENTS ────

Platycodi Radix (*jié gěng*)..............................6-9g
Schizonepetae Herba (*jīng jiè*).....................6-9g
Asteris Radix (*zǐ wǎn*)....................................6-9g
Stemonae Radix (*bǎi bù*) 6-90g
Cynanchi stauntonii Rhizoma (*bái qián*)......6-9g
Glycyrrhizae Radix (*gān cǎo*)...........................6g
Citri reticulatae Pericarpium (*chén pí*) 6g

Actions: stops coughing • transforms phlegm • disperses the exterior • disseminates the Lung qi

Main pattern: cough that occurs as the sequela to externally-contracted wind-cold

COMPOSITION

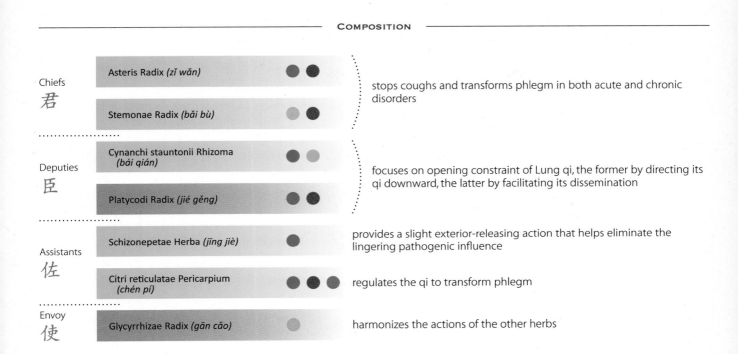

Chiefs
君

Asteris Radix *(zǐ wǎn)* — stops coughs and transforms phlegm in both acute and chronic disorders

Stemonae Radix *(bǎi bù)*

Deputies
臣

Cynanchi stauntonii Rhizoma *(bái qián)* — focuses on opening constraint of Lung qi, the former by directing its qi downward, the latter by facilitating its dissemination

Platycodi Radix *(jié gěng)*

Assistants
佐

Schizonepetae Herba *(jīng jiè)* — provides a slight exterior-releasing action that helps eliminate the lingering pathogenic influence

Citri reticulatae Pericarpium *(chén pí)* — regulates the qi to transform phlegm

Envoy
使

Glycyrrhizae Radix *(gān cǎo)* — harmonizes the actions of the other herbs

豬苓湯 （猪苓汤）
Polyporus Decoction
zhū líng tāng

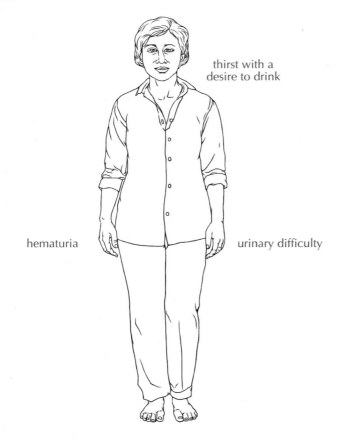

thirst with a desire to drink

hematuria

urinary difficulty

INGREDIENTS

Polyporus (*zhū líng*).. 9g
Poria (*fú líng*).. 9g
Alismatis Rhizoma (*zé xiè*) 9g
Talcum (*huá shí*)... 9-15g
Asini Corii Colla (*ē jiāo*).. 9g

Actions: promotes urination • clears heat • nourishes the yin

Main pattern: injury from cold entering the yang brightness or lesser yin warp where it transforms into heat

Key symptoms: hematuria • urinary difficulty • urination brings no relief

Secondary symptoms: fever • thirst with a desire to drink • diarrhea • cough • nausea • irritability • insomnia

Tongue: dark, dry body • white coating

Pulse: thin

Abdomen: fullness and tenderness on pressure in lower abdomen • focal distention in epigastrium

► CLINICAL NOTES

• This formula treats clumping of water and heat in the lower abdomen where heat has already damaged the yin. This is a combined excess/deficiency pattern. Key clinical markers include the following:

→ reduced urinary frequency, urinary difficulty, or incomplete voiding

→ signs of water excess such as edema, fullness, and resistance to pressure in the lower abdomen, diarrhea, and a white (but dry) tongue coating

→ signs that heat has damaged the yin such as a darkish red tongue, insomnia, and irritability

Contraindications: severe yin deficiency with dryness • pronounced dampness

► FORMULAS WITH SIMILAR INDICATIONS

Five-Ingredient Powder with Poria (*wǔ líng sǎn*): For water accumulation in the lower abdomen blocking qi transformation, presenting with signs of cold or rebellious ascent of qi and yang.

*Coptis and Ass-Hide Gelatin Decoction (*huáng lián ē jiāo tāng*): For heat damaging the yin where both pathogenic heat and yin deficiency are relatively pronounced. This presents with such symptoms as insomnia, focal distention in the epigastrium, abdominal pain, irritability and thirst, and palpitations.

COMPOSITION

Chief
君

Polyporus *(zhū líng)* ● ● — strongly reinforces the proper functioning of the water pathways and thereby promotes urination

Deputies
臣

Poria *(fú líng)* ● ● — promotes urination, benefits the Spleen, and harmonizes the Stomach

Alismatis Rhizoma *(zé xiè)* ● ● — promotes water metabolism and aids the chief ingredient in promoting urination

Assistants
佐

Talcum *(huá shí)* ● ● — clears heat and unblocks painful urinary dribbling

Asini Corii Colla *(ē jiāo)* ● — enriches the yin and prevents excessive urination and further injury to the yin

竹葉石膏湯（竹叶石膏汤）
Lophatherum and Gypsum Decoction
zhú yè shí gāo tang

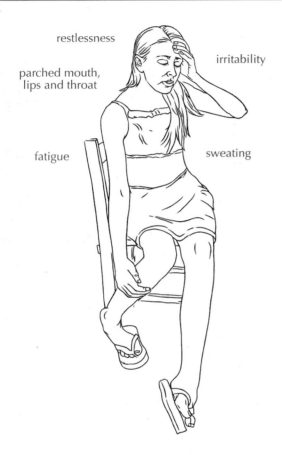

restlessness

irritability

parched mouth, lips and throat

fatigue

sweating

Main pattern: qi-level heat lingering in the Lungs and Stomach where it injures the qi and fluids

Key symptoms: irritability • restlessness • parched mouth, lips, and throat • sweating • fatigue

Secondary symptoms: lingering fever • nausea • vomiting • thirst • insomnia • choking cough • stifling sensation in the chest

Tongue: red body • scanty coating

Pulse: rapid • deficient

Abdomen: focal distention in the epigastrium

► CLINICAL NOTES

• This is a very versatile formula that can be used whenever there is evidence of excess heat in the Stomach that is accompanied by injury to the qi and yin. Typical examples are the later stages of a cold-damage disorder, acute summerheat damage patterns, Stomach heat patterns during pregnancy, recovery from surgery, weak children, or adults with chronic disorders.

• Important diagnostic pointers are Stomach heat-induced rebellious qi with nausea or vomiting and heat accumulating in the chest giving rise to irritability, restlessness, and insomnia.

Contraindications: febrile diseases where both the normal and pathogenic qi are abundant • when the fever remains high • when the qi and yin have not yet been injured

► FORMULAS WITH SIMILAR INDICATIONS

Clear Summerheat and Augment the Qi Decoction (*qīng shǔ yì qì tāng*): For damage of the Lung qi by summerheat manifesting with sweating and shortness of breath.

Sweet Wormwood and Soft-shelled Turtle Shell Decoction Version 1 (*qīng hāo biē jiǎ tāng*): For lingering fevers in the aftermath of warm pathogen disorders with heat constraint in the deep collaterals manifesting with night sweats, fever at night and coolness in the morning where the coolness in the morning occurs without sweating.

INGREDIENTS

Lophatheri Herba (*dàn zhú yè*)...................................... 6-15g
Gypsum fibrosum (*shí gāo*)... 30-50g
Ginseng Radix (*rén shēn*)... 6g
Ophiopogonis Radix (*mài mén dōng*) 15-20g
Pinelliae Rhizoma praeparatum (*zhì bàn xià*)...................... 9g
Glycyrrhizae Radix praeparata (*zhì gān cǎo*) 3-6g
Nonglutinous rice (*jīng mǐ*) 10-15g

Actions: clears heat • generates fluids • augments the qi • harmonizes the Stomach

COMPOSITION

Chief 君	Gypsum fibrosum (shí gāo)	clears lurking heat from the Lungs and Stomach, vents pathogenic heat to the exterior and helps to order the qi dynamic; generates fluids and stops thirst
	Lophatheri Herba (dàn zhú yè)	enters the collaterals, tracks down pathogens, and actively clears heat from the deepest yin aspect of the body
Deputies 臣	Ginseng Radix (rén shēn)	moistens the Lungs and nourishes the yin, benefits the Stomach and generates fluids, clears heat from the Heart, and eliminates irritability
	Ophiopogonis Radix (mài mén dōng)	
Assistant 佐	Pinelliae Rhizoma praeparatum (zhì bàn xià)	directs rebellious qi downward and thereby stops the vomiting
Envoys 使	Glycyrrhizae Radix praeparata (zhì gān cǎo)	tonifies the qi; harmonizes the middle burner and nourishes the Stomach
	Nonglutinous rice (jīng mǐ)	

左歸丸（左归丸）
Restore the Left [Kidney] Pill
zǔo guī wán

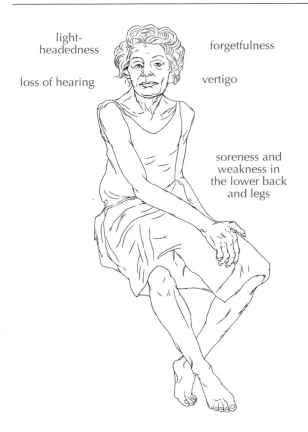

light-headedness

forgetfulness

loss of hearing

vertigo

soreness and weakness in the lower back and legs

Main pattern: Kidney yin deficiency with damaged essence and marrow

Key symptoms: light-headedness • vertigo • loss of hearing • forgetfulness • soreness and weakness in the lower back and legs

Secondary symptoms: tinnitus • spontaneous and night sweats • heat in the palms and chest • dry mouth and throat • thirst • spontaneous and nocturnal emissions • insomnia

Tongue: red body • scanty coating

Pulse: thin • rapid

Abdomen: no specific signs

▶ CLINICAL NOTES

• This formula strongly tonifies the essence and marrow rather than just the yin fluids. It does not contain any herbs for treating excess symptoms such as fire or dampness. It is therefore best suited for Kidney deficiency patterns where deficiency symptoms clearly outweigh those of excess, even if there is a small amount of heat from deficiency.

Contraindications: Spleen and Stomach deficiency • heat excess

▶ FORMULAS WITH SIMILAR INDICATIONS

Six-Ingredient Pill with Rehmannia (*liù wèi dì huáng wán*): For Kidney yin deficiency patterns with more pronounced signs of deficiency heat or some presence of phlegm.

─────── INGREDIENTS ───────

Rehmanniae Radix praeparata (*shú dì huáng*) 12-24g
Dioscoreae Rhizoma (*shān yào*) 12g
Lycii Fructus (*gǒu qǐ zǐ*) 12g
Corni Fructus (*shān zhū yú*) 12g
Cyathulae Radix (*chuān niú xī*) 9g
Cuscutae Semen (*tù sī zǐ*) 12g
Cervi Cornus Colla (*lù jiǎo jiāo*) 12g
Testudinis Plastri Colla (*guī bǎn jiāo*) 12g

Preparation notes: Most commonly taken in pill form.

Actions: nourishes the yin • enriches the Kidneys • fills the essence • augments the marrow

COMPOSITION

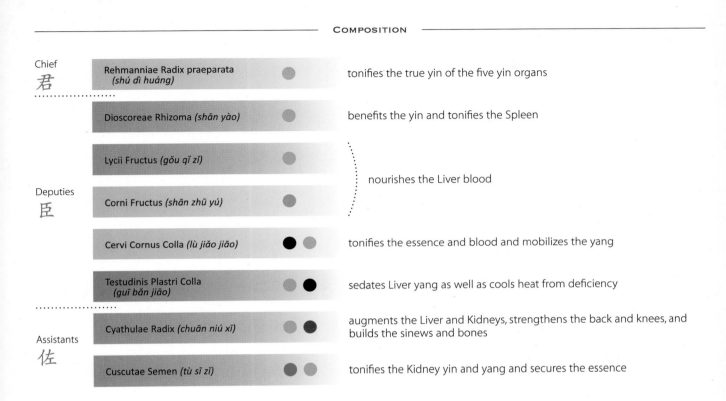

Chief 君	Rehmanniae Radix praeparata (shú dì huáng)	tonifies the true yin of the five yin organs
	Dioscoreae Rhizoma (shān yào)	benefits the yin and tonifies the Spleen
Deputies 臣	Lycii Fructus (gǒu qǐ zǐ)	nourishes the Liver blood
	Corni Fructus (shān zhū yú)	
	Cervi Cornus Colla (lù jiǎo jiāo)	tonifies the essence and blood and mobilizes the yang
	Testudinis Plastri Colla (guī bǎn jiāo)	sedates Liver yang as well as cools heat from deficiency
Assistants 佐	Cyathulae Radix (chuān niú xī)	augments the Liver and Kidneys, strengthens the back and knees, and builds the sinews and bones
	Cuscutae Semen (tù sī zǐ)	tonifies the Kidney yin and yang and secures the essence

Index of Formulas by Pinyin

Principal entries for each of the main formulas are shown as a page spread (e.g., 34-35). Other formulas that are discussed under the main entries, but are not themselves main formulas, are preceded with an asterisk (*).

· ·

bā zhēn tāng (Eight-Treasure Decoction) ······ 2-3, 252

bā zhèng sǎn (Eight-Herb Powder for Rectification) ······ 4-5, 80, 276, 290

bǎi hé gù jīn tāng (Lily Bulb Decoction to Preserve the Metal) ······ 6-7, 23, 195

*bái hǔ jiā rén shēn tāng (White Tiger plus Ginseng Decoction) ······ 131, 214, 346

bái hǔ tāng (White Tiger Decoction) ······ 8-9, 140, 182, 293, 324

bái tóu wēng tāng (Pulsatilla Decoction) ······ 10-11, 114

bàn xià bái zhú tiān má tāng (Pinellia, White Atractylodes, and Gastrodia Decoction) ······ 12-13, 93

bàn xià hòu pò tāng (Pinellia and Magnolia Bark Decoction) ······ 14-15, 195, 349

bàn xià xiè xīn tāng (Pinellia Decoction to Drain the Epigastrium) ······ 15, 16-17, 164, 201, 362

bǎo chǎn wú yōu fāng (Worry-Free Formula to Protect Birth) ······ 18-19

bǎo hé wán (Preserve Harmony Pill) ······ 20-21, 154, 228, 278, 306

bèi mǔ guā lóu sǎn (Fritillaria and Trichosanthes Fruit Powder) ······ 7, 22-23

bì xiè fēn qīng yǐn/bēi xiè fēn qīng yǐn (Tokoro Drink to Separate the Clear) ······ 4, 24-25

bīng péng sǎn (Borneal and Borax Powder) ······ 26-27

*bǔ fèi ē jiāo tāng (Tonify the Lungs Decoction with Ass-Hide Gelatin) ······ 6

bǔ fèi tāng (Tonify the Lungs Decoction) ······ 28-29

*bǔ pí wèi xiè yīn huǒ shēng yáng tāng (Tonify Spleen-Stomach, Drain Yin Fire, and Raise Yang Decoction) ······ 70

bǔ yáng huán wǔ tāng (Tonify the Yang to Restore Five [-Tenths] Decoction) ······ 30-31

bǔ zhōng yì qì tāng (Tonify the Middle to Augment the Qi Decoction) ······ 32-33, 70, 106, 122, 123, 315

cāng ér zǐ sǎn (Xanthium Powder) ······ 34-35, 47

chái gé jiě jī tāng (Bupleurum and Kudzu Decoction to Release the Muscle Layer) ······ 36-37 *chái hú dá yuán yǐn (Bupleurum Drink to Reach the Source) ⸱⸱⸱⸱⸱⸱ 66

chái hú guì jiāng tāng (Bupleurum, Cinnamon Twig, and Ginger Decoction) ⸱⸱⸱⸱⸱⸱ 38-39

*chái hú guì zhī tāng (Bupleurum and Cinnamon Twig Decoction) ⸱⸱⸱⸱⸱⸱ 38

chái hú jiā lóng gǔ mǔ lì tāng (Bupleurum Plus Dragon Bone and Oyster Shell Decoction) ⸱⸱⸱⸱⸱⸱ 39, 40, 55

*chái hú jiā máng xiāo tāng (Bupleurum Decoction plus Mirabilite) ⸱⸱⸱⸱⸱⸱ 55

chái hú qīng gān tāng (Bupleurum Decoction to Clear the Liver) ⸱⸱⸱⸱⸱⸱ 42-43, 202

chái hú shū gān sǎn (Bupleurum Powder to Dredge the Liver) ⸱⸱⸱⸱⸱⸱ 44-45, 260

chuān xiōng chá tiáo sǎn (Chuanxiong Powder to Be Taken with Green Tea) ⸱⸱⸱⸱⸱⸱ 35, 46-47

cōng bái qī wèi yǐn (Scallion Drink with Seven Ingredients) ⸱⸱⸱⸱⸱⸱ 48-49

cōng chǐ tāng (Scallion and Prepared Soybean Decoction) ⸱⸱⸱⸱⸱⸱ 50-51

dà bǔ yīn wán (Great Tonify the Yin Pill) ⸱⸱⸱⸱⸱⸱ 52-53, 138, 210, 276

dà chái hú tāng (Major Bupleurum Decoction) ⸱⸱⸱⸱⸱⸱ 41, 54-55, 58, 101, 309

dà chéng qì tāng (Major Order the Qi Decoction) ⸱⸱⸱⸱⸱⸱ 56-57, 60, 115, 132, 141

*dà dìng fēng zhū (Major Arrest Wind Pearls) ⸱⸱⸱⸱⸱⸱ 177

dà huáng fù zǐ tāng (Rhubarb and Aconite Accessory Root Decoction) ⸱⸱⸱⸱⸱⸱ 58-59, 288

dà huáng mǔ dān tāng (Rhubarb and Moutan Decoction) ⸱⸱⸱⸱⸱⸱ 57, 60-61

*dà jiàn zhōng tāng (Major Construct the Middle Decoction) ⸱⸱⸱⸱⸱⸱ 58, 315

dà qín jiāo tāng (Major Large Gentian Decoction) ⸱⸱⸱⸱⸱⸱ 62-63, 321

dà qīng lóng tāng (Major Bluegreen Dragon Decoction) ⸱⸱⸱⸱⸱⸱ 64-65

dá yuán yǐn (Reach the Source Drink) ⸱⸱⸱⸱⸱⸱ 66-67

dān shēn yǐn (Salvia Drink) ⸱⸱⸱⸱⸱⸱ 68-69, 120, 256, 335

dāng guī bǔ xuè tāng (Tangkuei Decoction to Tonify the Blood) ⸱⸱⸱⸱⸱⸱ 2, 9, 70-71, 310

*dāng guī liù huáng tāng (Tangkuei and Six-Yellow Decoction) ⸱⸱⸱⸱⸱⸱ 70

dāng guī lóng huì wán (Tangkuei, Gentian, and Aloe Pill) ⸱⸱⸱⸱⸱⸱ 72-73, 185

dāng guī niān tòng tāng (Tangkuei Decoction to Pry Out Pain) ⸱⸱⸱⸱⸱⸱ 74-75, 332

dāng guī sháo yào sǎn (Tangkuei and Peony Powder) ⸱⸱⸱⸱⸱⸱ 76-77, 128, 129, 236, 271, 287, 323

*dāng guī sì nì jiā wú zhū yú shēng jiāng tāng (Frigid Extremities plus Evodia and Fresh Ginger) ⸱⸱⸱⸱⸱⸱ 78, 303

dāng guī sì nì tāng (Tangkuei Decoction for Frigid Extremities) ⸱⸱⸱⸱⸱⸱ 78-79, 142

*dāng guī yǐn zi (Tangkuei Drink) ⸱⸱⸱⸱⸱⸱ 310

dǎo chì sǎn (Guide Out the Red Powder) ⸱⸱⸱⸱⸱⸱ 4, 5, 80-81

dì huáng yǐn zi (Rehmannia Drink) ⸱⸱⸱⸱⸱⸱ 82-83

dìng chuǎn tāng (Arrest Wheezing Decoction) ⸱⸱⸱⸱⸱⸱ 84-85, 213, 324 *dīng xiāng shī dì tāng (Clove and Persimmon Calyx Decoction) ······ 164, 303

dìng zhì wán (Settle the Emotions Pill) ······ 86-87

dú huó jì shēng tāng (Pubescent Angelica and Taxillus Decoction) ······ 88-89, 166, 206, 247

*ē jiāo jī zi huáng tāng (Ass-Hide Gelatin and Egg Yolk Decoction) ······ 177

èr chén tāng (Two-Aged Herb Decoction) ······ 92-93, 366

èr miào sǎn (Two-Marvel Powder) ······ 94-95, 138, 150, 276

èr xiān tāng (Two-Immortal Decoction) ······ 96-97

èr zhì wán (Two-Solstice Pill) ······ 98-99, 293

*èr zhú tāng (Two Atractylodes Decoction) ······ 107

fáng fēng tōng shèng sǎn (Saposhnikovia Powder that Sagely Unblocks) ······ 100-101

fáng jǐ huáng qí tāng (Stephania and Astragalus Decoction) ······ 104-105, 293, 298

fú líng wán (Poria Pill) ······ 106-107

gān cǎo gān jiāng fú líng bái zhú tāng (Licorice, Ginger, Poria, and White Atractylodes Decoction) ······ 108-109, 150, 174

gān lù xiāo dú dān (Sweet Dew Special Pill to Eliminate Toxin) ······ 110-111, 173, 202, 227, 341

gān mài dà zǎo tāng (Licorice, Wheat, and Jujube Decoction) ······ 15, 112-113, 269

gé gēn huáng qín huáng lián tāng (Kudzu, Scutellaria, and Coptis Decoction) ······ 10, 114-115, 144

gé gēn tāng (Kudzu Decoction) ······ 35, 37, 47, 116-117, 131, 187

*gé gēn tāng (Kudzu Decoction) plus chuān xiōng (Chuanxiong Rhizoma) and xīn yí (Magnoliae flos) ······ 328

gé huā jiě chéng sǎn (Kudzu Flower Powder to Relieve Hangovers) ······ 118-119

gé xià zhú yū tāng (Drive Out Stasis Below the Diaphragm Decoction) ······ 68, 120-121

gù chòng tāng (Stabilize Gushing Decoction) ······ 122-123, 124, 127

gù jīng wán (Stabilize the Menses Pill) ······ 123, 124-125

*guì líng gān lù yǐn (Cinnamon and Poria Sweet Dew Drink) ······ 182

*guī lù èr xiān jiāo (Tortoise Shell and Deer Antler Two-Immortal Syrup) ······ 82

guī pí tāng (Restore the Spleen Decoction) ······ 2, 33, 70, 122, 126-127, 178, 266, 274

guì zhī fú líng wán (Cinnamon Twig and Poria Pill) ······ 76, 128-129, 271

*guì zhī jiā hòu pò xìng zǐ tāng (Cinnamon Twig Decoction plus Magnolia Bark and Apricot Kernel) ······ 190

*guì zhī jiā lóng gǔ mǔ lì tāng (Cinnamon Twig Decoction plus Dragon Bone and Oyster Shell) ······ 285

*guì zhī rén shēn tāng (Cinnamon Twig and Ginseng Decoction) ······ 303

*guì zhī sháo yào zhī mǔ tāng (Cinnamon Twig, Peony, and Anemarrhena Decoction) ······ 75

guì zhī tāng (Cinnamon Twig Decoction) ······ 35, 50, 68, 116, 130-131, 152, 162, 344

gǔn tán wán (Flushing Away Roiling Phlegm Pill) ······ 132-133 *hāo qín qīng dǎn tāng* (Sweet Wormwood and Scutellaria Decoction to Clear the Gallbladder) ⋯⋯ 134, 309

hòu pò wēn zhōng tāng (Magnolia Bark Decoction for Warming the Middle) ⋯⋯ 136-137, 137, 171

hǔ qían wán (Hidden Tiger Pill) ⋯⋯ 52, 138-139

huáng lián ē jiāo tāng (Coptis and Ass-Hide Gelatin Decoction) ⋯⋯ 269, 368

huáng lián jiě dú tāng (Coptis Decoction to Resolve Toxicity) ⋯⋯ 9, 140-141, 150

huáng lián tāng (Coptis Decoction) ⋯⋯ 17

huáng qí guì zhī wǔ wù tāng (Astragalus and Cinnamon Twig Five-Substance Decoction) ⋯⋯ 142-143

huáng qín tāng (Scutellaria Decoction) ⋯⋯ 10, 114, 144-145

huáng tǔ tāng (Yellow Earth Decoction) ⋯⋯ 11, 127

huò xiāng zhèng qì sǎn (Patchouli/Agastache Powder to Rectify the Qi) ⋯⋯ 146-147, 172, 201

jì chuān jiān (Benefit the River [Flow] Decoction) ⋯⋯ 148-149

jī míng sǎn (Powder to Take at Cock's Crow) ⋯⋯ 150-151

jiā wèi xiāng sū sǎn (Augmented Cyperus and Perilla Leaf Powder) ⋯⋯ 50, 131, 152-153, 187

jiā wèi xiāo yáo sǎn (Augmented Rambling Powder) ⋯⋯ 12, 39, 158, 185

jiàn líng tāng (Construct Roof Tiles Decoction) ⋯⋯ 31

jiàn pí wán (Strengthen the Spleen Pill) ⋯⋯ 20, 154-155, 362

jiāo ài tāng (Ass-Hide Gelatin and Mugwort Decoction) ⋯⋯ 287

jīn huáng sǎn/jīn huáng gāo (Golden-Yellow Plaster) ⋯⋯ 156-157, 280

jīn líng zǐ sǎn (Melia Toosendan Powder) ⋯⋯ 68, 158-159

jīn suǒ gù jīng wán (Metal Lock Pill to Stabilize the Essence) ⋯⋯ 160-161

jīng jiè lián qiào tang (Schizonepeta and Forsythia Decoction) ⋯⋯ 328

jiǔ wèi qiāng huó tāng (Nine-Herb Decoction with Notopterygium) ⋯⋯ 162-163, 206, 227

jú pí zhú rú tāng (Tangerine Peel and Bamboo Shavings Decoction) ⋯⋯ 164-165

juān bì tāng (Remove Painful Obstruction Decoction) ⋯⋯ 89, 166-167, 247

kǔ shēn tāng (Sophora Root Wash) ⋯⋯ 168-169

lǐ zhōng wán (Regulate the Middle Pill) ⋯⋯ 137, 170-171, 258, 263, 295, 303

lián pò yǐn (Coptis and Magnolia Bark Drink) ⋯⋯ 111, 146, 172-173

liáng fù wán (Galangal and Cyperus Pill) ⋯⋯ 137

liáng gé sǎn (Cool the Diaphragm Powder) ⋯⋯ 101

líng guì zhú gān tāng (Poria, Cinnamon Twig, Atractylodes, and Licorice Decoction) ⋯⋯ 108, 174-175, 293, 356

líng jiǎo gōu téng tāng (Antelope Horn and Uncaria Decoction) ⋯⋯ 176-177, 272, 355

liù jūn zǐ tāng (Six-Gentlemen Decoction) ⋯⋯ 13, 93, 137, 178-179, 228, 243, 292, 306 *liù wèi dì huáng wán* (Six-Ingredient Pill with Rehmannia) ······ 13, 52, 98, 180-181, 372

liù yī săn (Six-to-One Powder) ······ 182-183

lóng dăn xiè gān tāng (Gentian Decoction to Drain the Liver) ······ 73, 184-185

má huáng tāng (Ephedra Decoction) ······ 110, 152, 186-187

má huáng xì xīn fù zĭ tāng (Ephedra, Asarum, and Aconite Accessory Root Decoction) ······ 35, 188-189, 350

má xìng shí gān tāng (Ephedra, Apricot Kernel, Gypsum, and Licorice Decoction) ······ 9, 65, 84, 190-191, 213, 324

má zĭ rén wán (Hemp Seed Pill) ······ 148, 192-193, 224

mài mén dōng tāng (Ophiopogonis Decoction) ······ 23, 164, 190, 194-195

mŭ lì săn (Oyster Shell Powder) ······ 196-197

mù xiāng bīng láng wán (Aucklandia and Betel Nut Pill) ······ 198-199, 360

píng wèi săn (Calm the Stomach Powder) ······ 17, 146, 200-201, 306

pŭ jì xiāo dú yĭn (Universal Benefit Drink to Eliminate Toxin) ······ 111, 202-203

*qĭ pí wán (Open the Spleen Pill) ······ 21

qiān zhèng săn (Lead to Symmetry Powder) ······ 63, 204-205

qiāng huó shèng shī tāng (Notopterygium Decoction to Overcome Dampness) ······ 106, 206-207

*qín jiāo biē jiă săn (Large Gentian and Soft-Shelled Turtle Shell Powder) ······ 211

qīng dài săn (Indigo Powder) ······ 156, 208-209

*qīng gŭ săn (Cool the Bones Powder) ······ 210

qīng hāo biē jiă tāng (Sweet Wormwood and Soft-Shelled Turtle Shell Decoction [Version 1]) ······ 210-211, 370

qīng qì huà tán wán (Clear the Qi and Transform Phlegm Pill) ······ 212-213, 319

qīng shŭ yì qì tāng (Clear Summerheat and Augment the Qi Decoction) ······ 214-215, 370

qīng wèi săn (Clear the Stomach Powder) ······ 216-217, 326

*qīng xīn lián zĭ yĭn (Clear the Heart Drink with Lotus Seed) ······ 4, 80, 185

qīng yíng tāng (Clear the Nutritive Level Decoction) ······ 218-219

qīng zào jiù fèi tāng (Clear Dryness and Rescue the Lungs Decoction) ······ 6, 23, 195, 220-221, 233, 234

rén shēn bài dú săn (Ginseng Powder to Overcome Pathogenic Influences) ······ 222-223

*rén shēn yăng róng tāng (Ginseng Decoction to Nourish Luxuriance) ······ 252

rùn cháng wán (Moisten the Intestines Pill from *Master Shen's Book*) ······ 192, 224-225

sān rén tāng (Three-Seed Decoction) ······ 111, 226-227

sān zĭ yăng qīn tāng (Three-Seed Decoction to Nourish One's Parents) ······ 20, 228-229

sāng jú yĭn (Mulberry Leaf and Chrysanthemum Drink) ······ 230-231, 232, 341

*sāng piāo xiāo săn (Mantis Egg-Case Powder) ······ 24, 160

sāng xìng tāng (Mulberry Leaf and Apricot Kernel Decoction) ······ 22, 220, 230, 232-233, 330

shā shēn mài mén dōng tāng (Glehnia and Ophiopogonis Decoction) ······ 221, 234-235

shào fù zhú yū tāng (Drive Out Stasis from the Lower Abdomen Decoction) ······ 236-237

sháo yào gān cǎo tāng (Peony and Licorice Decoction) ······ 238-239

*sháo yào tāng (Peony Decoction) ······ 10, 114, 144

shēn fù tang (Ginseng and Aconite Accessory Root Decoction) ······ 240-241, 250, 263

shēn líng bái zhú sǎn (Ginseng, Poria, and White Atractylodes Powder) ······ 242-243

shèn qì wán (Kidney Qi Pill) ······ 13, 24, 96, 109, 244-245, 342, 357

*shēn sū yǐn (Ginseng and Perilla Leaf Drink) ······ 223

shēn tōng zhú yū tāng (Drive Out Stasis from a Painful Body Decoction) ······ 246-247

shēng huà tāng (Generating and Transforming Decoction) ······ 248-249, 256

shēng mài sǎn (Generate the Pulse Powder) ······ 250-251, 359

shí quán dà bǔ tāng (All-Inclusive Great Tonifying Decoction) ······ 2, 252-253

*shí shén tāng (Ten Divine Decoction) ······ 152

shí wèi bài dú sǎn (Ten-Ingredient Powder to Overcome Toxicity) ······ 254-255

shī xiào sǎn (Sudden Smile Powder) ······ 68, 248, 256-257

sì jūn zǐ tāng (Four-Gentlemen Decoction) ······ 33, 171, 178, 242, 258-259, 306

sì nì sǎn (Frigid Extremities Powder) ······ 39, 45, 68, 76, 79, 260-261, 295, 323, 336

sì nì tāng (Frigid Extremities Decoction) ······ 79, 171, 189, 240, 251, 262-263, 303, 357

sì shén wán (Four-Miracle Pill) ······ 264-265

sì wù tāng (Four-Substance Decoction) ······ 127, 266-267, 310

suān zǎo rén tāng (Sour Jujube Decoction) ······ 86, 112, 127, 268-269

*Taìshān pán shí sǎn (Taishan Bedrock Powder) ······ 18

táo hé chéng qì tāng (Peach Pit Decoction to Order the Qi) ······ 56, 129, 236, 270-271, 335

tiān má gōu téng yǐn (Gastrodia and Uncaria Drink) ······ 12, 177, 272-273, 355

tiān wáng bǔ xīn dān (Emperor of Heaven's Special Pill to Tonify the Heart) ······ 274-275

tōng guān wán (Open the Gate Pill) ······ 5, 95, 276-277

tòng xiè yào fāng (Important Formula for Painful Diarrhea) ······ 278-279

*tòu nóng sǎn (Discharge Pus Powder) ······ 70

tuō lǐ xiāo dú yǐn (Support the Interior and Eliminate Toxin Drink) ······ 280-281, 301, 304

wěi jīng tāng (Reed Decoction) ······ 282-283

wēn dǎn tāng (Warm Gallbladder Decoction) ······ 93, 132, 284-285 *wēn jīng tāng* (Flow-Warming Decoction) ⸱⸱⸱⸱⸱⸱ 96, 128, 129, 236, 248, 286-287

wēn pí tāng (Warm the Spleen Decoction) ⸱⸱⸱⸱⸱⸱ 288-289

wǔ lín sǎn (Powder for Five Types of Painful Urinary Dribbling) ⸱⸱⸱⸱⸱⸱ 290-291

wǔ líng sǎn (Five-Ingredient Powder with Poria) ⸱⸱⸱⸱⸱⸱ 9, 292-293, 298, 317, 368

wū méi wán (Mume Pill) ⸱⸱⸱⸱⸱⸱ 171, 294-295

wǔ pí sǎn (Five-Peel Powder) ⸱⸱⸱⸱⸱⸱ 104, 298-299

*wǔ rén wán (Five-Seed Pill) ⸱⸱⸱⸱⸱⸱ 193

wǔ wèi xiāo dú yǐn (Five-Ingredient Drink to Eliminate Toxin) ⸱⸱⸱⸱⸱⸱ 254, 300-301, 304

*wū yào shùn qì sǎn (Lindera Powder to Smooth the Flow of Qi) ⸱⸱⸱⸱⸱⸱ 31

wú zhū yú tāng (Evodia Decoction) ⸱⸱⸱⸱⸱⸱ 302-303

xiān fāng huó mìng yǐn (Immortals' Formula for Sustaining Life) ⸱⸱⸱⸱⸱⸱ 202, 254, 280, 301, 304-305

xiāng shā liù jūn zǐ tāng (Six-Gentlemen Decoction with Aucklandia and Amomum) ⸱⸱⸱⸱⸱⸱ 201, 306-307, 349

*xiāng sū sǎn (Cyperus and Perilla Leaf Powder) ⸱⸱⸱⸱⸱⸱ 152

xiǎo chái hú tāng (Minor Bupleurum Decoction) ⸱⸱⸱⸱⸱⸱ 54, 135, 261, 308-309

*xiǎo chéng qì tāng (Minor Order the Qi Decoction) ⸱⸱⸱⸱⸱⸱ 56

xiāo fēng sǎn (Eliminate Wind Powder from *Orthodox Lineage*) ⸱⸱⸱⸱⸱⸱ 310-311

xiǎo huó luò dān (Minor Invigorate the Collaterals Special Pill) ⸱⸱⸱⸱⸱⸱ 312-313

xiǎo jiàn zhōng tāng (Minor Construct the Middle Decoction) ⸱⸱⸱⸱⸱⸱ 314-315

xiǎo qīng lóng tāng (Minor Bluegreen Dragon Decoction) ⸱⸱⸱⸱⸱⸱ 65, 85, 190, 293, 316-317

xiǎo xiàn xiōng tāng (Minor Decoction [for Pathogens] Stuck in the Chest) ⸱⸱⸱⸱⸱⸱ 318-319

xiǎo xù mìng tāng (Minor Extend Life Decoction) ⸱⸱⸱⸱⸱⸱ 62, 320-321

xiāo yáo sǎn (Rambling Powder) ⸱⸱⸱⸱⸱⸱ 45, 76, 322-323, 336, 349

xiè bái sǎn (Drain the White Powder from
    Craft of Medicinal Treatment for Childhood Disease Patterns) ⸱⸱⸱⸱⸱⸱ 9, 84, 190, 324-325

xiè huáng sǎn (Drain the Yellow Powder) ⸱⸱⸱⸱⸱⸱ 216, 326-327

*xiè xīn tāng (Drain the Epigastrium Decoction) ⸱⸱⸱⸱⸱⸱ 4, 141

xīn yí qīng fèi yǐn (Magnolia Flower Drink to Clear the Lungs) ⸱⸱⸱⸱⸱⸱ 328-329

*xīn yí sǎn (Magnolia Flower Powder) ⸱⸱⸱⸱⸱⸱ 35

xìng sū sǎn (Apricot Kernel and Perilla Leaf Powder) ⸱⸱⸱⸱⸱⸱ 232, 330-331, 366

xuān bì tāng (Disband Painful Obstruction Decoction) ⸱⸱⸱⸱⸱⸱ 332-333

*xuán fù dài zhě tāng (Inula and Haematite Decoction) ⸱⸱⸱⸱⸱⸱ 165

xuè fǔ zhú yū tāng (Drive Out Stasis from the Mansion of Blood Decoction) ⸱⸱⸱⸱⸱⸱ 334-335 *yǎng yīn qīng fèi tāng (Nourish the Yin and Clear the Lungs Decoction) ······ 352

*yì gān sǎn (Restrain the Liver Powder) ······ 41, 323

yī guàn jiān (Linking Decoction) ······ 336-337

*yì yǐ fù zǐ sǎn (Coix and Aconite Powder) ······ 365

yīn chén hāo tāng (Virgate Wormwood Decoction) ······ 338-339

yín qiáo sǎn (Honeysuckle and Forsythia Powder) ······ 110, 230, 340-341

yòu guī wán (Restore the Right [Kidney] Pill) ······ 245, 342-343

*yù nū jiān (Jade Woman Decoction) ······ 216

yù píng fēng sǎn (Jade Windscreen Powder) ······ 28, 104, 196, 248, 344-345

yù quán wán (Jade Spring Pill) ······ 346-347

yuè jū wán (Escape Restraint Pill) ······ 14, 322, 348-349

zài zào sǎn (Renewal Powder) ······ 188, 350-351

zēng yè tāng (Increase the Fluids Decoction) ······ 352-353

zhèn gān xī fēng tāng (Sedate the Liver and Extinguish Wind Decoction) ······ 177, 273, 354-355

*zhēn rén yǎng zàng tāng (True Man's Decoction to Nourish the Organs) ······ 264

zhēn wǔ tāng (True Warrior Decoction) ······ 30, 108, 174, 245, 263, 295, 356-357

*zhī bái dì huáng wán (Anemarrhena, Phellodendron, and Rehmannia Pill) ······ 4, 52, 96, 185

zhì gān cǎo tāng (Prepared Licorice Decoction) ······ 126, 251, 274, 358-359

zhǐ shí dǎo zhì wán (Unripe Bitter Orange Pill to Guide Out Stagnation) ······ 199, 360-361

zhǐ shí xiāo pǐ wán (Unripe Bitter Orange Pill to Reduce Focal Distention) ······ 154, 362-363

zhǐ shí xiè bái guì zhī tāng (Unripe Bitter Orange, Chinese Garlic, and Cinnamon Twig Decoction) ······ 68, 364-365

zhǐ sòu sǎn (Stop Coughing Powder) ······ 330, 366-367

*zhī zǐ chǐ tāng (Gardenia and Prepared Soybean Decoction) ······ 48, 80, 269, 285

zhū líng tāng (Polyporus Decoction) ······ 95, 185, 293, 368-369

zhú yè shí gāo tang (Lophatherum and Gypsum Decoction) ······ 195, 214, 285, 370-371

zuǒ guī wán (Restore the Left [Kidney] Pill) ······ 181, 372-373

*zuǒ jīn wán (Left Metal Pill) ······ 158, 284

Index of Formulas by English Common Name

Principal entries for each of the main formulas are shown as a page spread (e.g., 34-35). Other formulas that are discussed under the main entries, but are not themselves main formulas, are preceded with an asterisk (*).

. . . .

All-Inclusive Great Tonifying Decoction *(shí quán dà bǔ tāng)* ······ 2, 252–253

*Anemarrhena, Phellodendron, and Rehmannia Pill *(zhī bǎi dì huáng wán)* ······ 4, 52, 96, 185

Antelope Horn and Uncaria Decoction *(líng jiǎo gōu téng tāng)* ······ 176–177, 272, 355

Apricot Kernel and Perilla Leaf Powder *(xìng sū sǎn)* ······ 232, 330–331, 366

Arrest Wheezing Decoction *(dìng chuǎn tāng)* ······ 84–85, 213, 324

*Ass-Hide Gelatin and Egg Yolk Decoction *(ē jiāo jī zi huáng tāng)* ······ 177

*Ass-Hide Gelatin and Mugwort Decoction *(jiāo ài tāng)* ······ 287

Astragalus and Cinnamon Twig Five-Substance Decoction *(huáng qí guì zhī wǔ wù tāng)* ······ 142

Aucklandia and Betel Nut Pill *(mù xiāng bīng láng wán)* ······ 198–199, 360

Augmented Cyperus and Perilla Leaf Powder *(jiā wèi xiāng sū sǎn)* ······ 50, 131, 152–153, 187

*Augmented Rambling Powder *(jiā wèi xiāo yáo sǎn)* ······ 12, 39, 158, 185

Benefit the River [Flow] Decoction *(jì chuān jiān)* ······ 148–149

Borneal and Borax Powder *(bīng péng sǎn)* ······ 26–27

*Bupleurum and Cinnamon Twig Decoction *(chái hú guì zhī tāng)* ······ 38

Bupleurum and Kudzu Decoction to Release the Muscle Layer *(chái gé jiě jī tāng)* ······ 36

*Bupleurum Decoction plus Mirabilite *(chái hú jiā máng xiāo tāng)* ······ 55

Bupleurum Decoction to Clear the Liver *(chái hú qīng gān tāng)* ······ 42–43, 202

*Bupleurum Drink to Reach the Source *(chái hú dá yuán yǐn)* ······ 66

Bupleurum plus Dragon Bone and Oyster Shell Decoction *(chái hú jiā lóng gǔ mǔ lì tāng)* ······ 39, 40–41, 55

Bupleurum Powder to Dredge he Liver *(chái hú shū gān sǎn)* ······ 44–45

Bupleurum, Cinnamon Twig, and Ginger Decoction *(chái hú guì jiāng tāng)* ······ 38–39

Calm the Stomach Powder (*píng wèi săn*) ⋯⋯ 17, 146, 200–201, 306

Chuanxiong Powder to be Taken with Green Tea (*chuān xiōng chá tiáo săn*) ⋯⋯ 35, 46–47

*Cinnamon and Poria Sweet Dew Drink (*guì líng gān lù yǐn*) ⋯⋯ 182

*Cinnamon Twig and Ginseng Decoction (*guì zhī rén shēn tāng*) ⋯⋯ 303

Cinnamon Twig and Poria Pill (*guì zhī fú líng wán*) ⋯⋯ 76, 128–129, 271

Cinnamon Twig Decoction (*guì zhī tang*) ⋯⋯ 3, 50, 116, 130–131, 152, 344

*Cinnamon Twig Decoction plus Dragon Bone and Oyster Shell (*chái hú jiā lóng gǔ mǔ lì tāng*) ⋯⋯ 285

*Cinnamon Twig Decoction plus Magnolia Bark and Apricot Kernel (*guì zhī jiā hòu pò xìng zǐ tāng*) ⋯⋯ 190

*Cinnamon Twig, Peony, and Anemarrhena Decoction (*guì zhī sháo yào zhī mǔ tāng*) ⋯⋯ 75

Clear Dryness and Rescue the Lungs Decoction (*qīng zào jiù fèi tāng*) ⋯⋯ 6, 23, 195, 220–221, 233, 234

Clear Summerheat and Augment the Qi Decoction (*qīng shǔ yì qì tāng*) ⋯⋯ 214–215, 370

*Clear the Heart Drink with Lotus Seed (*qīng xīn lián zǐ yǐn*) ⋯⋯ 4, 80, 185

Clear the Nutritive Level Decoction (*qīng yíng tāng*) ⋯⋯ 218–219

Clear the Qi and Transform Phlegm Pill (*qīng qì huà tán wán*) ⋯⋯ 212–213, 319

Clear the Stomach Powder (*qīng wèi săn*) ⋯⋯ 216–217, 326

*Clove and Persimmon Calyx Decoction (*dīng xiāng shì dì tāng*) ⋯⋯ 164, 303

*Coix and Aconite Powder (*yì yǐ fù zǐ săn*) ⋯⋯ 365

*Construct Roof Tiles Decoction (*jiàn líng tāng*) ⋯⋯ 31

*Cool the Bones Powder (*qīng gǔ săn*) ⋯⋯ 210

*Cool the Diaphragm Powder (*liáng gé săn*) ⋯⋯ 101

*Coptis and Ass-Hide Gelatin Decoction (*huáng lián ē jiāo tāng*) ⋯⋯ 269, 368

Coptis and Magnolia Bark Drink (*ián pò yǐn*) ⋯⋯ 111, 146, 172–173

*Coptis Decoction (*huáng lián tāng*) ⋯⋯ 17

Coptis Decoction to Resolve Toxicity (*huáng lián jiě dú tāng*) ⋯⋯ 9, 140–141

*Cyperus and Perilla Leaf Powder (*xiāng sū săn*) ⋯⋯ 152

Disband Painful Obstruction Decoction (*xuān bì tāng*) ⋯⋯ 75, 332–333

*Discharge Pus Powder (*tòu nóng săn*) ⋯⋯ 70

*Drain the Epigastrium Decoction (*xiè xīn tāng*) ⋯⋯ 4, 141

Drain the White Powder from *Craft of Medicinal Treatment for Childhood Disease Patterns* (*xiè bái săn*) ⋯⋯ 9, 84, 190, 324–325

Drain the Yellow Powder (*xiè huáng săn*) ⋯⋯ 216, 326–327

Drive Out Stasis Below the Diaphragm Decoction (*gé xià zhú yū tāng*) ⋯⋯ 68, 120–121

Drive Out Stasis from a Painful Body Decoction (shēn tōng zhú yū tāng) ······ 246–247

Drive Out Stasis from the Lower Abdomen Decoction (shào fù zhú yū tāng) ······ 236–237

Drive Out Stasis from the Mansion of Blood Decoction (xuè fǔ zhú yū tāng) ······ 334–335

Eight-Herb Powder for Rectification (bā zhèng sǎn) ······ 4–5, 80, 276, 290

Eight-Treasure Decoction (bā zhēn tāng) ······ 2–3, 252

Eliminate Wind Powder from Orthodox Lineage (xiāo fēng sǎn) ······ 310–311

Emperor of Heaven's Special Pill to Tonify the Heart (tiān wáng bǔ xīn dān) ······ 274–275

Ephedra Decoction (má huáng tāng) ······ 65, 116, 131, 152, 186–187

Ephedra, Apricot Kernel, Gypsum, and Licorice Decoction (má xìng shí gān tāng) ······ 9, 65, 84, 190–191, 213, 324

Ephedra, Asarum, and Aconite Accessory Root Decoction (má huáng xì xīn fù zǐ tāng) ······ 35, 188–189, 350

Escape Restraint Pill (yuè jū wán) ······ 14–15, 322, 348–349

Evodia Decoction (wú zhū yú tāng) ······ 302–303

Five-Ingredient Drink to Eliminate Toxin (wǔ wèi xiāo dú yǐn) ······ 254, 300–301, 304

Five-Ingredient Powder with Poria (wǔ líng sǎn) ······ 9, 292–293, 317, 368

Five-Peel Powder (wǔ pí sǎn) ······ 104, 298–299

*Five-Seed Pill (wǔ rén wán) ······ 193

Flow-Warming Decoction (wēn jīng tāng) ······ 96, 129, 248, 286–287

Flushing Away Roiling Phlegm Pill (gǔn tán wán) ······ 132–133

Four-Gentlemen Decoction (sì jūn zǐ tāng) ······ 33, 171, 242, 258–259, 306

Four-Miracle Pill (sì shén wán) ······ 264–265

Four-Substance Decoction (sì wù tāng) ······ 127, 266–267

Frigid Extremities Decoction (sì nì tāng) ······ 79, 171, 189, 240, 251, 262–263, 295, 303, 323, 336, 357

*Frigid Extremities plus Evodia and Fresh Ginger (dāng guī sì nì jiā wú zhū yú shēng jiāng tāng) ······ 78, 303

Frigid Extremities Powder (sì nì sǎn) ······ 39, 45, 76, 79, 260–261

Fritillaria and Tricosanthes Fruit Powder (bèi mǔ guā lóu sǎn) ······ 7, 22–23

*Galangal and Cyperus Pill (iáng fù wán) ······ 137

*Gardenia and Phellodendron Decoction (zhī zǐ bǎi pí tāng) ······ 338

*Gardenia and Prepared Soybean Decoction (zhī zǐ chǐ tāng) ······ 48, 80, 269, 285

Gastrodia and Uncaria Drink (tiān má gōu téng yǐn) ······ 12, 177, 272–273, 355

Generate the Pulse Powder (shēng mài sǎn) ······ 250–251, 359

Generating and Transforming Decoction (shēng huà tāng) ······ 248–249, 256

Gentian Decoction to Drain the Liver (lóng dǎn xiè gān tāng) ······ 73, 184–185

Ginseng and Aconite Accessory Root Decoction *(shēn fù tāng)* ······ 240–241, 250, 263

*Ginseng and Perilla Leaf Drink *(shēn sū yǐn)* ······ 223

*Ginseng Decoction to Nourish Luxuriance *(rén shēn yǎng róng tāng)* ······ 252

Ginseng Powder to Overcome Pathogenic Influences *(rén shēn bài dú sǎn)* ······ 222–223

Ginseng, Poria, and White Atractylodes Macrocephala Powder
   (shēn líng bái zhú sǎn) ······ 178, 242–243, 258, 264, 278

Glehnia and Ophiopogonis Decoction *(shā shēn mài mén dōng tāng)* ······ 221, 234–235

Golden-Yellow Plaster *(jīn huáng sǎn/jīn huáng gāo)* ······ 156–157, 208

Great Tonify the Yin Pill *(dà bǔ yīn wán)* ······ 52–53, 138, 210, 276

Guide Out the Red Powder *(dǎo chì sǎn)* ······ 5, 80–81

Hemp Seed Pill *(má zǐ rén wán)* ······ 148, 192–193, 224

Hidden Tiger Pill *(hǔ qián wán)* ······ 52, 138–139

Honeysuckle and Forsythia Powder *(yín qiáo sǎn)* ······ 230, 340–341

Immortals' Formula for Sustaining Life *(xiān fāng huó mìng yǐn)* ······ 202, 254, 280, 301, 304–305

Important Formula for Painful Diarrhea *(tòng xiè yào fāng)* ······ 278–279

Increase the Fluids Decoction *(zēng yè tāng)* ······ 352–353

Indigo Powder *(qīng dài sǎn)* ······ 156, 208–209

*Inula and Haematite Decoction *(xuán fù dài zhě tāng)* ······ 165

Jade Spring Pill *(yù quán wán)* ······ 346–347

Jade Windscreen Powder *(yù píng fēng sǎn)* ······ 28, 104, 196, 344–345

*Jade Woman Decoction *(yù nǚ jiān)* ······ 216

Kidney Qi Pill *(shèn qì wán)* ······ 13, 24, 96, 109, 244–245, 342, 357

Kudzu Decoction *(gé gēn tāng)* ······ 35, 37, 47, 116–117, 131, 187

*Kudzu Decoction *(gé gēn tāng)* plus Chuanxiong Rhizoma *(chuān xiōng)* and Magnoliae flos *(xīn yí)* ······ 328

Kudzu Flower Powder to Relieve Hangovers *(gé huā jiě chéng sǎn)* ······ 118–119

Kudzu, Scutellaria, and Coptis Decoction *(gé gēn huáng qín huáng lián tāng)* ······ 10, 114–115, 145

*Large Gentian and Soft-Shelled Turtle Shell Powder *(qín jiāo biē jiǎ sǎn)* ······ 211

Lead to Symmetry Powder *(qiān zhèng sǎn)* ······ 63, 204–205

*Left Metal Pill *(zuǒ jīn wán)* ······ 158, 284

Licorice, Ginger, Poria, and White Atractylodes Decoction
   (gān cǎo gān jiāng fú líng bái zhú tāng) ······ 108–109, 150, 174

Licorice, Wheat, and Jujube Decoction *(gān mài dà zǎo tāng)* ······ 15, 112–113, 269

Lily Bulb Decoction to Preserve the Metal *(bǎi hé gù jīn tāng)* ⋯⋯ 6–7, 23, 195

*Lindera Powder to Smooth the Flow of Qi *(wū yào shùn qì sǎn)* ⋯⋯ 31

Linking Decoction *(yī guàn jiān)* ⋯⋯ 336–337

Lophatherum and Gypsum Decoction *(zhú yè shí gāo tang)* ⋯⋯ 195, 214, 285, 370–371

Magnolia Bark Decoction for Warming the Middle *(hòu pò wēn zhōng tāng)* ⋯⋯ 136–137, 171

Magnolia Flower Drink to Clear the Lungs *(xīn yí qīng fèi yǐn)* ⋯⋯ 328–329

*Magnolia Flower Powder *(xīn yí sǎn)* ⋯⋯ 35

*Major Arrest Wind Pearls *(dà dìng fēng zhū)* ⋯⋯ 177

Major Bluegreen Dragon Decoction *(dà qīng lóng tāng)* ⋯⋯ 64–65

Major Bupleurum Decoction *(dà chái hú tāng)* ⋯⋯ 41, 54–55, 57, 58, 101, 309

*Major Construct the Middle Decoction *(dà jiàn zhōng tāng)* ⋯⋯ 58, 315

Major Large Gentian Decoction *(dà qín jiāo tāng)* ⋯⋯ 62–63, 321

Major Order the Qi Decoction *(dà chéng qì tāng)* ⋯⋯ 56–57, 60, 115, 132, 141

*Mantis Egg-Case Powder *(sāng piāo xiāo sǎn)* ⋯⋯ 24, 160

Melia Toosendan Powder *(jīn líng zǐ sǎn)* ⋯⋯ 158–159

Metal Lock Pill to Stabilize the Essence *(jīn suǒ gù jīng wán)* ⋯⋯ 160–161

Minor Bluegreen Dragon Decoction *(xiǎo qīng lóng tāng)* ⋯⋯ 65, 84–85, 190, 293, 316–317

Minor Bupleurum Decoction *(xiǎo chái hú tāng)* ⋯⋯ 54, 135, 261, 308–309

Minor Construct the Middle Decoction *(xiǎo jiàn zhōng tāng)* ⋯⋯ 314–315

Minor Decoction [for Pathogens] Stuck in the Chest *(xiǎo xiàn xiōng tāng)* ⋯⋯ 318–319

Minor Extend Life Decoction *(xiǎo xù mìng tāng)* ⋯⋯ 63, 320–321

Minor Invigorate the Collaterals Special Pill *(xiǎo huó luò dān)* ⋯⋯ 312–313

*Minor Order the Qi Decoction *(xiǎo chéng qì tāng)* ⋯⋯ 56

Moisten the Intestines Pill from *Master Shen's Book* *(rùn cháng wán)* ⋯⋯ 193, 224–225

Mulberry Leaf and Apricot Kernel Decoction *(sāng xìng tāng)* ⋯⋯ 22, 220, 230, 232–233, 330

Mulberry Leaf and Chrysanthemum Drink *(sāng jú yǐn)* ⋯⋯ 50, 230–231, 232, 341

Mume Pill *(wū méi wán)* ⋯⋯ 171, 294–296

Nine-Herb Decoction with Notopterygium *(jiǔ wèi qiāng huó tāng)* ⋯⋯ 162–163, 206, 227

Notopterygium Decoction to Overcome Dampness *(qiāng huó shèng shī tāng)* ⋯⋯ 106, 206–207

*Nourish the Yin and Clear the Lungs Decoction *(yǎng yīn qīng fèi tāng)* ⋯⋯ 352

Open the Gate Pill *(tōng guān wán)* ⋯⋯ 5, 95, 276–277

*Open the Spleen Pill *(qǐ pí wán)* ⋯⋯ 21

Ophiopogonis Decoction *(mài mén dōng tāng)* ⋯⋯ 23, 190, 194–195

Oyster Shell Powder *(mǔ lì sǎn)* ⋯⋯ 196–197

Patchouli/Agastache Powder to Rectify the Qi *(huò xiāng zhèng qì sǎn)* ⋯⋯ 146, 172, 201

Peach Pit Decoction to Order the Qi *(táo hé chéng qì tāng)* ⋯⋯ 56, 129, 236, 270–271, 335

Peony and Licorice Decoction *(sháo yào gān cǎo tāng)* ⋯⋯ 238–239

*Peony Decoction *(sháo yào tāng)* ⋯⋯ 10, 114, 144

Pinellia and Magnolia Bark Decoction *(bàn xià hòu pò tāng)* ⋯⋯ 14–15, 195, 349

Pinellia Decoction to Drain the Epigastrium *(bàn xià xiè xīn tāng)* ⋯⋯ 15, 16–17, 201, 319, 362

Pinellia, White Atractylodes, and Gastrodia Decoction *(bàn xià bái zhú tiān má tāng)* ⋯⋯ 12–13, 93

Polyporus Decoction *(zhū líng tāng)* ⋯⋯ 95, 293, 368–369

Poria Pill *(fú líng wán)* ⋯⋯ 106–107

Poria, Cinnamon Twig, Atractylodes, and Licorice Decoction *(líng guì zhú gān tāng)* ⋯⋯ 108, 174–175, 293, 356

Powder for Five types of Urinary Dribbling *(wǔ lín sǎn)* ⋯⋯ 290–291

Powder to Take at Cock's Crow *(jī míng sǎn)* ⋯⋯ 150–151

Prepared Licorice Decoction *(zhì gān cǎo tāng)* ⋯⋯ 126–127, 251, 274, 358

Preserve Harmony Pill *(bǎo hé wán)* ⋯⋯ 20–21, 154, 228, 278, 306

Pubescent Angelica and Taxillus Decoction *(dú huó jì shēng tāng)* ⋯⋯ 88–90, 166, 206, 247

Pulsatilla Decoction *(bái tóu wēng tāng)* ⋯⋯ 10–11, 114

Rambling Powder *(xiāo yáo sǎn)* ⋯⋯ 45, 76, 322–323, 336, 349

Reed Decoction *(wěi jīng tāng)* ⋯⋯ 282–283

Regulate the Middle Pill *(lǐ zhōng wán)* ⋯⋯ 137, 170–171, 258, 263, 295, 303

Rehmannia Drink *(dì huáng yǐn zi)* ⋯⋯ 82–83

Remove Painful Obstruction Decoction *(juān bì tāng)* ⋯⋯ 89, 166–167, 247

Renewal Powder *(zài zào sǎn)* ⋯⋯ 188–189, 350–351

Restore the Left (Kidney) Pill *(zuǒ guī wán)* ⋯⋯ 181, 372–373

Restore the Right (Kidney) Pill *(yòu guī wán)* ⋯⋯ 245, 342–343

Restore the Spleen Decoction *(guī pí tāng)* ⋯⋯ 2, 33, 70, 122–123, 126–127, 178, 266, 274

*Restrain the Liver Powder *(yì gān sǎn)* ⋯⋯ 41, 323

Rhubarb and Aconite Accessory Root Decoction *(dà huáng fù zǐ tāng)* ⋯⋯ 58–59, 288

Rhubarb and Moutan Decoction *(dà huáng mǔ dān tāng)* ⋯⋯ 57, 60–61

Salvia Drink *(dān shēn yǐn)* ⋯⋯ 68–69, 120, 256

Saposhnikovia Powder that Sagely Unblocks *(fáng fēng tōng shèng sǎn)* ⋯⋯ 100–101

Scallion and Prepared Soybean Decoction *(cōng chǐ tāng)* ······ 50–51

Scallion Drink with Seven Ingredients *(cōng bái qī wèi yǐn)* ······ 48–49

*Schizonepeta and Forsythia Decoction *(jīng jiè lián qiào tang)* ······ 328

Scutellaria Decoction *(huáng qín tāng)* ······ 10, 114, 144–145

Sedate the Liver and Extinguish Wind Decoction *(zhèn gān xī fēng tāng)* ······ 177, 273, 354–355

Settle the Emotions Pill *(dìng zhì wán)* ······ 86–87

Six-Gentlemen Decoction *(liù jūn zǐ tāng)* ······ 13, 137, 178–179, 243

Six-Gentlemen Decoction with Aucklandia and Amomum *(xiāng shā liù jūn zǐ tāng)* ······ 201, 306–307, 349

Six-Ingredient Pill with Rehmannia *(liù wèi dì huáng wán)* ······ 13, 52, 98, 180–181, 372

Six-to-One Powder *(liù yī sǎn)* ······ 182–183

Sophora Root Wash *(kǔ shēn tāng)* ······ 168–169

Sour Jujube Decoction *(suān zǎo rén tāng)* ······ 86, 112, 127, 268–269

Stabilize Gushing Decoction *(gù chòng tāng)* ······ 122–123, 124, 127

Stabilize the Menses Pill *(gù jīng wán)* ······ 123, 124–125

Stephania and Astragalus Decoction *(fáng jǐ huáng qí tāng)* ······ 104–105, 293, 298

Stop Coughing Powder *(zhǐ sòu sǎn)* ······ 330, 366–367

Strengthen the Spleen Pill *(jiàn pí wán)* ······ 20, 154–155, 362

Sudden Smile Powder *(shī xiào sǎn)* ······ 68, 248, 256–257

Support the Interior and Eliminate Toxin Drink *(tuō lǐ xiāo dú yǐn)* ······ 280–281, 301, 304

Sweet Dew Special Pill to Eliminate Toxin *(gān lù xiāo dú dān)* ······ 110–111, 173, 202, 227, 341

Sweet Wormwood and Scutellaria Decoction to Clear the Gallbladder *(hāo qín qīng dǎn tāng)* ······ 134–135, 309

Sweet Wormwood and Soft-Shelled Turtle Shell Decoction [Version 1] *(qīng hāo biē jiǎ tang)* ······ 210–211, 370

*Taishan Bedrock Powder *(Tàishān pán shí sǎn)* ······ 18

Tangerine Peel and Bamboo Shavings Decoction *(jú pí zhú rú tāng)* ······ 164–165

Tangkuei and Peony Powder *(dāng guī sháo yào sǎn)* ······ 76–77, 129, 236, 271, 287, 323

*Tangkuei and Six-Yellow Decoction *(dāng guī liù huáng tāng)* ······ 70

Tangkuei Decoction for Frigid Extremities *(dāng guī sì nì tāng)* ······ 78–79, 142

Tangkuei Decoction to Pry Out Pain *(dāng guī niān tòng tāng)* ······ 74–75, 332

Tangkuei Decoction to Tonify the Blood *(dāng guī bǔ xuè tāng)* ······ 2, 9, 70–71

*Tangkuei Drink *(dāng guī yǐn zi)* ······ 310

Tangkuei, Gentian, and Aloe Pill *(dāng guī lóng huì wán)* ······ 72–73, 185

*Ten Divine Decoction *(shí shén tāng)* ······ 152

Ten-Ingredient Powder to Overcome Toxicity *(shí wèi bài dú sǎn)* ······ 254–255

Three-Seed Decoction *(sān rén tāng)* ······ 163, 226–227

Three-Seed Decoction to Nourish One's Parents *(sān zǐ yǎng qīn tāng)* ······ 20–21, 111, 228–229

Tokoro Drink to Separate the Clear *(bì xiè fēn qīng yǐn/bēi xiè fēn qīng yǐn)* ······ 24–25

*Tonify Spleen-Stomach, Drain Yin Fire, and Raise Yang Decoction *(bǔ pí wèi xiè yīn huǒ shēng yáng tāng)* ······ 70

Tonify the Lungs Decoction *(bǔ fèi tāng)* ······ 28–29

*Tonify the Lungs Decoction with Ass-Hide Gelatin *(bǔ fèi ē jiāo tāng)* ······ 6

Tonify the Middle to Augment the Qi Decoction *(bǔ zhōng yì qì tāng)* ······ 32–33, 70, 106, 123, 315

Tonify the Yang to Restore Five (-Tenths) Decoction *(bǔ yáng huán wǔ tāng)* ······ 30–31

*Tortoise Shell and Deer Antler Two-Immortal Syrup *(guī lù èr xiān jiāo)* ······ 82

*True Man's Decoction to Nourish the Organs *(zhēn rén yǎng zàng tāng)* ······ 264

True Warrior Decoction *(zhēn wǔ tāng)* ······ 108, 174–175, 245, 263, 295, 356–357

*Two Atractylodes Decoction *(èr zhú tāng)* ······ 107

Two-Aged Herb Decoction *(èr chén tāng)* ······ 92–93

Two-Immortal Decoction *(èr xiān tāng)* ······ 96–97

Two-Marvel Powder *(èr miào sǎn)* ······ 94–95, 139, 276

Two-Solstice Pill *(èr zhì wán)* ······ 98–99

Universal Benefit Drink to Eliminate Toxin *(pǔ jì xiāo dú yǐn)* ······ 111, 202–203

Unripe Bitter Orange Pill to Guide out Stagnation *(zhǐ shí dǎo zhì wán)* ······ 199, 360–361

Unripe Bitter Orange Pill to Reduce Focal Distention *(zhǐ shí xiāo pǐ wán)* ······ 154, 362–363

Unripe Bitter Orange, Chinese Garlic, and Cinnamon Twig Decoction *(zhǐ shí xiè bái guì zhī tāng)* ······ 364–365

Virgate Wormwood Decoction *(yīn chén hāo tāng)* ······ 338

Warm Gallbladder Decoction *(wēn dǎn tāng)* ······ 93, 132, 284–285

Warm the Spleen Decoction *(wēn pí tāng)* ······ 288–289

White Tiger Decoction *(bái hǔ tāng)* ······ 8–9, 140, 293, 324

*White Tiger plus Ginseng Decoction *(bái hǔ jiā rén shēn tāng)* ······ 131, 214, 346

Worry-Free Formula to Protect Birth *(bǎo chǎn wú yōu fāng)* ······ 18–19

Xanthium Powder *(cāng ér zǐ sǎn)* ······ 34–35, 47

*Yellow Earth Decoction *(huáng tǔ tāng)* ······ 11, 127

Index of Patterns and Key Symptoms

—A

abdomen
  cold excess in, 58
  distention and fullness, 44, 200, 298
  focal distention in, 362
  fullness or distention in, 20
  stifling sensation in, 348
  upper, stifling sensation in, 12
abdominal distention, 110, 170, 306
  and fullness, 136
  and pain, 260
  focal, 154
  slight, 338
abdominal fullness, and epigastric distention, 100
abdominal guarding, 60
abdominal masses, palpable, 120
abdominal pain, 10, 144, 278, 288, 294, 306, 308
  acute, 58
  and distention, 56
  due to Liver/Spleen disharmony, 76
  increased with pressure, 56
  lower, 60
  periodic, 136
  spasmodic, 314
absentmindedness, 112
achy limbs, 110
acne, 10
agitation, mental, 270
alcohol consumption, damp-heat in yang brightness due to, with Spleen deficiency, 118
alternating fever and chills, 54
  at irregular intervals, 66

anger, 40
  arising from frustration, 44
  propensity to, 72
anus, burning sensation around, 10, 114
anxiety, 86, 284
  with irritability, 260
appetite
  emaciation without loss of, 210
  increased, 346
  lack of, 32, 214, 228, 362
  loss of, 178
  reduced, 2, 118, 126, 242, 258, 306
    with indigestion, 154
arm pain, 246
  bilateral, 106
arms and legs, inability to move, 62
ascendant Liver yang, leading to internal Liver wind, 272
asymmetry, facial, 320
atrophy, of lower limbs, 30
atrophy disorder, due to Liver and Kidney deficiency, 138

—B

back and waist, painful obstruction, 108
back pain, 206
back weakness, 244
backache, 236
bad breath, 326
behavior, inability to control, 112
belching, 306
  foul-smelling, 20
bending, difficult, 108
bitter fluids, spitting up, 134

bitter taste, 144, 184, 308
Bladder damp-heat, Eight-Herb Powder for Rectification in, 4
Bladder qi transformation, heat obstructing, 276
bleeding
    chronic, 126
    due to middle burner yang deficiency, 170
    uterine, with thin and pale blood, 122
bloating, 154
blood
    in stool, 288
    Spleen unable to govern, 126
blood and qi stasis, in chest, with impairment of blood flow above diaphragm, 334
blood buildup, in lower burner, due to blood stasis/heat accumulation, 270
blood circulation, cold obstructing with deficiency, 78
blood congestion, in brain, 354
blood deficiency, 238
    and stagnation, 266
    cold obstructing blood circulation with, 78
    from long-term illness, 70
    Liver constraint and frail Spleen with, 322
blood flow, impairment above diaphragm, 334
blood loss, qi abandonment from, 70
blood painful obstruction, 142
blood stagnation, postpartum, due to cold and blood deficiency, 248
blood stasis
    accumulation in lower burner, 270
    and qi stagnation in middle burner, 68
    and water accumulation, 272
    below diaphragm, 120
    cold-induced accumulation in lower abdomen, 236
    in lower abdomen, 128
    Liver wind stirring with, 272
    Lung abscess from, 282
    obstruction of channels by, 312
    with deficiency cold of Conception and Penetrating vessels, 286
    with qi constraint, 348
blood-streaked sputum, 282
blurred vision, 98
body aches, generalized, 74, 316
boils, 300
bones and joints, migrating pain in, 312

borborygmus, 278
    after eating, 200
brain, congestion of blood in, 354
breast pain and distention, 322
breathing
    difficult, 212
    labored, 84
burning sensation, around anus, 10, 114

— C

calves
    heavy and weak, 150
    numbness, cold or pain in, 150
carbuncles, 100, 300
    early-stage, 304
channel stroke, sequelae of, 204
channels, wind-dampness lodging in, 206
channels and collaterals
    middle burner phlegm overflowing into, 106
    obstruction by wind-cold-dampness, blood stasis, and phlegm, 312
    painful obstruction due to damp-heat in, 332
    painful obstruction due to qi/blood stasis in, 246
cheeks, flushed, 42
chest
    blood and qi stasis in, with impairment of blood flow above diaphragm, 334
    clumping of heat and phlegm in, 318
    distention in, 298, 308
    focal distention in, 118, 228, 362, 364
        worse pressure, 318
    fullness in, 40, 212, 298
    fullness or pain in, 364
    irritability and warmth in, 294
    irritability with heat in, 80
    pain in, 334
    stifling sensation in, 12, 110, 134, 150, 172, 174, 178, 226, 242, 316, 348
chest discomfort, difficult to describe, 268
chest fullness, 54
chest pain, 58, 158, 308, 336
chest painful obstruction, 364
chills
    alternating with fever, 54
    fever with slight, 340

followed by aversion to heat, 340
mild, alternating with pronounced fever, 134
severe fever and, 64
slight, 50
  with fever, 230
strong with slight fever, 350
without sweating, 330
clear, loss of ability to ascend, 308
clear and turbid, loss of ability to ascend and descend, 308
clear liquid, vomiting of, 136
clots
  dark menstrual blood with, 236
  uterine bleeding with dark purple, 124
cloudy vision, 32
clumping, of qi and phlegm, 14
cold
  as trigger for headaches, 302
  in exterior with interior heat from constraint, 64
  in lower body, 244, 286
  injuring yang brightness or lesser yin warp, transforming into heat, 368
  interior deficiency, 262
  obstructing blood circulation with blood deficiency, 78
  pain in lower abdomen/extremities from, 78
  sensation of internal, 356
  sensitivity to, 76, 78, 266
  tendency to feel, 128
cold aversion, 88, 262, 302, 342
cold below, with heat above, 294
cold damage
  at greater yang stage, 186
  interior deficiency with, 314
cold excess, in flanks and abdomen, causing qi stagnation and clumping of fluids, 58
cold extremities, 78, 356
cold feet, with facial flushing, 82
cold hands and feet, 170, 294
cold pathogen, constraining lesser yang warp, 308
cold sensation, in exterior of body, 188
common cold, 152
complexion
  lusterless, 314
  pale, 76
  pallid, 2, 258, 350
  pallid and wan, 126, 242
  sallow, 2

shiny, pale, 344
concentration, difficult, 180, 274
Conception vessel
  deficiency cold with blood stasis and deficiency heat, 286
  heat due to Liver qi constraint, with yin deficiency, 124
  weakness in, 18
concurrent disorders, greater yang and yang brightness stage, 36
confusion, 132
connective tissue weakness, 32
consciousness, sudden loss of, 354
constipation, 100, 132, 148, 288, 352, 358
  due to fluid exhaustion, 352
  due to Kidney deficiency, 148
  from dessicated intestines, 224
  with dry stools, 224
  with flatulence or foul-smelling diarrhea, 56
  with hard stool, difficult to expel, 192
  with smooth urination, 270
constraint, from dampness transforming into heat, 74
consumptive deficiency, 314
  with qi and blood deficiency, manifesting as functional Heart disorders, 358
consumptive disorders, qi and blood deficiency in, 252
cool extremities, 342
cool-dryness, externally-contracted, 330
coolness, morning, with nighttime fever, 210
cough, 28, 190, 194, 228, 230, 316, 324, 330, 366
  and wheezing, with thick, viscous sputum, 132
  as sequela to externally-contracted wind-cold, 366
  dry or hacking, 232
  hacking, 234
  productive, with yellow, viscous sputum, 212
  unproductive hacking, 220
  with deep-seated sputum, 22
  with foul-smelling sputum, 282
  with scanty, thick, sticky sputum, 232
  with scanty sputum, 234
  with wheezing, 84
crying, without reason, 112

— D

damp leg qi, from damp-cold, 150
damp rash, 310
damp-cold

damp leg qi from, 150
  stagnating in middle burner, 306
damp-heat
  accumulating in yang brightness channels, due to alcohol
    consumption and Spleen deficiency, 118
  and phlegm turbidity, in lesser yang channels, 134
  Eight-Herb Powder for Rectification in, 4
  in Bladder, 4
  lodged in lower burner, 94
  obstructing middle burner, 16
  smoldering in middle burner, 172
  with bloody painful urinary dribbling, 290
damp-heat excess, in Liver and/or Gallbladder channels,
  184
damp-heat food stagnation, obstructing Stomach and
  Intestines, 360
damp-heat skin disorders, 208
damp-warmth epidemic disorder, early stage
  flooding all three burners, 110
  with dampness predominating, 226
dampness
  and stagnation in middle burner, 146
  constraint from, 74
  qi constraint with, 348
  Spleen qi deficiency leading to, 242
  stagnating in Spleen and Stomach, 200
daybreak diarrhea, 264
deep breaths
  difficulty taking, 308
  to relieve tension, 44
deficiency cold
  in middle burner, 302
  of Spleen and Kidney, 264
  with upward rebellion of turbid yin, 302
deficiency fire, yin deficiency with, 52
deficiency heat, with deficiency cold of Conception and
  Penetrating vessels, 286
deficiency irritability, 268
deficiency overwork, 268
deficient constitution, toxic sores with, 280
delivery, difficult, 18
deviation, of mouth and eyes, 62, 204
diaphragm
  blood stasis below, 120
  focal distention in chest and, 118
  fullness in chest and, 212

impairment of blood flow above, 334
  qi stagnation in, 228
diarrhea, 16, 38, 242
  chronic, 294
  circumfluent, 56
  daybreak, 264
  foul-smelling, 56
  from heat constraint in lesser yang, 144
  from insufficient fire at gate of vitality, 264
  heat clumping with circumfluent, 56
  painful, due to Spleen deficiency and overcontrolling
    Liver, 278
  with pain, 278
  with watery stools, 170
  yellow, 172
difficult bending, 108
difficult breathing, 212
difficult concentration, 180
difficult delivery, 18
digestion, sensitive, 258
distention
  abdominal, 44, 56, 110, 260, 306
  epigastric and abdominal, with fullness, 136
  focal, 92, 348
  focal in chest and epigastrium, painful when pressed, 318
  in breast, 322
  in chest and epigastrium, 242, 298
  in epigastrium and abdomen, 200
  in flanks, 308, 322
  lower abdominal, 60
  slight abdominal, 338
dizziness, 12, 86, 98, 118, 174, 176, 272, 284, 322, 354
downcast feeling, 308
drafts
  aversion to, 130, 344
  slight aversion to, 230
dream-disturbed sleep, 98, 284
dreams, strange, 132, 284
dry eyes, 266
dry heaves, 164
dry lips, 326
dry mouth, 48, 194, 224, 250, 326, 346
dry nails, 224
dry retching, 308
dry skin, 266, 358
dry throat, 22, 144, 194, 234, 308, 322, 330, 336, 352

dry tongue, 250
dryness, injury to Lungs, Stomach, fluids from, 234
dysenteric disorder
    chronic, 294
    due to heat toxin searing Stomach and Intestines, 10
    from heat constraint in lesser yang, 144
    heat-type, 114
    with pus or blood in stool, 288

— E

edema
    superficial, 104
    superficial in extremities, 64
    superficial with dry skin, aches, no sweating, 64
    upper body, 298
    with urinary difficulty, 244
emaciation, without appetite loss, 210
emotional instability, 40
emotional stress, symptoms worse under, 14
epidemic disorders, early stage damp-warmth, 110
epigastric distention, 200
    and abdominal fullness, 100
    and fullness, 136
    focal, 154
epigastric focal distention, 16
epigastric fullness, 14
epigastric pain, 68, 336
    when hungry, 140
epigastrium
    distention and stifling sensation in, 242
    focal distention in, 364
    focal distention worse pressure, 318
    fullness or distention in, 20
    irritability and warmth in, 294
    spasmodic pain in, 314
    stifling sensation in, 172, 174, 178
    thin mucus in, 174, 316
erosion, 208
erythema
    faint and indistinct, 218
    localized with swelling, heat, pain, 300
essence damage, from Kidney yin deficiency, 372
excess fire, with chronic phlegm, 132
exhaustion, 38, 356
    from long-term illness, 342

inability to sleep despite, 268
    physical, 244
exterior cold, with heat from interior constraint, 64
exterior deficiency, with weak and unstable protective qi, 344
extremities
    burning pain in, 94
    cold, 78, 356
    constraint from dampness/heat pouring into, 74
    cool, 342
    deep aching and heaviness in, 356
    extremely cold, 262
    fatigued, 2
    paresthesia in, 142
    red, hot, swollen, painful, 94
    soreness and pain in, 222
    swelling and pain of lower, 74
    twitching and spasms in, 176
    yang failing to reach, 260
eye pain, 36
eyes
    deviation of, 204
    dry, 266
    red, 72

— F

face
    pain in, 216
    redness, swelling, burning pain of, 202
    sequelae of channel stroke, 204
facial asymmetry, 320
facial flushing, 8, 80, 140, 270
    as if intoxicated, 254
facial paralysis, 30
    sudden, 204
fatigue, 38, 96, 118, 178, 226, 258, 274, 370
    in extremities, 2
    inability to sleep despite, 268
    symptoms worse with, 32
    with desire to lie down, 350
    with desire to sleep, 188
fear, 40
febrile disorder, due to seasonal epidemic toxin, 202
feet
    cold, with flushed face, 82

heavy and weak, with difficulty walking, 150
numbness, cold or pain in, 150
red, hot, swollen, painful, 94
fever, 110, 114, 140, 144, 182, 214, 220, 234
  afternoon, 226
  alternating with chills, 54
  high, 8
    worse at night, 218
  low-grade, 210
  mild, 50
  mild chills alternating with pronounced, 134
  moderate, 232
  of unexplained origin, 66
  of unknown origin, 308
  persistent high, 176
  qi deficiency type, 32
  slight
    with or without sweating, 190
    with severe chills, 188
    with strong chills, 350
  strong with decreasing chills, 36
  strong with lesser chills, 222
  triggered by wind-cold, 130
  with aversion to drafts, 48
  with chills or aversion to drags, 12
  with slight chills, 48, 340
fever and chills, 320
  alternating, 308
  chills predominant, 162, 186, 316
  severe, 64
  strong, 202
  without sweating, 116, 316
fevers, worse early evening, gone in morning, 334
fingers and toes, cold and clammy, with warm body and head, 160
fire
  excess, with chronic phlegm, 132
  lurking due to constrained heat in Lungs, 324
  lurking in Spleen, 326
  with qi constraint, 348
fire toxin
  clumping in mouth and throat, 42
  in any or all burners, 140
fixed Kidney disorder, 108
flank pain, 44, 308, 322
flanks, cold excess in, 58

flatulence, constipation and, 56
fluids
  clumping of, 58
  constipation due to exhaustion of, 352
  injury from dryness, 234
  injury to, 238
flushing, 52
  facial, 80, 140, 270
    with cold feet, 82
focal distention, 92, 172, 178, 198, 348
  and pain, in chest and hypochondrium, 134
  epigastric and abdominal, 154
  in chest and abdomen, 362
  in chest and diaphragm, 118, 228
    painful with pressure, 318
  in chest and epigastrium, 364
food, disinterest in, 308
food accumulation, obstructing middle burner, 198
food and drink, reduced intake, 308
food aversion, 20
food stagnation
  obstructing Stomach and Intestines, 360
  transforming to heat, 154
  with qi constraint, 348
forgetfulness, 86, 126, 274, 370
foul turbidity, entering via nose and mouth, 66
frustration, leading to anger, 44
fullness
  abdominal, 170
  after eating little, 306
  epigastric, 14
  in chest and epigastrium, 298
  in chest with pain in flanks, 308
  in epigastrium or abdomen, 20, 198, 200
  with slight or no pain, 16
furuncles, 100

—G

Gallbladder channel, damp-heat excess in, 184
Gallbladder heat
  accosting Stomach, 308
  with Spleen cold, 38
gate of essence, instability, 160
gate of vitality
  diarrhea due to insufficient fire at, 264

flaring of fire at, 96
insufficient fire at, 244
Kidney yang deficiency with waning fire at, 342
greater yang stage disorder
    concurrent with yang brightness stage, 36
    externally-contracted wind-cold, 116, 130
    water buildup in context of, 292
    wind-cold attacking exterior, 186
groin pain, 336
gum soreness, 216
gynecological disorders, pain and masses associated with, 128

— H

hair loss, premature, 98
hands and feet
    cold, 179
    lack of sensation in, 62
head
    massive febrile disorder, 202
    redness, swelling, burning pain of, 202
    sequelae of channel stroke, 204
headache, 12, 36, 42, 46, 72, 118, 152, 162, 272, 354
    from externally-contracted wind, 46
    migraine-like, 302
    vertex, 302
hearing loss, 72, 370
Heart and Kidneys, failing to communicate, 274
Heart disorders, functional, 358
Heart failing to nourish spirit, 126
Heart heat, 80
    collecting in lower burner, 4
    Eight-Herb Powder for Rectification in, 4
    flowing to Small Intestine, 4
Heart qi deficiency and constraint, due to phlegm turbidity, 86
heat, 208
    accumulation in lower burner, 270
    constrained in Lungs, 324
    deficiency, 286
    depleting yin and fluids, 210
    from interior constraint, 64
    in joints, 332
    in nutritive level, 218
    in palms and soles, 180, 274

intermittent flushing, 358
internal accumulation, with externally-contracted wind-cold-dampness, 162
Liver constraint transforming into, 158
lodged in Lungs, obstructing qi flow, 190
Lung atrophy due to, 194
lurking in yin aspects, 210
upward flushing of, 286
with localized erythema, 300
heat above, with cold below, 294
heat accumulation, in Stomach, 216
heat and phlegm, clumping in chest, 318
heat aversion, 8, 100
    after slight chills, 340
heat clumping, with circumfluent diarrhea, 56
heat constraint, in lesser yang, overcoming Stomach and Intestines, 144
heat excess
    in interior and exterior, 100, 114
    in Liver channel, with stirring of internal wind, 176
    in yang brightness organs, 56
    overwhelming, in any or all burners, 140
heat inversion, 56
heat toxin
    flushing through exterior body, 254
    searing Stomach and Intestines, 19
heat-dryness, blocking movement of fluids in Spleen, 192
heaviness
    and aching of entire body, 64
    at fixed locations in lower back and extremities, 88
    bodily, 40
    generalized, 166, 316
    in feet and calves, with difficulty walking, 150
    of limbs, 214
heavy sensation, 226
hematuria, 368
hemiplegia, 30, 320
hernial pain, 158
hiccup, 164
hot flushes, 96, 174
    intermittent, 358
    upward, 286
hot food, epigastric and abdominal pain worse, 158
hot sensation, in muscles, 70
hot-type inversion, due to internal constraint of yang qi, 260

hypochondria
    fixed pain in, 120
    focal distention and pain in, 134
    fullness in chest and, 54
    pain in, 334
hypochondriac pain, 58, 336

— I

impotence, 160
insomnia, 36, 98, 126, 132, 284. *See also* sleep
    with dream-disturbed sleep, 272
interior deficiency, with cold damage, 314
interior deficiency cold, 262
intermittent symptoms, 294
intestinal abscess, early-stage, with interior clumping of
    heat and blood, 60
Intestines
    dryness in, 148
    Spleen cold from yang deficiency with accumulation in,
    288
intestines, constipation due to dessicated, 224
inversion
    from roundworms, 294
    yang- or hot-type, 260
irritability, 8, 36, 38, 40, 52, 56, 64, 70, 74, 96, 140, 182,
    184, 214, 218, 220, 232, 274, 302, 334, 346, 354, 370
    and restlessness, 308
    and warmth in chest and epigastrium, 294
    deficiency, 268
    with anxiety, 260
    with heat in chest, 80
itching, 208
itchy throat, 366

— J

jaundice
    with tangerine coloration, 338
    yang-type, 338
joints
    constraint from dampness transforming into heat, 74
    generalized aches and pains in, 74
    heat and pan in, 332
    pain, swelling, or stiffness in, 104

— K

Kidney deficiency
    constipation due to, 148
    leading to gate of essence instability, 160
Kidney disorder, fixed, 108
Kidney yang deficiency
    with insufficient fire at gate of vitality, 244
    with retention of pathogenic water, 356
    with waning fire at gate of vitality, 342
Kidney yin and yang deficiency
    with flaring of fire at gate of vitality, 96
    with upward-flaring of deficient yang and phlegm
    turbidity, 82
Kidney yin deficiency, with damaged essence and marrow,
    372
Kidneys, unable to transform fluids, with dryness in
    Intestines, 148
knees
    aching and weakness in, 342
    red, hot, swollen, painful, 94
    soreness and weakness, 180
    weakness and aching, 138

— L

labored breathing, 84
lassitude, 96
laughing, without reason, 112
leg pain, 246
leg qi, damp, 150
legs
    soreness and weakness, 372
    tight, 138
lesions. *See* skin lesions
lesser yang brightness warp disorder, concurrent with yang
    brightness disorder, 54
lesser yang channel
    clumping of fire toxin in, 42
    damp-heat and phlegm turbidity in, 134
lesser yang constraint, with heat affecting spirit, 40
lesser yang warp
    cold pathogen constraining, 308
    constraint with fluids clumping, 38
    diarrhea from heat contraint in, overcoming Stomach
    and Intestines, 144

lesser yin warp, cold transforming into heat in, 368
lesser yin warp disorders, 262
   with water excess, 356
lethargy, 110
   with constant desire to sleep, 262
lightheadedness, 2, 180, 372
limbs
   achy, 110
   heavy, 214
   weakness in, 258
lips
   dry, 286, 326
   parched, 370
Liver, over-controlling, 278
Liver and Gallbladder qi, constraint and clumping of, 72
Liver and Gallbladder qi constraint, with Gallbladder heat
 accosting Stomach, and Liver qi invading Spleen, 308
Liver and Kidney deficiency
   atrophy disorder due to, 138
   painful obstruction with, 88
Liver and Kidney yin deficiency, 18, 98
   with Liver qi stagnation, 336
Liver and Spleen disharmony, abdominal pain from, 76
Liver channel
   damp-heat excess in, 184
   heat excess in, 176
Liver constraint, transforming into heat, 158
Liver qi constraint
   and clumping, 44
   in context of yin deficiency, 124
   with blood deficiency and frail Spleen, 322
   with Liver and Kidney yin deficiency, 336
Liver qi invading Spleen, 308
Liver wind
   ascendant Liver yang leading to, 272
   with blood stasis and water accumulation, 272
lochia, retention of, 248
long-term illness
   blood deficiency from, 70
   exhaustion from, 342
   qi and blood deficiency in, 252
loose stools, 38, 172, 242
loss of consciousness, sudden, 354
lower abdomen
   acute pain in, 270
   blood stasis in, 128

cold-induced blood stasis accumulation in, 236
distention intensifying with onset of menstruation, 236
pain aggravated by pressure, 270
pain in, 128, 236
   relieved by warmth, 248
palpable masses in, 236
retention of static blood in, 256
lower back
   aching and weakness in, 342
   burning pain in, 94
   cold and pain, 108
   heaviness and pain at fixed locations, 88
   pain in, 246
   soreness and weakness, 180, 372
   tight, 138
   weakness and aching, 138
lower backache, 148
lower body, cold and pain in, 286
lower burner
   accumulation of blood stasis and heat in, 270
   blood buildup in, 270
   damp-heat lodged in, 94
   deficiency cold in, 24
   heat obstructing Bladder qi transformation in, 276
   thin mucus in, 292
lower extremities
   chronic pain, weakness, numbness, due to wind-stroke, 312
   heaviness and pain at fixed locations, 88
   swelling and pain of, 74
   weakness of, 82, 244
   weakness or atrophy, 94
lower limb atrophy, 30
Lung abscess, 282
Lung and Kidney yin deficiency, 6
   Lily Bulb Decoction to Preserve the Metal in, 6
Lung atrophy, due to heat, 194
Lung dryness
   from Lung/Kidney yin deficiency with deficiency heat, 6
   injuring fluids and producing phlegm, 22
   Lily Bulb Decoction to Preserve the Metal in, 6
Lung heat, leading to nasal congestion, 328
Lung qi and yin deficiency, 250
Lung qi deficiency, 28
Lungs
   heat lodged in, obstructing qi flow, 190

injury from dryness, 234
lurking fire due to constrained heat in, 324
phlegm clogging, with qi stagnation in middle burner/
  diaphragm, 228
wind-heat invading, 230
wind-heat toxins invading, 340
Lungs and Stomach, qi-level heat lingering in, 370
lurking fire
  in Lungs, 324
  in Spleen, 326
lusterless complexion, 314
lusterless skin, 224

— M

malpositioned fetus, 18
mania, 132
marrow, damage from Kidney yin deficiency, 372
masses
  palpable abdominal, 120
  palpable in lower abdomen, 236
membrane source, foul turbidity lodging in, 66
menstrual blood, dark with clots, 236
menstrual pain, 158, 336
menstruation, lower abdominal pain intensifying with, 236
mental agitation, 270
middle burner
  blood stasis and qi stagnation in, 68
  damp-cold stagnating in, 306
  damp-heat obstructing, 16
  damp-heat smoldering in, 172
  dampness and stagnation in, 146
  deficiency cold in, 170, 302
  food accumulation obstructing, 198
  phlegm tarrying in, overflowing to channels and
    collaterals, 106
  qi stagnation in, 228
  upward rebellion of turbid yin in, 302
middle burner qi sinking, 32
middle burner yang deficiency, bleeding due to, 170
migraines, 302
migrating pain, in bones and joints, 312
miscarriage, tendency to, 18
mobility, reduced, 332
mood swings, 40, 322

mouth
  deviation of, 62, 204
  dry, 48, 224, 250, 286, 326, 346
  dry and parched, 336
  inflammation, 42
  parched, 370
mouth sores, 80
mouth ulcers, 326
moving difficulty, 166
mucus, overflowing thin, 64
muscle layer
  accumulated water and dampness overflowing into, 292
  wind-dampness lodging in, 206
muscle spasms/cramps, 238
muscle weakness, 32
muscles, hot sensation in, 70
muscular tension, 44

— N

nails
  brittle, 266
  dry, 224
nasal congestion/discharge, 34, 46
  Lung heat leading to, 328
  sticky, 328
nasal discharge, unrelenting, 34
nasal obstruction, 34, 152
nasal passages, dryness in, 36
nausea, 16, 92, 164, 172, 284, 302, 308
neck and upper back, stiff and rigid, 116
neck pain, or stiffness, 114
neck stiffness, 36, 162, 206
  or pain, 114
night sweats, 52, 196, 210
  due to constrained heat at nutritive qi level, 196
nodules, focal distention with or without, 318
numbness, 62, 142
nutritive and protective qi, imbalance of, 130
nutritive level, heat in, 218

— O

orbital pain, 36
overwork, deficiency, 268

— P

pain, 208
abdominal, 10, 144, 260, 278, 288, 294, 306, 308
acute abdominal, 58
acute in lower abdomen, 256
and masses with gynecological disorders, 128
at fixed locations in low back and extremities, 88
bodily, 64
chest, 58, 336
chronic, 246
diarrhea with, 278
epigastric, 68, 336
faint or indistinct burning, 336
when hungry, 140
eye and orbital, 36
facial, 216
fixed, in hypochondria, 120
flank, 44
from wind-dampness, 320
generalized bodily, 74, 162
hernial, 158
hypochondriac, 58, 336
in arms, 246
in back, 206
in both arms or shoulders, 106
in breast, 322
in chest, 158, 334
in chest and hypochondrium, 134
in epigastrium and abdomen, 198
in extremities, 222
in extremities from cold, 78
in groin and lower abdomen, 336
in hypochondria, 334
in joints, 332
in legs, 246
in Liver channel, 336
in lower abdomen from cold, 78
in lower body, 286
in shoulder, 246
increased with pressure, 60
intermittent epigastric and abdominal, 158
lower abdominal, 4, 76, 128
menstrual, 158, 336
migrating in bones and joints, 312
neck, 114

periodic abdominal, 136
recurrent spasmodic, 238
spasmodic abdominal, 314
with localized erythema, 300
painful diarrhea, with Spleen deficiency and over-
controlling Liver, 278
painful obstruction
blood, 142
due to damp-heat in channels and collaterals, 332
due to qi and blood stasis, in channels and collaterals,
246
in chest, 364
of back and waist, 108
with Liver and Kidney deficiency, 88
with qi and blood deficiency, 166
pale complexion, 76
pallid complexion, 2, 76, 258, 350
pallor, 266
palms and soles, hot, 180, 274
palpitations, 86, 126, 132, 174, 274, 284, 358
paralysis
facial, 30
of lower limbs, 30
sudden facial, 204
paresthesia, in extremities, 142
pathogenic water, retention of, 356
Penetrating vessel
deficiency cold with blood stasis and deficiency heat, 286
heat due to Liver qi constraint, with yin deficiency, 124
instability of, 122
weakness in, 18
phlegm
and heat clumping in chest, 318
clogging Lungs, with qi stagnation in middle burner/
diaphragm, 228
due to lung dryness injuring fluids, 22
excess fire with chronic, 132
in middle burner, overflowing to channels and
collaterals, 106
Lung abscess from, 282
obstruction of channels by, 312
Spleen qi deficiency with, 178
Stomach and Lung yin deficiency with, 194
with qi constraint, 348
phlegm obstruction, 222

phlegm turbidity
    Heart qi deficiency and constraint from, 86
    in lesser yang channels, constraining qi dynamic, 134
    upward flaring of, 82
phlegm-dampness
    due to failure of Spleen and Lung to transport fluids, 92
    in seasonal febrile epidemic disorder, 202
phlegm-heat
    internal clumping of, 212
    obstructing qi dynamic, 284
    smoldering in interior, 84
plum-pit qi, 14
postpartum blood stagnation, in uterus, 248
premature graying, 98
pressure
    focal distention worse from, 318
    spasmodic pain better from, 314
protective and qi levels, pathogenic influences at, 226
protective qi
    unstable, 196
    weak and unstable, 344
    wind-heat toxin invading upper-burner, 340
purpura, faint and indistinct, 218
pus
    in stool, 288
    sores not leaking, 280

— Q

qi abandonment, from blood loss, 70
qi and blood deficiency
    consumptive condition with, 358
    Eight-Treasure Decoction for, 2
    in consumptive/long-term disorders, 252
    leading to weakness in Penetrating and Conception
        vessels, 18
    painful obstruction with, 166
qi and blood imbalance, 130
qi and blood stasis, in channels and collaterals, 246
qi and fluids, injury from lingering qi-level heat, 370
qi and phlegm, clumping of, 14
qi and yang deficiency, externally-contracted wind-cold
    with, 350
qi and yin deficiency, of Lungs, 250
qi constraint, with dampness, phlegm, fire, blood stasis, or
    food stagnation, 348

qi deficiency, with static blood obstructing channels, 30
qi dynamic, contraint from damp-heat and phlegm
    turbidity, in lesser yang channels, 134
qi flowing sensation, from flanks to heart area, 364
qi level heat, White Tiger Decoction for, 8–9
qi stagnation
    and blood stasis in middle burner, 68
    cold excess causing, 58
    in Liver channel, 336
    in middle burner and diaphragm, 228
    with wind-cold-dampness, 222
qi stagnation and constraint, due to long-term Stomach
    deficiency, 164
qi-level heat, lingering in Lungs and Stomach, 370

— R

range of motion, reduced due to wind-cold-damp painful
    obstruction, 312
rashes
    damp-type, 310
    dry, scaly, itchy, 168
    wet, papular, 94
    wind-type, 310
rebellious Stomach qi, 14
    Stomach and Lung yin deficiency with, 194
rebound tenderness, 60
red eyes, 72
red face, 70
    and eyes, 72
restless fetus, 18
restless organ disorder, 112
restless sleep, 334
restlessness, 38, 56, 72, 218, 370
    and irritability, 308
retching, dry, 308
rice-water urine, 24
rigidity, in neck and upper back, 116
roundworms, inversion from, 294
runny nose, 152

— S

saliva, spitting up, 194
scabbing skin disorders, 168
sensation, lacking in hands and feet, 62

short temper, 184

shortness of breath, 28, 194, 250

shoulder pain, 246
   bilateral, 106

shoulder stiffness, 166

sighing, 308
   to relieve tension, 44

skin
   dry, 266, 358
   lusterless, 224

skin conditions
   damp-heat related, 208
   with localized swelling, redness, pain, 100

skin disorders, scabbing, 168

skin edema, 298

skin lesions
   deep-rooted and hard, 300
   red, hot, swollen, painful, 304
   weepy, itchy, red, 310

skin sores, superficial, 26

sleep
   constant desire to, 262
   dream-disturbed, 98, 284
   inability despite fatigue and exhaustion, 268
   restless, 276, 334

sore throat, with swelling, 26

soreness, in extremities, 222

sores, 94
   early-stage, 304
   in throat, mouth, or outer ear, 26
   non-suppurating, 280
   slow healing, 280

sour fluids, spitting up, 134

source qi deficiency, with sudden collapse of yang qi, 240

spasms
   better warmth and pressure, 314
   in extremities, 176
   recurrent, 238

speech
   difficulty due to tongue stiffness, 62
   slow and slurred, 320

spermatorrhea, chronic, 160

spirit, Heart failing to nourish, 126

spitting up, bitter or sour fluids, 134

Spleen
   frail with Liver constraint and blood deficiency, 322

heat-dryness blocking movement of fluids in, 192
   Liver qi invading, 308
   lurking fire in, 326

Spleen and Heart qi and blood deficiency, 126

Spleen and Kidney, deficiency cold of, 264

Spleen and Kidney yang deficiency, with retention of
   pathogenic water, 356

Spleen and Lung qi, failure to transport fluids, 92

Spleen and Stomach
   dampness stagnating in, 200
   disruption in ascending and descending functions, 172

Spleen and Stomach deficiency cold, with damp-heat
   obstructing middle burner, 16

Spleen and Stomach qi deficiency
   food stagnation transforming to heat with, 154
   with damp-cold stagnating in middle burner, 306
   with inability to raise the clear, 32

Spleen bind, 192

Spleen cold, from yang deficiency with accumulation in
   Intestines, 288

Spleen deficiency
   damp-heat in yang brightness channels, due to alcohol
      consumption with, 118
   with accumulation and stagnation, 362
   with internal accumulation of water and dampness,
      overflowing into muscles and skin, 292
   with over-controlling Liver, 278

Spleen qi deficiency, 258
   leading to internal dampness, 242
   with phlegm, 178

Spleen unable to govern blood, 126

spontaneous sweating, 28
   due to unstable protective qi, 196

sputum
   blood-streaked, 282
   copious, 228
      thick, yellow, 84
      watery, white, 316
   cough with foul-smelling, 282
   difficult to expectorate, 366
   expectoration of watery, 330
   little or difficult to expectorate, 324
   scanty, thick, sticky, 232
   thick, viscous, 132
   yellow, viscous, difficult to expectorate, 212

stamina, lack of physical/mental, 32

static blood
  obstructing channels, 30
  retention obstructing lower abdomen vessels, 256
stiff neck, 36, 162, 166, 206
stiffness
  bodily, 40
  in joints, 104
  in neck and upper back, 116
stifling sensation
  in chest, 110, 134, 150
  in chest and epigastrium, 172, 178
  in chest and hypochondria, 14
  in chest or upper abdomen, 12, 226
Stomach
  Gallbladder heat accosting, 308
  heat accumulation in, 216
  injury from dryness, 234
Stomach and Intestines
  damp-heat food stagnation obstructing, 360
  dysenteric disorder overcoming, 144
  heat toxin searing, 10
Stomach and Lung yin deficiency, with phlegm and
  rebellious qi, 194
Stomach deficiency, qi stagnation and constraint due to
  long-term, 164
Stomach qi
  injury due to vomiting, diarrhea, 164
  rebellious, 14
Stomach-Gallbladder disharmony, with phlegm-heat
  obstructing qi dynamic, 284
stools
  diarrhea with watery, 170
  foul-smelling, 114
  hard and difficult to expel, 192
  loose, 172, 242
  pus or blood in, 288
  thin or unformed, 179
stretching, frequent, 112
summerheat
  injuring qi and fluids, 214
  obstructing Triple Burner, 182
summerheat-warmth, dampness predominating, 226
superficial edema, 104
swallowing difficulty, 42
sweating, 96, 104, 114, 182, 292, 370
  absence of, 50, 64, 152, 162, 186, 222

  in superficial edema, 64
  chills without, 330
  daytime or nighttime, 130
  fever and chills without, 316
  from palms, soles, or head, 56
  nighttime, 52, 210
  profuse, 8, 56, 214
  spontaneous, 28, 250, 344
    due to unstable protective qi, 196
swelling, 208
  hot, red, 156
  red, itchy, 168
  with localized erythema, 300

—T

tachycardia, 174, 358
tenesmus, 10
terminal yin warp disorder, 294
  water buildup in context of, 292
thin mucus
  accumulating in epigastrium, 316
  in epigastrium, 174
  in lower burner, 292
  internal accumulation of, 316
think, inability to, 274
thirst, 10, 38, 190, 214, 234, 292, 346, 352
  absence of, 276
  lack of, 362
  severe, 8
  with desire for warm beverages, 70
throat
  dry, 22, 144, 234, 308, 322, 330
    with constipation, 352
  inflammation, 42
  itchy, 366
  parched, 370
  redness, swelling, burning pain of, 202
  something caught in, 14
  sore, 48
  sore and swollen, 26
throat obstruction, 194
tidal fever, in afternoon, 52
tightness, with slight or no pain, 16
tinnitus, 72, 132, 354

tongue
   dry, 250
   red with scanty coating, 234
tongue sores, 80
tongue stiffness
   difficult speech due to, 62
   with inability to speak, 82
toothache, 216
toxic sores
   initial stages of hot/painful, 254
   with deficient constitution, 280
toxic swelling, red, hot without head, 156
Triple Burner, summerheat obstructing, 182
trunk, difficulty bending/rotating, 206
turbid, loss of ability to descend, 308
turbid yin, upward rebellion of, 302
twitching
   in extremities, 176
   of facial muscles, 204

— U

umbilicus, spasmodic pain in, 314
upper abdomen, stifling sensation in, 150, 226
upper back stiffness, 166
upper burner, wind-heat toxin invading protective qi of, 340
upward qi surging, wind-stroke due to, 354
upward-flaring, of deficient yang and phlegm turbidity, 82
urinary difficulty, 182, 292, 298, 338, 368
   with edema, 244
urinary dribbling
   cloudy and painful, 24
   damp-heat painful bloody, 290
   due to lower burner deficiency cold, 24
urinary frequency, 24, 346
urinary obstruction, 276
   due to heat in lower burner, 276
urinary retention, 4
urination
   dark
      and scant, 134
      scanty, rough, painful, 80
      turbid, scanty, difficult, and painful, 4
   discomfort during of after, 290
   excessive, 244

increased, 160
inhibited, 118
normal to frequent, 192
rough and painful, 276, 290
smooth with constipation, 270
without relief, 368
urine
   clear and copious, 148
   dark, scanty, 110
   greasy, 24
   rice-water, 24
   scanty
      dark, 184
      yellow, 94
uterine bleeding
   with deep red blood or dark purple clots, 124
   with thin and pale blood, 122
uterus, postpartum blood stagnation in, 248

— V

vaginal discharge, thick, yellow, foul-smelling, 94
vertex headaches, 302
vertigo, 2, 12, 72, 132, 176, 180, 322, 354, 370
vision
   blurred, 98
   impaired/cloudy, 32
vitality, lack of physical/mental, 32
voice, weak, 350
vomiting, 16, 92, 118, 170, 172, 284, 302, 308
   of clear liquid, 136

— W

walking difficulty, 138
   with heaviness and weakness in feet and calves, 150
warm beverages, thirst for, 70
warm pathogen disorder, early stage, 230, 340
warm-dryness, attacking Lungs, with damage to qi and yin, 220
warm-heat pathogen disease, later stages, 210
warmth
   attraction to, 88
   spasmodic pain better from, 314
wasting and thirsting disorder, 346

water buildup, in context of greater yang/terminal yin
 warp disorder, 292
water excess, lesser yin warp patterns with, 356
weakness, in limbs, 258
weeping, 208
wheezing, 28, 190, 220, 228, 316, 324
  cough and, with thick, viscous sputum, 132
  from wind-cold constraining exterior, with phlegm-heat
   smoldering in interior, 84
wind
  headache from externally-contracted, 46
  stirring of internal, 176
wind attack, externally-contracted, at greater yang stage,
 130
wind edema, with deficient exterior, 104
wind rash, 310
wind-cold
  attacking exterior, 186
  constraining exterior, with phlegm-heat smoldering in
   interior, 84
  cough as sequela to externally-contracted, 366
  early stage externally-contracted, 50
  exterior, with pre-existing yang deficiency, 188
  externally-contracted
    at greater yang stage, 130
    penetrating to greater yang head and neck channels,
     116
    with concurrent middle burner dampness and
     stagnation, 146
    with constitutional yin deficiency, 48
    with internal accumulation of thin mucus, 316
    with preexisting qi and yang deficiency, 350
  transforming into heat, 36
  unresolved exterior with constraint, 36
wind-cold-damp painful obstruction, reduced range of
 motion due to, 312
wind-cold-dampness
  externally-contracted
    with concurrent internal heat accumulation, 162
    with qi deficient constitution, 222
  obstruction of channels by, 312
wind-dampness
  lodging in exterior, 206
  pain from, 320
  with deficient exterior, 104
wind-heat

early stage externally-contracted, 50
in seasonal febrile disorder, 202
invading Lungs, 230
invading protective qi and Lungs, due to damage of yin
 and fluids, 48
wind-heat toxin
  invading Lungs and upper burner protective qi, 340
  Lung abscess from, 282
wind-phlegm, upward disturbance by, 12
wind-stroke
  chronic pain, weakness, numbness due to, 312
  due to exterior invasion into channels, 320
  early- or middle-stage, 62
  from excessive upward surging of qi, 354

worrying, unwarranted, 126

—Y

yang abandonment, 240
yang brightness channels
  cold transforming into heat in, 368
  damp-heat due to alcohol and Spleen deficiency, 118
yang brightness organs, heat excess in, 56
yang brightness stage disorder
  concurrent with greater yang, 36
  concurrent with lesser yang, 54
yang brightness warp, blazing fire in, 8
yang brightness warp disorder, 114
yang deficiency
  exterior wind-cold with preexisting, 188
  with accumulation impeding Intestines, 288
yang failing to reach extremities, 260
yang qi
  internal constraint of, 260
  sudden collapse of, 240
yang-type inversion, 260
yang-type jaundice, 338
yawning, frequent, 112
yin and blood deficiency, leading to restless mind, 274
yin and yang imbalance, 130
yin deficiency
  externally-contracted wind-cold with, 48
  heat in Penetrating and Conception vessels with, 124
  of Liver and Kidneys, with Liver qi stagnation, 336
  with flourishing deficiency fire, 52